Advances in Bariatric and Metabolic Endoscopy

Editors

VIOLETA POPOV
SHELBY SULLIVAN

GASTROINTESTINAL ENDOSCOPY CLINICS OF NORTH AMERICA

www.giendo.theclinics.com

Consulting Editor
ASHLEY L. FAULX

October 2024 • Volume 34 • Number 4

ELSEVIER

1600 John F. Kennedy Boulevard • Suite 1800 • Philadelphia, Pennsylvania, 19103-2899

http://www.theclinics.com

GASTROINTESTINAL ENDOSCOPY CLINICS OF NORTH AMERICA Volume 34, Number 4
October 2024 ISSN 1052-5157, ISBN-13: 978-0-443-12901-8

Editor: Kerry Holland
Developmental Editor: Malvika Shah

Photocopying
Single photocopies of single articles may be made for personal use as allowed by national copyright laws. Permission of the Publisher and payment of a fee is required for all other photocopying, including multiple or systematic copying, copying for advertising or promotional purposes, resale, and all forms of document delivery. Special rates are available for educational institutions that wish to make photocopies for non-profit educational classroom use. For information on how to seek permission visit www.elsevier.com/permissions or call: (+44) 1865 843830 (UK)/(+1) 215 239 3804 (USA).

Derivative Works
Subscribers may reproduce tables of contents or prepare lists of articles including abstracts for internal circulation within their institutions. Permission of the Publisher is required for resale or distribution outside the institution. Permission of the Publisher is required for all other derivative works, including compilations and translations (please consult www.elsevier.com/permissions).

Electronic Storage or Usage
Permission of the Publisher is required to store or use electronically any material contained in this periodical, including any article or part of an article (please consult www.elsevier.com/permissions). Except as outlined above, no part of this publication may be reproduced, stored in a retrieval system or transmitted in any form or by any means, electronic, mechanical, photocopying, recording or otherwise, without prior written permission of the Publisher.

Notice
No responsibility is assumed by the Publisher for any injury and/or damage to persons or property as a matter of products liability, negligence or otherwise, or from any use or operation of any methods, products, instructions or ideas contained in the material herein. Because of rapid advances in the medical sciences, in particular, independent verification of diagnoses and drug dosages should be made.

Although all advertising material is expected to conform to ethical (medical) standards, inclusion in this publication does not constitute a guarantee or endorsement of the quality or value of such product or of the claims made of it by its manufacturer.

Gastrointestinal Endoscopy Clinics of North America (ISSN 1052-5157) is published quarterly by Elsevier Inc., 360 Park Avenue South, New York, NY 10010-1710. Months of issue are January, April, July, and October. Business and Editorial Offices: 1600 John F. Kennedy Blvd., Suite 1800, Philadelphia, PA, 19103-2899. Periodicals postage paid at New York, NY and additional mailing offices. Subscription prices are $392.00 per year for US individuals, $100.00 per year for US and Canadian students/residents, $432.00 per year for Canadian individuals, $516.00 per year for international individuals, and $245.00 per year for international students/residents. For institutional access pricing please contact Customer Service via the contact information below. To receive student/resident rate, orders must be accompanied by name of affiliated institution, date of term, and the *signature* of program/residency coordinator on institution letterhead. Orders will be billed at individual rate until proof of status is received. Foreign air speed delivery is included in all *Clinics* subscription prices. All prices are subject to change without notice. Orders, claims, and journal inquiries: Please visit our Support Hub page https://service.elsevier.com for assistance.

Reprints. For copies of 100 or more, of articles in this publication, please contact the Commercial Reprints Department, Elsevier Inc., 360 Park Avenue South, New York, NY 10010-1710. Tel. 212-633-3874; Fax: 212-633-3820; E-mail: reprints@elsevier.com.

Gastrointestinal Endoscopy Clinics of North America is covered in *Excerpta Medica, MEDLINE/PubMed (Index Medicus), and MEDLINE/MEDLARS.*

Contributors

CONSULTING EDITOR

ASHLEY L. FAULX, MD, MASGE, FACG
Professor of Medicine, Case Western Reserve University School of Medicine, University Hospitals Cleveland Medical Center, Louis Stokes Veterans Affairs Medical Center, Cleveland, Ohio, USA

EDITORS

VIOLETA POPOV, MD, PhD, DABOM
Director of Bariatric Endoscopy, VA NY Harbor Healthcare System, NYU Langone Health Systems, New York, New York, USA

SHELBY SULLIVAN, MD
Professor of Medicine, Director of Metabolic and Bariatric Endoscopy, Center for Digestive Health, Dartmouth Hitchcock Medical Center, Lebanon, New Hampshire, USA

AUTHORS

BARHAM K. ABU DAYYEH, MD, MPH
Professor of Medicine, Department of Gastroenterology and Hepatology, Mayo Clinic, Rochester, Minnesota, USA

ANDRES ACOSTA, MD, PhD
Assistant Professor, Precision Medicine for Obesity Program, Division of Gastroenterology and Hepatology, Department of Medicine, Mayo Clinic, Rochester, Minnesota, USA

JOSÉ O. ALEMÁN, MD, PhD
Assistant Professor, Holman Division of Endocrinology, New York University Langone Health, Attending Physician, Department of Medicine, Margaret Corbin Campus of the VA New York Harbor Health Care System, Head, Laboratory of Translational Obesity Research, NYU Langone Health, New York, New York, USA

ALEXANDRE MORAES BESTETTI, MD
Gastrointestinal Endoscopy Division, Instituto D'Or de Pesquisa e Ensino (IDOR), Hospital Vila Nova Star, Gastrointestinal Endoscopy Unit, Department of Gastroenterology, Hospital das Clínicas da Faculdade de Medicina da Universidade de São Paulo, São Paulo, Brazil

IVO BOŠKOSKI, MD, PhD, FESGE
Assistant Professor of Gastroenterology, Digestive Endoscopy Unit, Fondazione Policlinico Unversitario Agostino Gemelli IRCCS, Università Cattolica del Sacro Cuore, Roma, Italy

VITOR BRUNALDI, MD, PhD
Research Collaborator, Department of Gastroenterology and Hepatology, Mayo Clinic, Rochester, Minnesota, USA

SARAH CHOKSI, MD
Postdoctoral Research Fellow, Department of Surgery, Lenox Hill Hospital, Northwell Health, New York, New York, USA

D.T.H. DE MOURA, MD, MSc, PhD, POST-PhD
Associate Professor, Gastrointestinal Endoscopy Unit, Department of Gastroenterology, Hospital das Clínicas da Faculdade de Medicina da Universidade de São Paulo, Gastrointestinal Endoscopy Division, Instituto D'Or de Pesquisa e Ensino (IDOR), Hospital Vila Nova Star, São Paulo, Brazil

KHUSHBOO GALA, MBBS
Fellow, Precision Medicine for Obesity Program, Division of Gastroenterology and Hepatology, Department of Medicine, Mayo Clinic, Rochester, Minnesota, USA

WISSAM GHUSN, MD
Post-Doctorate Research Fellow, Precision Medicine for Obesity Program, Division of Gastroenterology and Hepatology, Department of Medicine, Mayo Clinic, Rochester, Minnesota, USA; Department of Internal Medicine, Boston University Medical Center, Boston, Massachusetts, USA

MARK A. GROMSKI, MD
Interventional Endoscopist, Assistant Professor of Medicine, Department of Gastroenterology and Hepatology, Indiana University Health, Indiana University School of Medicine, Indianapolis, Indiana, USA

LOREDANA GUALTIERI, MD
Resident, Digestive Endoscopy Unit, Fondazione Policlinico Unversitario Agostino Gemelli IRCCS, Università Cattolica del Sacro Cuore, Roma, Italy

ELIZABETH HEGEDUS, BS
Medical Student, Department of Pediatrics, Children's Hospital Los Angeles and Keck School of Medicine of USC, Center for Endocrinology, Diabetes and Metabolism, Los Angeles, California, USA

PICHAMOL JIRAPINYO, MD, MPH
Director, Bariatric Endoscopy Fellowship, Division of Gastroenterology, Hepatology and Endoscopy, Brigham and Women's Hospital, Assistant Professor of Medicine, Harvard Medical School, Boston, Massachusetts, USA

KATE E. JOHNSON, BA
Researcher, Division of Gastroenterology and Hepatology, Department of Medicine, Weill Cornell Medicine, New York, New York, USA

GABRIELA JORDAN, MD
Fellow, Department of Medicine, Margaret Corbin Campus of the VA New York Harbor Health Care System, Laboratory of Translational Obesity Research, NYU Langone Health, New York, New York, USA

JAMIE KANE, MD
Associate Professor of Medicine, Department of General Internal Medicine, Section of Obesity Medicine, Northwell Health, Northwell Center for Weight Management, Great Neck, New York, USA

ROHIT KOHLI, MBBS, MS
Professor, Department of Pediatrics, Division of Gastroenterology, Children's Hospital Los Angeles and Keck School of Medicine of USC, Los Angeles, California, USA

ROSHNI KOHLI
Undergraduate Student, Department of Pediatrics, Children's Hospital Los Angeles and Keck School of Medicine of USC, Center for Endocrinology, Diabetes and Metabolism, Los Angeles, California, USA

VLADIMIR KUSHNIR, MD
Professor, Division of Gastroenterology, Washington University School of Medicine, Washington University, St Louis, Missouri, USA

ALI LAHOOTI, BS
Student, Division of Gastroenterology and Hepatology, Department of Medicine, Weill Cornell Medicine, New York, New York, USA

DOUGLAS C. LAMBERT, MD, MPH
Assistant Professor of Medicine, Department of General Internal Medicine, Section of Obesity Medicine, Northwell Health, Northwell Center for Weight Management, Great Neck, New York, USA

JANESE LASTER, MD
Gastroenterology, Nutrition, Obesity Medicine, and Bariatric Endoscopist, Gut Theory Total Digestive Care, Georgetown University Hospital, Washington, DC, USA

MARIA VALERIA MATTEO, MD, PhD Candidate
Digestive Endoscopy Unit, Fondazione Policlinico Unversitario Agostino Gemelli IRCCS, Università Cattolica del Sacro Cuore, Roma, Italy

MADELINE MAYER, BS
Medical Student, Department of Pediatrics, Children's Hospital Los Angeles and Keck School of Medicine of USC, Center for Endocrinology, Diabetes and Metabolism, Los Angeles, California, USA

RAMZI MULKI, MD
Interventional Endoscopist, Assistant Professor of Medicine, Department of Gastroenterology and Hepatology, The University of Alabama, Heersink School of Medicine, Birmingham, Alabama, USA

CAROLYN NEWBERRY, MD
Assistant Professor of Medicine, Director of GI Nutrition, Division of Gastroenterology and Hepatology, Innovative Center for Health and Nutrition in Gastroenterology (ICHANGE), Weill Cornell Medicine, New York, New York, USA

MARIANNA PAPADEMETRIOU, MD
Gastronteroloigst, Director of Endoscopy, Georgetown University Medical Center, Washington DC VA Medical Center, Washington, DC, USA

AURORA DAWN PRYOR, MD, MBA
Surgeon in Chief, Long Island Jewish Medical Center, System Director for Bariatric Surgery, Northwell Health, Professor of Surgery, Donald and Barbara Zucker School of Medicine at Hofstra/Northwell, New Hyde Park, New York, USA

RUBEN D. SALAS-PARRA, MD
Chief Resident, Department of Surgery, Long Island Jewish Medical Center and North Shore University Hospital, Northwell, New Hyde Park, New York, USA

SERGIO A. SÁNCHEZ-LUNA, MD, ABOM-D
Interventional Endoscopist, Assistant Professor of Medicine, Division of Gastroenterology and Hepatology, Department of Internal Medicine, Basil I. Hirschowitz Endoscopic Center

of Excellence, The University of Alabama at Birmingham Heersink School of Medicine, Birmingham, Alabama, USA

ALLISON R. SCHULMAN, MD, MPH, FASGE
Associate Professor of Medicine and Surgery, Chief of Endoscopy, Director of Bariatric Endoscopy, Division of Gastroenterology and Hepatology, Department of Surgery, University of Michigan, Ann Arbor, Michigan, USA

REEM Z. SHARAIHA, MD, MSc
Associate Professor, Division of Gastroenterology and Hepatology, Department of Medicine, Weill Cornell Medicine, New York, New York, USA

ABHISHEK SHENOY, MD, MSc
Fellow Physician, Division of Gastroenterology and Hepatology, University of Michigan, Ann Arbor, Michigan, USA

ADRIANA FERNANDES SILVA, MD
Gastrointestinal Endoscopy Unit, Department of Gastroenterology, Hospital das Clínicas da Faculdade de Medicina da Universidade de São Paulo, São Paulo, Brazil

CAROLINE SMOLKIN, MD
Resident, Department of Surgery, Long Island Jewish Medical Center and North Shore University Hospital, Northwell, New Hyde Park, New York, USA

DANIEL SZVARCA, MD
Fellow, Division of Gastroenterology, Hepatology, and Endoscopy, Brigham and Women's Hospital, Harvard Medical School, Boston, Massachusetts, USA

CHRISTOPHER C. THOMPSON, MD
Director of Endoscopy, Division of Gastroenterology, Hepatology and Endoscopy, Co-Director, Center for Weight Management and Wellness, Brigham and Women's Hospital, Professor, Department of Medicine, Harvard Medical School, Boston, Massachusetts, USA

ALAINA P. VIDMAR, MD
Assistant Professor, Department of Pediatrics, Children's Hospital Los Angeles and Keck School of Medicine of USC, Center for Endocrinology, Diabetes and Metabolism, Los Angeles, California, USA

TRENT WALRADT, MD
Fellow, Division of Gastroenterology, Hepatology and Endoscopy, Brigham and Women's Hospital, Harvard Medical School, Boston, Massachusetts, USA

MEGAN E. WHITE, MD
Fellow, Division of Gastroenterology, Washington University School of Medicine, Washington University, Barnes Jewish Hospital, St Louis, Missouri, USA

SUJANI YADLAPATI, MD
Advanced Endoscopy Fellow, Visitng Clinical Lecturer in Medicine, Department of Gastroenterology and Hepatology, Indiana University Health, Indiana University School of Medicine, Indianapolis, Indiana, USA

SIGRID YOUNG, MD
Resident Physician, Department of Medicine, Margaret Corbin Campus of the VA New York Harbor Health Care System, Laboratory of Translational Obesity Research, NYU Langone Health, New York, New York, USA

Contents

Lifestyle management of obesity includes nutritional therapy, physical activity, and several intermittent fasting therapies. Effective nutrition therapies include optimized low-fat diets, high-quality ketogenic diets, and energy-restricted diets. Adherence to dietary change remains the most substantial barrier to success; therefore, patients engaging in lifestyle changes require intensive support and resources. Physical activity is shown to have benefits to body composition and disease risk beyond the effects on weight loss. Patients should be guided toward a regimen that is appropriate for their capacity for movement. Multiple intermittent fasting strategies have now been shown to cause substantial weight loss and metabolic health improvement.

The rising prevalence of obesity is of major concern. There are currently 5 Food and Drug Administration-approved medications for the treatment of obesity: orlistat, phentermine/topiramate, naltrexone/bupropion, liraglutide 3.0 mg, and semaglutide 2.4 mg. Surgical options such as bariatric surgery and endoscopic surgery induce more durable weight loss than pharmacotherapy or lifestyle interventions alone. However, patients often experience weight regain and weight loss plateau after surgery. The addition of multimodal or multihormonal pharmacotherapy is a promising tool to address these challenges. The optimal timing of obesity pharmacotherapy with surgical and endoscopic interventions requires further investigation.

Bariatric surgery has evolved and gained in popularity as it has been recognized as the most sustainable and effective treatment for obesity and related diseases. These related diseases are significant causes of obesity related morbidity and mortality. Most bariatric procedures incorporate some component of gastric restriction with or without intestinal bypass, but the full mechanism of these procedures has yet to be elucidated. The most popular surgical procedure remains the sleeve gastrectomy

Video content accompanies this article at http://www.giendo.
theclinics.com.

Obesity is escalating, projected to affect 17.5% of adults globally and af-
flict 400 million children by 2035. Managing this intricate and chronic condition demands personalized, multidisciplinary approaches. While dietary
changes, lifestyle modifications, and medications yield short-term results,
long-term outcomes are often poor, with bariatric surgery standing out as
the most effective option. However, only a small fraction undergoes surgery due to various barriers. Intragastric balloon (IGB) emerges as a minimally invasive alternative, approved by major regulatory bodies. This
review adresses the pivotal role of IGB in obesity management, delving
into its history and technological evolution.

The small bowel has a crucial role in metabolic homeostasis. Small bowel endoscopic bariatric metabolic treatments (EBMTs) include several devices
aimed at providing minimally invasive approaches for the management of
metabolic disorders. The aim of this review is to provide an updated and ex-
haustive overview of the EBMTs targeting the small bowel developed to date,
including the duodenal mucosa resurfacing, the duodenal-jejunal bypass lin-
ers, gastro-jejunal bypass sleeve, and the incisioneless magnetic anastomosis system, as well as to mention the future perspectives in the field.

 Video content accompanies this article at http://www.giendo.
theclinics.com.

Endoscopic suturing has been described in many applications, including
the approximation of tissue defects, anchoring stents, hemostasis, and
primary and secondary bariatric interventions. Primary endobariatric procedures use endoscopic suturing for gastric remodeling with the intention
of weight loss. Currently, the only commercially available device in the
United States is the OverStitch endoscopic suturing system (Apollo Endosurgery). We describe devices of potential that are currently in design and/
or trials as devices for weight loss by gastric remodeling, including USGI
incisionless operating platform used for the primary obesity surgery endoluminal 2.0 procedure, Endomina used for the Endomina endoscopic
sleeve gastroplasty, and EndoZip.

The obesity epidemic continues to worsen in the United States with currently 40% of adults with obesity. While lifestyle changes, pharmacologic

and surgical treatments are the mainstay of therapy, they often are either inadequate to meet desired weight loss or underutilized due to patient preference. Endoscopic bariatric treatment can fill these gaps. Combination of endoscopic therapy with pharmacologic therapy can help narrow the gap between endoscopic and surgical bariatric treatment, as well as treat weight recidivism, inadequate weight loss, or further improve associated medical comorbidities in patients who have undergone or are undergoing endoscopic bariatric treatment.

In the last decade there has been significant development of novel devices and techniques in the field of endoscopic bariatric and metabolic therapies (EBMTs). Bariatric endoscopy fulfills an unmet need within the current paradigm of obesity management. The expansion of this field is an important step in offering complete care to patients with obesity and metabolic disease. Nevertheless, information, mentorship and guidance through starting a practice in EBMTs are limited. We discuss important considerations when beginning a practice in obesity care with a focus on endobariatrics in a variety of practice settings.

Obesity is a multi-factorial disease that is influenced by genetic, epigenetic, and environmental factors. Precision medicine is a practice wherein prevention and treatment strategies take individual variability into account. It involves using a variety of factors including deep phenotyping using clinical, physiologic, and behavioral characteristics, 'omics assays (eg, genomics, epigenomics, transcriptomics, and microbiomics among others), and environmental factors to devise practices that are individualized to subsets of patients. Personalizing the therapeutic modality to the individual can lead to enhanced effectiveness and tolerability. The authors review advances in precision medicine made in the field of bariatrics and discuss future avenues and challenges.

Pediatric obesity continues to be an omnipresent disease; 1 in 5 children and adolescents have obesity in the United States. The comorbidities associated with youth-onset obesity tend to have a more severe disease progression in youth compared to their adult counterparts with the same obesity-related condition. A comorbidity of focus in this study is metabolism-associated steatotic liver disease (MASLD), which has rapidly evolved into the most common liver disease seen in the pediatric population. A direct association exists between the treatment of MASLD and the treatment of pediatric obesity. The current evidence supports that obesity treatment is safe and effective.

Ali Lahooti, Kate E. Johnson, and Reem Z. Sharaiha

With the growing global burden of obesity, the field of endobariatrics has emerged as a promising alternative, filling the void between lifestyle interventions with modest efficacy and more invasive surgical procedures. This article explores the latest advancements in endobariatric therapies, encompassing endoscopic sleeve gastroplasty (ESG), intragastric balloons (IGB), endoscopic metabolic therapies, and promising pharmacologic and surgical combination approaches that integrate multiple therapeutic modalities. It also outlines the critical factors and strategic considerations necessary for the successful integration of endobariatric interventions into clinical practice.

GASTROINTESTINAL ENDOSCOPY CLINICS OF NORTH AMERICA

SERIES OF RELATED INTEREST

Gastroenterology Clinics
(www.gastro.theclinics.com)
Clinics in Liver Disease
(www.liver.theclinics.com)

THE CLINICS ARE AVAILABLE ONLINE!
Access your subscription at:
www.theclinics.com

Foreword

Endobariatrics and Obesity Medicine: Present Status and Future Directions

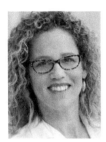

Ashley L. Faulx, MD, MASGE, FACG
Consulting Editor

Obesity continues to be a growing public health epidemic in the United States. For most patients, this is a chronic health condition and requires a multidisciplinary approach to manage. In this issue, two leaders in the field of endoscopic bariatrics and obesity medicine, Drs Violeta Popov and Shelby Sullivan, have assembled an outstanding group of experts to discuss obesity management options, how to build an endobariatrics program, novel devices and approaches to obesity, as well as surgical management. The field of endobariatrics has grown exponentially in the past few years. Endoscopic sleeve gastroplasty has emerged as a less-invasive modality for gastric remodeling compared with a surgical approach. Gastric balloons to reduce gastric capacity are indicated for obese patients with lower body mass index, and emerging small bowel therapies are promising weight loss options for our patients. Anti-obesity medications, most notably the GLP-1 agonists, will also play an important role in the management of these patients, and the challenge will be how the gastroenterologist will incorporate these into a bariatrics practice.

This comprehensive review covers all of these aspects of obesity management, emphasizing a team approach needed to successfully and safely manage patients with obesity, including options for children and adolescents. There is also a discussion of the future direction of endobariatrics, in addition to the utilization of precision medicine in bariatric procedures. All gastroenterologists will benefit from reading this issue,

Gastrointest Endoscopy Clin N Am 34 (2024) xiii–xiv
https://doi.org/10.1016/j.giec.2024.07.004
1052-5157/24/Published by Elsevier Inc.

giendo.theclinics.com

as it lays out the armamentarium available to gastroenterologists in managing this challenging disease.

Ashley L. Faulx, MD, MASGE, FACG
Case Western Reserve University
School of Medicine
UH Cleveland Medical Center
Louis Stokes VAMC
11100 Euclid Avenue, Wearn 2nd Floor
Cleveland, OH 44106, USA

E-mail address:
Ashley.faulx@uhhospitals.org

Preface

Why Bariatric and Metabolic Endoscopy Matters Today

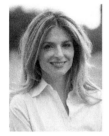
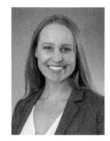

Violeta Popov, MD, PhD, DABOM   Shelby Sullivan, MD

Editors

The obesity pandemic causes an estimated 300,000 deaths per year in the United States.[1] Particularly worrisome is the rise in childhood and adolescent obesity, foreshadowing continued need for both prevention and effective therapies. Seven years have passed since the 2017 issue of *Gastrointestinal Endoscopy Clinics of North America* focused on Advances in Bariatric and Metabolic Endoscopy. This gap coincides with the approval of new anti-obesity medications, new bariatric surgical techniques, and new endoscopic metabolic and bariatric therapies that have the potential to significantly impact the obesity pandemic; however, there continues to be a critical unmet need for access to these therapies. Moreover, a knowledge gap still exists within the physician community, both with respect to the new therapies that are available and with how best to use them. Far from pharmacotherapy replacing endobariatric options, we show that these therapies can be synergistically combined to maximize patient results.

We planned this current issue of *Gastrointestinal Endoscopy Clinics of North America* to highlight the innovation and review comprehensively current obesity management from the standpoint of the gastroenterologist. Gastroenterologists are accustomed to treating GI-related metabolic comorbidities, such as gastroesophageal reflux and metabolic-associated steatotic liver disease. Weight loss remains the cornerstone of treatment for these conditions. The emergence of bariatric and metabolic endoscopic technologies empowers gastroenterologists to take a more prominent role in managing not only obesity but also diabetes, one of the costliest diseases in health care. This issue's goal is to broaden our knowledge of the behavioral, medical, surgical, and endoscopic options for treating this critical public health concern.

Our field is exploding with innovation. Endoscopic Gastric Remodeling techniques, including endoscopic sleeve gastroplasty (ESG), have emerged as a game-changer.

ESG offers additional advantages: greater durability, expanded treatment indications, the ability to be repeated, and even reversed, making it suitable for a broader patient population.

Novel small bowel metabolic procedures present a unique opportunity to explore the duodenum's role in glucose metabolism. Early trials are yielding promising results for treating both diabetes and obesity. Furthermore, an adjustable-volume gastric balloon and a fully procedureless balloon have joined the treatment armamentarium, enhancing tolerability and weight-loss outcomes.

While endoscopy takes center stage in this issue, we acknowledge the significant momentum in anti-obesity pharmacotherapy. The arrival of trendsetting GLP-1 agonists, semaglutide and tirzepatide, represents a major leap forward, although recent studies show that ESG remains significantly more cost-effective.[2] Dedicated articles address the use of the most common weight-loss medications in both adults and children, along with a guide for their integration into a bariatric endoscopy practice.

This expansion of treatment options empowers gastroenterologists to emerge as primary providers for obesity management. Their expertise allows them to deliver minimally invasive therapies, along with a staged approach that reserves more aggressive interventions for suitable patients later. This influx of qualified providers will significantly improve access to care, broaden treatment choices, and ultimately, benefit patients. However, it's crucial to note that despite these advancements in medical solutions, effective public health action remains a critical missing piece in addressing the obesity epidemic.

DISCLOSURES

S. Sullivan discloses a research grant from Microtech Endoscopy, Inc.

Contracted Research: Allurion Technologies, RebiotixConsulting: Biolinq, Endo Tools Therapeutics, Fractyl Health, Olympus, and Pentax.

Violeta Popov, MD, PhD, DABOM
VA NY Harbor Healthcare System
NYU Langone Health Systems
423 East 23 Street
11 North Gastroenterology
New York, NY 10010, USA

Shelby Sullivan, MD
Center for Digestive Health
Dartmouth Hitchcock Medical Center
Lebanon, NH, USA

E-mail addresses:
Violeta.popov@nyulangone.org (V. Popov)
shelby53549@live.com (S. Sullivan)

REFERENCES

1. Allison DB, Fontaine KR, Manson JE, et al. Annual deaths attributable to obesity in the United States. JAMA 1999;282(16):1530–8.
2. Haseeb M, Chhatwal J, Xiao J, et al. Semaglutide vs endoscopic sleeve gastroplasty for weight loss. JAMA Netw Open 2024;7(4):e246221.

Lifestyle Therapy for Obesity

Douglas C. Lambert, MD, MPH[a],*, Jamie Kane, MD[a],
Carolyn Newberry, MD[b]

KEYWORDS

• Obesity • Nutrition • Weight loss • Diet • Physical activity • Intermittent fasting

KEY POINTS

• High-quality low-fat, ketogenic, and energy-restricted diets are effective nutrition therapies for obesity.
• Adherence to dietary change remains the primary barrier to successful nutrition therapy.
• Intensive support is needed for patients beginning nutrition therapy for weight loss.
• Physical activity combined with dietary change can enhance weight loss and further improve disease risk.
• A variety of intermittent fasting therapies have been shown to cause weight loss and cardiometabolic improvement regardless of dietary change.

NUTRITION THERAPY FOR OBESITY

Introduction

Patients receive an array of conflicting nutrition advice from media and online social media sources that may, alongside food preferences, lead to entrenched beliefs about effective nutritional strategies for weight loss. It is imperative that clinicians build trust with the patient while also providing clear, convincing, and unambiguous guidance for effective dietary approaches to weight loss.

Successful weight loss from dietary change relies on a patient's capacity to create a sustained caloric deficit in metabolizable energy from food. This can be achieved through 2 approaches[1] not mutually exclusive: (1) deliberate restriction of calories through counting and tracking and (2) altering food quality to promote caloric reduction without conscious calorie tracking. This second approach is referred to as "ad libitum" dieting, which translates to "eating as much as desired" (**Table 1**).

[a] Department of General Internal Medicine, Section of Obesity Medicine, Northwell Health, Northwell Center for Weight Management, 865 Northern Boulevard, Suite 102, Great Neck, NY 11021, USA; [b] Division of Gastroenterology and Hepatology, Innovative Center for Health and Nutrition in Gastroenterology (ICHANGE), Weill Cornell Medicine, 420 East 70th Street, #442, New York, NY 10021, USA
* Corresponding author.
E-mail address: dlambert1@northwell.edu

Gastrointest Endoscopy Clin N Am 34 (2024) 577–589
https://doi.org/10.1016/j.giec.2024.03.003
1052-5157/24/© 2024 Elsevier Inc. All rights reserved.
giendo.theclinics.com

Table 1	
Nutrition therapy for obesity	
Caloric Restriction	**AD Libitum Diets**
Very low-calorie diets	Low fat
Low-calorie diets	• Conventional low fat/omnivorous
Caloric restriction/energy restriction	• Plant based
	Moderate fat
	• Mediterranean diet
	• High-protein diets (Zone, Paleo)
	High fat low carbohydrate/ketogenic

CALORIC RESTRICTION

Very low-calorie diets (VLCDs), where daily calories are reduced to approximately 25% of energy needs over several weeks to months, have been extensively studied and are demonstrated to lead to weight loss of approximately 10% to 20% total body weight loss over 1 to 3 months.[2,3] High rates of weight regain following VLCDs[4] have led overtime to an examination of more moderate caloric restriction (CR) regimens termed low-calorie diets (LCDs), where calories are reduced to approximately 50% of energy needs.[5] In long-term studies, VLCDs and LCDs are shown to have similar weight loss outcomes.[5] More modest CR of approximately 25% to 30% of energy needs is commonly used and studied up to the present.[6,7]

Key Research Findings

The most studied research question has been whether the macronutrient composition (% fat, carbohydrate, and protein) or glycemic index (GI)/load (GL) of a CR diet affects weight loss or risk factor reductions. Multiple studies have demonstrated and ultimately confirmed that macronutrient composition has no effect on weight loss results over 3+ months.[8,9] Research has also concluded that the GI or GL of a diet is largely unrelated to the degree of weight loss under CR or ad libitum conditions.[10] However, diet quality may be an important factor in greater weight loss during CR.[11] Weight loss from nutrient-dense diets characterized by unrefined foods, plant-based protein, fiber, and unsaturated fat may be superior to diets higher in added sucrose, refined starch, and animal-sourced foods.[6,7] A persistent concern with CR is whether long-term adherence is possible for most people. Many intervention studies have now shown that ad libitum approaches can have similar or superior results compared to CR.[12-18]

AD LIBITUM DIETS

Ad libitum approaches can be divided into (1) low fat (~10%–30% fat), (2) moderate fat (~35%–45% fat), and (3) high fat/low carbohydrate, or ketogenic (55%–70% fat) diets. Mechanisms through which ad libitum diets reduce metabolizable energy intake are not entirely defined but likely include (1) reduced caloric density of meals[19]; (2) greater satiety and satiation from whole foods[20]; (3) reduced gastrointestinal absorption of food energy[21]; (4) greater thermic effect of digestion[22]; and (5) reduced hedonic food qualities,[23] preventing passive overconsumption of calories.

Low-fat Diets

Low-fat diets (10%–30% fat) are, by nature, typically higher in carbohydrate, as carbohydrate-rich foods (grains, bread, potatoes, legumes) tend to be very low in fat.

However, increasing protein calories alone can modestly reduce dietary fat, for example, when lower versus higher fat animal-sourced foods are chosen.

Mechanisms of weight loss

Fat is calorically dense (9 calories/gram) compared to carbohydrate (4 calories/gram) and protein (4 calories/gram), which may contribute to passive overconsumption of food energy for a given weight of food, as demonstrated in many short-term[24] and long-term[25] intervention studies. Carbohydrate stores in the body are tightly regulated compared to fat, such that carbohydrate is preferentially oxidized for energy in response to consumption of mixed meals under ad libitum conditions, with excess stored as glycogen.[26] In contrast, excess fat calories in a mixed meal under ad libitum conditions are stored as fat[27–29] until a caloric deficit or strenuous exercise is initiated. In overfeeding experiments in humans, the contribution of excess carbohydrate-to-fat balance is minimal[27,28] except under conditions of chronic experimental overfeeding of refined carbohydrates unrepresentative of real-world conditions.[30] Carbohydrate compared to fat is also more satiating, as demonstrated in many controlled feeding studies.[24]

Due to these factors, overnutrition and fat gain appear to be incredibly unlikely on a diet sufficiently low in fat and high in carbohydrate.[31–33] And, contrary to popular belief, evidence does not support that carbohydrates are fattening under low-fat, ad libitum conditions. This is even true when diets are high in simple sugars[32–35]; in cases where no weight loss is intended[36,37]; and among normal weight subjects.[36–38] It is more accurate to say that carbohydrates as part of mixed meals are the preferred fuel for the body,[26] which permits weight gain on higher fat mixed diets composed of foods that promote overconsumption. Fat balance is consistently negative when carbohydrate quality is high on an ad libitum low-fat diet.[32,39–41] Even the partial addition of low-fat, whole foods to the diet has been shown to be sufficient to induce weight loss.[42]

Intervention results

Weight loss in low-fat diet interventions is highly variable. Among ad libitum interventions with a weight loss goal, percent weight loss varies from 3% to 12% total body weight over the course of 3 to 12 months.[15–18,40,43–49] Over longer study periods (2+ years), weight loss was shown to diminish substantially in some studies, even when weight loss was the intention.[18,47] Several long-term studies (18+ months) have demonstrated modest but significant weight loss of 2% to 5%.[44,45,50]

Reasons for variable weight loss

Variability of intervention intensity, weight loss intention, and food quality likely explain variable weight loss results. Typically, lower fat animal-sourced foods (low-fat dairy, poultry, lean beef)[50] and ultra-processed low-fat products (spreads, cheeses, crackers, muffins)[34,35] have been recommended as replacements for high-fat foods, rather than natural, low-fat whole foods such as grains, legumes, and tubers. In some interventions, primarily refined sugar (sucrose) and refined starch (flour) were used as carbohydrate replacements for fat.[34,35] These replacements by current nutrition standards are disadvantages for weight loss and health improvement.[20,34]

Low-fat plant-based diets

Results of several interventions comparing low-fat plant-based diets to conventional omnivorous diets, are suggestive of a relative benefit of plant-sourced versus animal-sourced foods on weight loss and health improvement.[17,51] Weight loss on low-fat, plant-based diets is consistently clinically significant, ranging from 6% to

12% total body weight over 4 to 12 months.[17,22,46,51,52] However, implementation of these diets requires a substantial degree of behavior change for most people. It is necessary to provide intensive counseling, support, and resources to patients making these changes.

Adherence

Several large and prominent randomized controlled studies have demonstrated a clear failure of low-fat diet participants to achieve their targeted reduction in dietary fat.[53] This makes the results of certain low-fat comparison studies difficult to interpret.[54] However, it is abundantly clear that adherence, regardless of dietary prescription, is the most important determinant of weight loss success.[32] It is notable that the majority of participants in the National Weight Control Registry report following a low-fat diet.[55]

Moderate Fat Diets

To promote weight loss through diet alone, the foods in a moderate-fat diet must promote a reduction in metabolizable energy greater the calories passively overconsumed from fat. Carbohydrate and protein sources that promote satiety without the addition of excess calories are likely to drive weight loss using a moderate-fat dietary approach.[56]

The Mediterranean diet

Meta-analyses of weight loss on the Mediterranean diet have not shown clinically relevant weight loss in the absence of CR or exercise.[57] In a randomized crossover study comparing a low-fat vegan diet to a Mediterranean diet, weight loss was demonstrated only on the low-fat vegan diet.[52] Thus, existing evidence does not support the Mediterranean diet, as traditionally formulated, as an ad libitum weight loss treatment. However, the cardiometabolic benefits of this diet may be relevant for patients focusing on other lifestyle measures for weight loss.

High-protein diets

Examples of moderate-fat and high-protein diets include the Zone diet (30% fat and 40% protein) and the Paleo diet (40% fat and 30% protein). In theory, a diet higher in protein has a weight loss advantage, as protein relative to carbohydrate is known to promote greater satiety, and requires more energy to digest, favoring a negative calorie balance. Additionally, a very modest benefit to lean mass retention is apparent under energy-restricted conditions.[58] However, long-term weight loss results are generally similar compared to low-fat, moderate carbohydrate, and moderate protein diets.[59] Adherence to high-protein diets appears to markedly wane overtime.[25,54,59]

High-fat/Ketogenic Diets

A strict ketogenic diet typically includes a reduction of carbohydrate to 20 to 50 g per day ($\sim$10%), allowing for a high percentage of dietary fat ($\geq$70%).[60] Following weight loss, depending on patient goals, carbohydrate may be reintroduced into the diet ($\sim$5 g each week) until a stable weight is reached.[48]

Mechanisms of weight loss

The high-fat content of the diet, together with a concomitant reduction in dietary carbohydrate, reduces insulin and liberates free fatty acids from adipose tissue stores. Free fatty acids are converted to ketones by the liver, which are utilized as the primary bodily fuel to meet energy needs.[60] While in nutritional ketosis, hunger does not substantially increase in response to CR, which may be due to the blunting of the increase in the hunger hormone ghrelin typically seen with CR.[61]

Intervention results

Ketogenic diets lead to 6% to 13% total body weight loss over 3 to 6 months,[12-14] which is superior to conventional low-fat diets over this timeframe. Moderate-to-substantial long-term weight loss (4%–7%) is seen after 1 year,[62] which is comparable to weight loss on high-quality low-fat diets.[48,62]

Adherence

Similar to low-fat interventions, there may be substantial decrements in adherence to ketogenic diets overtime,[63] and wide variability in adherence is seen relative to more moderate diets.[56] However, during 1998 to 2001, approximately 11% of participants in the National Weight Control Registry reported maintaining a greater than 10% weight loss over 3 years while following a ketogenic diet.[64] These patients reported a high adherence to carbohydrate restriction,[64] which likely promotes a sustained reduction in appetite favoring continued spontaneous CR.[61]

Clinics Care Points

- When first discussing dietary changes with patients, discuss the evidence-based options available to them, including optimized low-fat diets, ketogenic diets, and calorie restriction.
- If patients are resistant to making changes to diet, emphasize a position of nonjudgmental support and offer to guide them in the future when they are more motivated.
- If patients are having difficulty initiating changes, discuss small achievable goals and consider referring to a dietician who can help with incremental improvements to the diet.

PHYSICAL ACTIVITY

Physical activity is one of the cornerstones of obesity management in conjunction with dietary and behavioral modifications. Physical activity is defined as any movement that increases resting energy expenditure, of which exercise is a subtype that is planned, purposeful, and performed with a goal to increase physical fitness.[65] Exercise can be additionally characterized by its effect on the body, with aerobic exercises consisting of prolonged periods of movement that challenges and enhances oxygen delivery to large muscle groups, and strength training defined by rapid repetitive movements against resistance that fatigue muscles quickly.[66] A combination of activity is ideal for overall health and obesity management. These activities are associated with better weight loss maintenance, preservation, or expansion of lean body mass (LBM), and improvement in weight-related comorbidities and cardiovascular endurance.[67,68]

Although physical activity alone is unlikely to produce significant weight loss without an associated decrease in energy intake, it is associated with a reduction in body fat and an expansion of LBM, which are each associated with beneficial health outcomes.[69,70] Aerobic exercise is shown to reduce visceral fat, while strength training is shown to increase LBM.[71] Exercise additionally prevents weight regain after successful weight loss from dietary changes. A large meta-analysis assessing weight changes overtime in patients prescribed lifestyle modifications concluded that exercise combined with dietary change was superior to dietary change alone.[72]

Physical activity as part of a comprehensive behavioral modification plan can take a variety of forms and should consider a patient's existing exercise capacity as well as any physical limitations. Recent guidelines from the European Association for the Study of Obesity's Physical Activity Work Group suggest utilizing the 5 A's strategy (ask, assess, advise, agree, and assist) when developing an individualized exercise plan and again when refining longitudinal care and adjusting regimens.[71] Patients with higher classes of obesity may have limited aerobic capacities and develop fatigue and dyspnea with even short intervals of targeted physical activity. These patients may better tolerate isolated, shorter activity periods several times per day, an approach that can be also beneficial for the maintenance of weight loss and durability of practice. A total of 70 patients with limited mobility or joint pain related to osteoarthritis can participate in chair exercises and water aerobics, which reduce joint strain but can still provide cardiovascular benefit.[73,74]

In addition to a personalized approach, structured exercise programs are beneficial for patients, offering both educational opportunities and supervision of practice. Participation in such programs has been shown to increase fitness levels and reduce comorbid disease,[75,76] but access for patients may be limited by cost, availability, and time constraints. Current joint guidelines from the major obesity, endocrine, and cardiovascular societies in the United States suggest targeting at least 150 minutes of dedicated physical activity per week to promote weight loss in conjunction with a hypocaloric diet. A total of 68 recent literature suggest higher physical activity goals (ie, 200–300 minutes of activity per week) may be necessary to both induce and maintain lower weight in some individuals. This may reflect individual heterogeneity regarding exercise response, which is dependent on patient age, sex, degree of obesity, and body composition.[77] Adaptive effects of weight loss on resting energy expenditure may also be implicated, with a reduction in caloric utilization being associated with lower body mass overtime.[78]

Clinics Care Points

- When first discussing exercise with patients, assess patient exercise tolerance, mobility limitations, and interest in various forms of exercise, and make realistic, customized recommendations that are appropriate for each patient.
- When patients have lost weight from other measures, clinicians should discuss and encourage exercise to help them maintain weight and preserve lean mass.

INTERMITTENT FASTING
Background

The practice of fasting dates back millennia. Over the past several decades, studies have demonstrated longevity and health benefits to rodents when calorically restricted, due at least in part to improved glucose regulation and an enhanced response to metabolic and oxidative stresses, which supersede weight loss effects. While human studies have yet to replicate the magnitude and breadth of these results, intermittent fasting (IF) has been an increasingly popular area of study in recent years.[79,80]

Definition and Types of Intermittent Fasting

IF is a broad term, used for a variety of interventions, that encompasses various eating patterns involving continuous fasting lasting from 12 hours to several days.[81] In weight loss vernacular, this contrasts with chronic CR. There are several iterations of IF listed later (**Table 2**).

Table 2 Types of intermittent fasting	
If Sub-type	**Definition**
Alternate day fasting (ADF)	Rotating fasting or partial fasting day (as low as 500 kcal/day) with ad libitum feasting day
Periodic fasting	Multiple fast days per week or month with the majority of time in ad libitum state—fast can be consecutive days or divided (eg, 5 + 2 fasting)
Time-restricted eating	Eating during prescribed window each day followed by fasting (water, noncaloric liquid allowed) until next day's window

Mechanisms and Rationale

There are a few potential mechanisms that have been theorized and/or demonstrated to account for the efficacy of IF. First, a time limitation alone leads to spontaneous CR.[81] While feast days have some degree of caloric compensation, this phenomenon tends to be incomplete, rendering a net negative caloric balance of 10% to 30% on average.[81] Additionally, fasting presumably taps into evolutionary adaptations secondary to the induction of minor metabolic stress.[80] With substantial recovery built in, risks of long-term fasting and low-carbohydrate, high-fat diets might be mitigated. Patients involved in an IF program perhaps also benefit from transient states of ketosis after glycogen stores are depleted (a process taking anywhere from 12 to 36 hours).[79] Patients would convert to using fat for energy, a process maxed out after 18 to 24 hours.[82,83] Finally, animal models of IF have demonstrated improved circadian function[84] and gut microbiota profiles,[85] both of which could affect cardiometabolic outcomes.

Weight Loss and Body Composition

Alternate day fasting (ADF) and 5 : 2 diets have resulted in similar weight loss (4%–8% total body weight) from baseline after 8 to 12 weeks.[81] Longer studies of up to 52 weeks have demonstrated similar weight loss but have failed to show more substantial weight loss.[81] Time-restricted eating (TRE) studies have resulted in significant short-term weight loss of 3% to 4% (<5 kg), with longer term results currently lacking. Nonetheless, these human IF studies have demonstrated comparable weight loss to CR.[81] Human ADF and 5 : 2 trials demonstrate a comparable ratio of fat : lean mass loss (75% : 25%) compared to CR.[81] Some TRE studies have shown increased retention of lean mass, although it is unclear whether this is due to accompanying resistance training in these studies.[81]

Cardiometabolic Outcomes

A variety of IF studies have shown improvements in fasting insulin (11%–38%), but not in hemoglobin A1c in patients without type 2 diabetes mellitus.[81] While TRE trials have not consistently produced significant cardiometabolic risk reduction, early TRE (starting the eating window in the morning) has shown significant benefits to insulin sensitivity, beta cell responsiveness, blood pressure, and oxidative stress.[86] While overall ADF and IF studies have lowered lipids and blood pressure,[79,80] it is worth noting that, in a large study comparing ADF with CR, low-density lipoprotein cholesterol decreased by 5% in the CR group but increased by 10% in the ADF group, even in the presence of weight loss.[87] A variety of IF studies have failed to show improvements in inflammatory markers but have demonstrated reductions in oxidative stress,[81] even without accompanying weight loss. Participants in IF studies have generally not improved food quality (for instance, fiber, fruits, and vegetables) during the intervention, even when this was encouraged, a finding comparable to studies of CR.[81] While periodic fasting trials have a large amount of heterogeneity, studies on fasting mimicking diets have shown promise for improvement in a variety of cardiometabolic outcomes.[88]

Tolerability

While TRE is shown to have lower dropout rates than CR, possibly because of the relative ease of the intervention,[89] ADF subjects are more likely to drop out (38%) within a year compared to those following CR (29%),[87] possibly due to frustration over counting calories on fasting days.[81] Potential side effects of IF include hypoglycemia in at-risk patients with diabetes and changes in medication and caffeine clearance. An increase in disordered eating during fasting studies has not been observed; however, high-risk patients have been generally excluded from study participation.[90]

CLINICS CARE POINTS

- If patients are interested in fasting therapy, review the different forms of IF and guide them to books, phone apps, and online resources to help them initiate the practice.
- For patients who are motivated to try fasting therapy but are resistant to dietary change and exercise, discuss the limitations of this approach as a sole intervention while still providing nonjudgmental supportive care.

DISCLOSURE

D.C. Lambert reports no financial or other conflicts of interest. J. Kane reports being on the 2022 Eli Lilly Obesity Health System Advisory Board (no longer active). C. Newberry reports no financial or other conflicts of interest.

REFERENCES

1. Gonzalez-Campoy JM, St Jeor ST, Castorino K, et al. Clinical practice guidelines for healthy eating for the prevention and treatment of metabolic and endocrine diseases in adults: cosponsored by the American Association of Clinical Endocrinologists/the American College of Endocrinology and the Obesity Society. Endocr Pract 2013;19(Suppl 3):1–82.
2. Wadden TA, Stunkard AJ, Brownell KD. Very low calorie diets: their efficacy, safety, and future. Ann Intern Med 1983;99(5):675–84.
3. Castellana M, Conte E, Cignarelli A, et al. Efficacy and safety of very low calorie ketogenic diet (VLCKD) in patients with overweight and obesity: A systematic review and meta-analysis. Rev Endocr Metab Disord 2020;21(1):5–16.
4. Saris WH. Very-low-calorie diets and sustained weight loss. Obes Res 2001; 9(Suppl 4):295S–301S.
5. Tsai AG, Wadden TA. The evolution of very-low-calorie diets: an update and meta-analysis. Obesity 2006;14(8):1283–93.
6. Shai I, Schwarzfuchs D, Henkin Y, et al. Weight loss with a low-carbohydrate, Mediterranean, or low-fat diet. N Engl J Med 2008;359(3):229–41.
7. Schutte S, Esser D, Siebelink E, et al. Diverging metabolic effects of 2 energy-restricted diets differing in nutrient quality: a 12-week randomized controlled trial in subjects with abdominal obesity. Am J Clin Nutr 2022;116(1):132–50.

8. Golay A, Eigenheer C, Morel Y, et al. Weight-loss with low or high carbohydrate diet? Int J Obes Relat Metab Disord 1996;20(12):1067–72.
9. Sacks FM, Bray GA, Carey VJ, et al. Comparison of weight-loss diets with different compositions of fat, protein, and carbohydrates. N Engl J Med 2009; 360(9):859–73.
10. Chekima K, Yan SW, Lee SWH, et al. Low glycaemic index or low glycaemic load diets for people with overweight or obesity. Cochrane Database Syst Rev 2023; 6(6):CD005105.
11. Mihaylova MM, Chaix A, Delibegovic M, et al. When a calorie is not just a calorie: Diet quality and timing as mediators of metabolism and healthy aging. Cell Metabol 2023;35(7):1114–31.
12. Samaha FF, Iqbal N, Seshadri P, et al. A low-carbohydrate as compared with a low-fat diet in severe obesity. N Engl J Med 2003;348(21):2074–81.
13. Yancy WS Jr, Olsen MK, Guyton JR, et al. A low-carbohydrate, ketogenic diet versus a low-fat diet to treat obesity and hyperlipidemia: a randomized, controlled trial. Ann Intern Med 2004;140(10):769–77.
14. Westman EC, Yancy WS Jr, Mavropoulos JC, et al. The effect of a low-carbohydrate, ketogenic diet versus a low-glycemic index diet on glycemic control in type 2 diabetes mellitus. Nutr Metab 2008;5:36.
15. Shah M, Baxter JE, McGovern PG, et al. Nutrient and food intake in obese women on a low-fat or low-calorie diet. Am J Health Promot 1996;10(3):179–82.
16. Shah M, McGovern P, French S, et al. Comparison of a low-fat, ad libitum complex-carbohydrate diet with a low-energy diet in moderately obese women. Am J Clin Nutr 1994;59(5):980–4.
17. Barnard ND, Cohen J, Jenkins DJ, et al. A low-fat vegan diet improves glycemic control and cardiovascular risk factors in a randomized clinical trial in individuals with type 2 diabetes. Diabetes Care 2006;29(8):1777–83.
18. Jeffery RW, Hellerstedt WL, French SA, et al. A randomized trial of counseling for fat restriction versus calorie restriction in the treatment of obesity. Int J Obes Relat Metab Disord 1995;19(2):132–7.
19. James Stubbs R, Horgan G, Robinson E, et al. Diet composition and energy intake in humans. Philos Trans R Soc Lond B Biol Sci 2023;378(1888):20220449.
20. Hall KD, Ayuketah A, Brychta R, et al. Ultra-processed diets cause excess calorie intake and weight gain: an inpatient randomized controlled trial of ad libitum food intake. Cell Metabol 2019;30(1):67–77, e3.
21. Baer DJ, Gebauer SK, Novotny JA. Walnuts consumed by healthy adults provide less available energy than predicted by the atwater factors. J Nutr 2016; 146(1):9–13.
22. Kahleova H, Petersen KF, Shulman GI, et al. Effect of a low-fat vegan diet on body weight, insulin sensitivity, postprandial metabolism, and intramyocellular and hepatocellular lipid levels in overweight adults: a randomized clinical trial. JAMA Netw Open 2020;3(11):e2025454.
23. Hopkins M, Gibbons C, Caudwell P, et al. Differing effects of high-fat or high-carbohydrate meals on food hedonics in overweight and obese individuals. Br J Nutr 2016;115(10):1875–84.
24. Shah M, Garg A. High-fat and high-carbohydrate diets and energy balance. Diabetes Care 1996;19(10):1142–52.
25. McAuley KA, Smith KJ, Taylor RW, et al. Long-term effects of popular dietary approaches on weight loss and features of insulin resistance. Int J Obes 2006;30(2): 342–9.

26. Abbott WG, Howard BV, Christin L, et al. Short-term energy balance: relationship with protein, carbohydrate, and fat balances. Am J Physiol 1988;255(3 Pt 1): E332–7.

27. Flatt JP, Ravussin E, Acheson KJ, et al. Effects of dietary fat on postprandial substrate oxidation and on carbohydrate and fat balances. J Clin Invest 1985;76(3): 1019–24.

28. McDevitt RM, Bott SJ, Harding M, et al. De novo lipogenesis during controlled overfeeding with sucrose or glucose in lean and obese women. Am J Clin Nutr 2001;74(6):737–46.

29. Larson DE, Rising R, Ferraro RT, et al. Spontaneous overfeeding with a 'cafeteria diet' in men: effects on 24-hour energy expenditure and substrate oxidation. Int J Obes Relat Metab Disord 1995;19(5):331–7.

30. Acheson KJ, Schutz Y, Bessard T, et al. Glycogen storage capacity and de novo lipogenesis during massive carbohydrate overfeeding in man. Am J Clin Nutr 1988;48(2):240–7.

31. Astrup A, Grunwald GK, Melanson EL, et al. The role of low-fat diets in body weight control: a meta-analysis of ad libitum dietary intervention studies. Int J Obes Relat Metab Disord 2000;24(12):1545–52.

32. Aronica L, Landry MJ, Rigdon J, et al. Weight, insulin resistance, blood lipids, and diet quality changes associated with ketogenic and ultra low-fat dietary patterns: a secondary analysis of the DIETFITS randomized clinical trial. Front Nutr 2023; 10:1220020.

33. Kendall A, Levitsky DA, Strupp BJ, et al. Weight loss on a low-fat diet: consequence of the imprecision of the control of food intake in humans. Am J Clin Nutr 1991;53(5):1124–9.

34. Poppitt SD, Keogh GF, Prentice AM, et al. Long-term effects of ad libitum low-fat, high-carbohydrate diets on body weight and serum lipids in overweight subjects with metabolic syndrome. Am J Clin Nutr 2002;75(1):11–20.

35. Gerhard GT, Ahmann A, Meeuws K, et al. Effects of a low-fat diet compared with those of a high-monounsaturated fat diet on body weight, plasma lipids and lipoproteins, and glycemic control in type 2 diabetes. Am J Clin Nutr 2004;80(3): 668–73.

36. Raben A, Jensen ND, Marckmann P, et al. Spontaneous weight loss during 11 weeks' ad libitum intake of a low fat/high fiber diet in young, normal weight subjects. Int J Obes Relat Metab Disord 1995;19(12):916–23.

37. Prewitt TE, Schmeisser D, Bowen PE, et al. Changes in body weight, body composition, and energy intake in women fed high- and low-fat diets. Am J Clin Nutr 1991;54(2):304–10.

38. Kasim-Karakas SE, Almario RU, Mueller WM, et al. Changes in plasma lipoproteins during low-fat, high-carbohydrate diets: effects of energy intake. Am J Clin Nutr 2000;71(6):1439–47.

39. Hall KD, Guo J, Courville AB, et al. Effect of a plant-based, low-fat diet versus an animal-based, ketogenic diet on ad libitum energy intake. Nat Med 2021;27(2): 344–53.

40. Yadav V, Marracci G, Kim E, et al. Low-fat, plant-based diet in multiple sclerosis: A randomized controlled trial. Mult Scler Relat Disord 2016;9:80–90.

41. Hall KD, Bemis T, Brychta R, et al. Calorie for calorie, dietary fat restriction results in more body fat loss than carbohydrate restriction in people with obesity. Cell Metabol 2015;22(3):427–36.

42. Rebello CJ, Beyl RA, Greenway FL, et al. Low-energy dense potato- and bean-based diets reduce body weight and insulin resistance: a randomized, feeding, equivalence trial. J Med Food 2022;25(12):1155–63.

43. Djuric Z, Poore KM, Depper JB, et al. Methods to increase fruit and vegetable intake with and without a decrease in fat intake: compliance and effects on body weight in the nutrition and breast health study. Nutr Cancer 2002;43(2): 141–51.

44. Barnard ND, Cohen J, Jenkins DJ, et al. A low-fat vegan diet and a conventional diabetes diet in the treatment of type 2 diabetes: a randomized, controlled, 74-wk clinical trial. Am J Clin Nutr 2009;89(5):1588S–96S.

45. Chlebowski RT, Blackburn GL, Thomson CA, et al. Dietary fat reduction and breast cancer outcome: interim efficacy results from the Women's Intervention Nutrition Study. J Natl Cancer Inst 2006;98(24):1767–76.

46. Wright N, Wilson L, Smith M, et al. The BROAD study: A randomised controlled trial using a whole food plant-based diet in the community for obesity, ischaemic heart disease or diabetes. Nutr Diabetes 2017;7(3):e256.

47. Swinburn BA, Metcalf PA, Ley SJ. Long-term (5-year) effects of a reduced-fat diet intervention in individuals with glucose intolerance. Diabetes Care 2001;24(4): 619–24.

48. Gardner CD, Trepanowski JF, Del Gobbo LC, et al. Effect of low-fat vs low-carbohydrate diet on 12-month weight loss in overweight adults and the association with genotype pattern or insulin secretion: The DIETFITS randomized clinical trial. JAMA 2018;319(7):667–79.

49. Skov AR, Toubro S, Ronn B, et al. Randomized trial on protein vs carbohydrate in ad libitum fat reduced diet for the treatment of obesity. Int J Obes Relat Metab Disord 1999;23(5):528–36.

50. Sheppard L, Kristal AR, Kushi LH. Weight loss in women participating in a randomized trial of low-fat diets. Am J Clin Nutr 1991;54(5):821–8.

51. Turner-McGrievy GM, Davidson CR, Wingard EE, et al. Comparative effectiveness of plant-based diets for weight loss: a randomized controlled trial of five different diets. Nutrition 2015;31(2):350–8.

52. Barnard ND, Alwarith J, Rembert E, et al. A mediterranean diet and low-fat vegan diet to improve body weight and cardiometabolic risk factors: a randomized, cross-over trial. J Am Nutraceutical Assoc 2022;41(2):127–39.

53. Lapointe A, Weisnagel SJ, Provencher V, et al. Comparison of a dietary intervention promoting high intakes of fruits and vegetables with a low-fat approach: long-term effects on dietary intakes, eating behaviours and body weight in postmenopausal women. Br J Nutr 2010;104(7):1080–90.

54. Gardner CD, Kiazand A, Alhassan S, et al. Comparison of the Atkins, Zone, Ornish, and LEARN diets for change in weight and related risk factors among overweight premenopausal women: the A TO Z Weight Loss Study: a randomized trial. JAMA 2007;297(9):969–77.

55. Thomas JG, Bond DS, Phelan S, et al. Weight-loss maintenance for 10 years in the National Weight Control Registry. Am J Prev Med 2014;46(1):17–23.

56. Gardner CD, Landry MJ, Perelman D, et al. Effect of a ketogenic diet versus Mediterranean diet on glycated hemoglobin in individuals with prediabetes and type 2 diabetes mellitus: The interventional Keto-Med randomized crossover trial. Am J Clin Nutr 2022;116(3):640–52.

57. Estruch R, Ros E. The role of the Mediterranean diet on weight loss and obesity-related diseases. Rev Endocr Metab Disord 2020;21(3):315–27.

58. Wycherley TP, Moran LJ, Clifton PM, et al. Effects of energy-restricted high-protein, low-fat compared with standard-protein, low-fat diets: a meta-analysis of randomized controlled trials. Am J Clin Nutr 2012;96(6):1281–98.

59. Mellberg C, Sandberg S, Ryberg M, et al. Long-term effects of a Palaeolithic-type diet in obese postmenopausal women: a 2-year randomized trial. Eur J Clin Nutr 2014;68(3):350–7.

60. Gershuni VM, Yan SL, Medici V. Nutritional ketosis for weight management and reversal of metabolic syndrome. Curr Nutr Rep 2018;7(3):97–106.

61. Roekenes J, Martins C. Ketogenic diets and appetite regulation. Curr Opin Clin Nutr Metab Care 2021;24(4):359–63.

62. Tobias DK, Chen M, Manson JE, et al. Effect of low-fat diet interventions versus other diet interventions on long-term weight change in adults: a systematic review and meta-analysis. Lancet Diabetes Endocrinol 2015;3(12):968–79.

63. Iqbal N, Vetter ML, Moore RH, et al. Effects of a low-intensity intervention that prescribed a low-carbohydrate vs. a low-fat diet in obese, diabetic participants. Obesity 2010;18(9):1733–8.

64. Phelan S, Wyatt H, Nassery S, et al. Three-year weight change in successful weight losers who lost weight on a low-carbohydrate diet. Obesity 2007;15(10):2470–7.

65. Caspersen CJ, Powell KE, Christenson GM. Physical activity, exercise, and physical fitness: definitions and distinctions for health-related research. Public Health Rep-Apr 1985;100(2):126–31.

66. Knuttgen HG. Strength training and aerobic exercise: comparison and contrast. J Strength Condit Res 2007;21(3):973–8.

67. Bellicha A, van Baak MA, Battista F, et al. Effect of exercise training on weight loss, body composition changes, and weight maintenance in adults with overweight or obesity: An overview of 12 systematic reviews and 149 studies. Obes Rev 2021;22(Suppl 4):e13256.

68. Jensen MD, Ryan DH, Apovian CM, et al. 2013 AHA/ACC/TOS guideline for the management of overweight and obesity in adults: a report of the American College of Cardiology/American Heart Association Task Force on Practice Guidelines and The Obesity Society. Circulation 2014;129(25 Suppl 2):S102–38.

69. Ballor DL, Keesey RE. A meta-analysis of the factors affecting exercise-induced changes in body mass, fat mass and fat-free mass in males and females. Int J Obes 1991;15(11):717–26.

70. Oppert JM, Bellicha A, van Baak MA, et al. Exercise training in the management of overweight and obesity in adults: Synthesis of the evidence and recommendations from the European Association for the Study of Obesity Physical Activity Working Group. Obes Rev 2021;22(Suppl 4):e13273.

71. Ballor DL, Poehlman ET. Exercise-training enhances fat-free mass preservation during diet-induced weight loss: a meta-analytical finding. Int J Obes Relat Metab Disord 1994;18(1):35–40.

72. Miller WC, Koceja DM, Hamilton EJ. A meta-analysis of the past 25 years of weight loss research using diet, exercise or diet plus exercise intervention. Int J Obes Relat Metab Disord 1997;21(10):941–7.

73. Messier SP, Mihalko SL, Legault C, et al. Effects of intensive diet and exercise on knee joint loads, inflammation, and clinical outcomes among overweight and obese adults with knee osteoarthritis: the IDEA randomized clinical trial. JAMA 25 2013;310(12):1263–73.

74. Lim JY, Tchai E, Jang SN. Effectiveness of aquatic exercise for obese patients with knee osteoarthritis: a randomized controlled trial. Pharm Manag PM R 2010;2(8):723–31, quiz 793.
75. Andersen RE, Wadden TA, Bartlett SJ, et al. Effects of lifestyle activity vs structured aerobic exercise in obese women: a randomized trial. JAMA 27 1999; 281(4):335–40.
76. Dunn AL, Marcus BH, Kampert JB, et al. Comparison of lifestyle and structured interventions to increase physical activity and cardiorespiratory fitness: a randomized trial. JAMA 27 1999;281(4):327–34.
77. Stone T, DiPietro L, Stachenfeld NS. Exercise Treatment of Obesity. [Updated 2021 May 15]. In: Feingold KR, Anawalt B, Blackman MR, et al, editors. Endotext [Internet]. MDText.com, Inc.; South Dartmouth, MA. 2000. 1-9. Available at: https://www.ncbi.nlm.nih.gov/books/NBK278961/.
78. Muller MJ, Enderle J, Bosy-Westphal A. Changes in energy expenditure with weight gain and weight loss in humans. Curr Obes Rep 2016;5(4):413–23.
79. Anton SD, Moehl K, Donahoo WT, et al. Flipping the metabolic switch: understanding and applying the health benefits of fasting. Obesity 2018;26(2):254–68.
80. de Cabo R, Mattson MP. Effects of intermittent fasting on health, aging, and disease. N Engl J Med 2019;381(26):2541–51.
81. Varady KA, Cienfuegos S, Ezpeleta M, et al. Clinical application of intermittent fasting for weight loss: progress and future directions. Nat Rev Endocrinol 2022;18(5):309–21.
82. Klein S, Sakurai Y, Romijn JA, et al. Progressive alterations in lipid and glucose metabolism during short-term fasting in young adult men. Am J Physiol 1993; 265(5 Pt 1):E801–6.
83. Horne BD, Muhlestein JB, Anderson JL. Health effects of intermittent fasting: hormesis or harm? A systematic review. Am J Clin Nutr 2015;102(2):464–70.
84. Laermans J, Depoortere I. Chronobesity: role of the circadian system in the obesity epidemic. Obes Rev 2016;17(2):108–25.
85. Li L, Su Y, Li F, et al. The effects of daily fasting hours on shaping gut microbiota in mice. BMC Microbiol 24 2020;20(1):65.
86. Sutton EF, Beyl R, Early KS, et al. Early time-restricted feeding improves insulin sensitivity, blood pressure, and oxidative stress even without weight loss in men with prediabetes. Cell Metabol 2018;27(6):1212–1221 e3.
87. Trepanowski JF, Kroeger CM, Barnosky A, et al. Effect of alternate-day fasting on weight loss, weight maintenance, and cardioprotection among metabolically healthy obese adults: a randomized clinical trial. JAMA Intern Med 2017; 177(7):930–8.
88. Wei M, Brandhorst S, Shelehchi M, et al. Fasting-mimicking diet and markers/risk factors for aging, diabetes, cancer, and cardiovascular disease. Sci Transl Med 2017;9:377.
89. Rynders CA, Thomas EA, Zaman A, et al. Effectiveness of intermittent fasting and time-restricted feeding compared to continuous energy restriction for weight loss. Nutrients 2019;11(10).
90. Schaumberg K, Anderson DA, Reilly EE, et al. Does short-term fasting promote pathological eating patterns? Eat Behav 2015;19:168–72.

Weight Loss Pharmacotherapy
Current and Future Therapies

Gabriela Jordan, MD[a,b], Sigrid Young, MD[a,b],
José O. Alemán, MD, PhD[a,b,c],*

KEYWORDS

- Obesity • Pharmacotherapy • GLP-1 agonist • Weight loss • Bariatric surgery
- Endoscopic bariatric surgery

KEY POINTS

- There are currently 5 Food and Drug Administration-approved medications for the long-term treatment of obesity, including orlistat, phentermine/topiramate, naltrexone/bupropion, liraglutide 3.0 mg, and semaglutide 2.4 mg.
- New drugs, such as tirzepatide, retatrutide, and orforglipron, are currently being evaluated for their efficacy in weight loss management.
- Surgical options such as bariatric surgery have been shown to induce more durable weight loss than pharmacotherapy or lifestyle interventions alone, and even more recently, endoscopic bariatric surgery has offered a less invasive option for weight loss.
- The addition of pharmacotherapy has shown to be a promising tool to address the common issue of weight regain or weight loss plateau after surgical bariatric interventions.
- The optimal timing of obesity pharmacotherapy with surgical and endoscopic interventions requires further investigation.

INTRODUCTION

The prevalence of adults with obesity in the United States has increased to more than 30%.[1] This is of major concern as obesity contributes to cardiovascular risk factors, such as dyslipidemia, type 2 diabetes, hypertension, and sleep disorders[2] as well as an increased risk of osteoarthritis[3] and several major cancers.[4] Weight loss of 5% to 10% reduces complications related to obesity and improves quality of life.[5]

ª Department of Medicine, Margaret Corbin Campus of the VA New York Harbor Health Care System, New York, NY, USA; ᵇ Laboratory of Translational Obesity Research, NYU Langone Health, New York, NY, USA; ᶜ Holman Division of Endocrinology, New York University Langone Health, 423 East 23rd Street, Room 16-048W, New York, NY 10010, USA
* Corresponding author. Holman Division of Endocrinology, New York University Langone Health, 423 East 23rd Street, Room 16-048W, New York, NY 10010.
E-mail address: jose.aleman@nyulangone.org

Gastrointest Endoscopy Clin N Am 34 (2024) 591–608
https://doi.org/10.1016/j.giec.2024.06.006
1052-5157/24/Published by Elsevier Inc.
giendo.theclinics.com

Lifestyle interventions are currently the first-line therapy for weight loss[6]; however, weight loss is difficult to maintain with lifestyle intervention alone.[7] The emergence of various pharmacotherapies for weight loss has significantly changed the landscape of obesity management over the past decade. Most approved antiobesity medications result in 5% to 10% total body weight loss (TBWL)[8]; however, newer drugs, such as glucagon-like peptide-1 agonists (GLP-1 agonists), have been shown to result in up to 17.4% weight loss in individuals without diabetes.[9]

Similar to lifestyle interventions, of those who achieve at least 10% TBWL, many struggle to maintain this weight loss achieved by antiobesity medications.[10] Surgical options such as bariatric surgery induce more durable weight loss than pharmacotherapy or lifestyle interventions alone, and even more recently, endoscopic bariatric surgery, such as intragastric balloons (IGBs) and endoscopic sleeve gastroplasty (ESG), has offered a less invasive option for weight loss.[11] Similar to other interventions for weight loss, there remains a common issue of weight regain (WR) or weight loss plateau after surgical interventions. Studies examined the benefit of combination therapy with antiobesity pharmacotherapy and endoscopic interventions, which results in more effective weight loss.[10] There are currently 5 Food and Drug Administration (FDA)-approved medications for the long-term treatment of obesity, including orlistat, phentermine/topiramate, naltrexone/bupropion, liraglutide 3.0 mg, and semaglutide 2.4 mg, and their effectiveness in treating postbariatric WR remains an active area of investigation.[12] Herein, we present the pivotal trial evidence for each approved obesity pharmacotherapy agent, as well as the emerging data of its combination with available endoscopic procedures.

Orlistat

Orlistat was FDA-approved for the treatment of obesity in 1999.[12] It is widely available, both as an over-the-counter medication at up to 60 mg 3 times per day and at prescription doses up to 120 mg 3 times per day. Its mechanism of action is as a gastric and pancreatic lipase inhibitor, blocking absorption of 30% of ingested fat when eating a 30% fat diet.[8] In a large double-blinded trial of orlistat 120 mg tid or placebo for 1 year in conjunction with a hypocaloric diet followed by a eucaloric diet, the orlistat group lost more weight than the placebo group (10.2% vs 6.1%) at the end of the first year and regained half as much as weight as patients on placebo during the second year.[13] In both patients with impaired and normal glucose tolerance, it was also found to cause greater mean weight loss after 4 years of therapy compared to placebo (5.8 vs 3.0 kg).[14] Another randomized trial found a significant reduction in weight (4.65 vs 2.5 kg), body mass index (BMI), waist circumference, cholesterol, and low density lipoprotein (LDL) group compared to placebo.[15]

Orlistat can address weight loss plateaus after weight loss surgeries, such as adjustable gastric banding (AGB). The drug was associated with weight loss in a nonrandomized intervention study of 38 patients experiencing a weight loss plateau after AGB, with a mean weight loss of 9 ± 3 kg in study subjects compared to 3 ± 2 kg in the placebo group after 8 months of treatment with orlistat 120 mg tid.[16] It was thought that, perhaps, orlistat was effective particularly for the high-calorie liquid diet required after bariatric procedures, which is often high in fat. One limitation of Orlistat is its association with multiple side effects, particularly gastrointestinal (GI) symptoms such as oily stools, diarrhea, abdominal pain, and fecal spotting. Randomized controlled trials have shown that GI adverse effects are significantly more common in orlistat groups compared with placebo groups.[14] Due to its mechanism, it also interferes with the absorption of drugs such as warfarin, amiodarone, cyclosporine, thyroxine, and fat-soluble vitamins, which affects their effectiveness.[17] The only contraindications include pregnancy, breastfeeding, and cholestasis. However, despite these side effects, drug interactions and some contraindications, it remains a widely used and easily accessible therapy for weight loss.

Phentermine and Phentermine/Topiramate

Phentermine and phentermine/topiramate are currently approved for weight loss management in the United States and came to the market as combination therapy in 2012.[8] Phentermine is a sympathomimetic drug that reduces hunger through stimulation of the release of noradrenaline, serotonin, and dopamine in several areas of the brain, including the hypothalamus.[18] As monotherapy, it is only approved for short-term use (less than 3 months); however, in combination with topiramate, it is approved by the FDA for chronic weight management.[19] Topiramate is an antiepileptic that acts as a carbonic anhydrase inhibitor and gamma-aminobutyric acid-A (GABA-A) agonist[20] and was found to have weight loss as a side effect; however, its mechanism of contribution to weight loss is not yet clear. One proposed mechanism is neurotransmitter-mediated appetite suppression and enhancement of satiety.[21]

Three notable phase 3 trials of phentermine/topiramate that led to FDA approval demonstrated statistically significant weight loss compared to placebo. Subjects across the 3 trials of phentermine/topiramate 15/92 mg, 7.5/46 mg, and 3.375 mg lost 10.6%, 8.4%, and 5.1%, respectively, of their baseline weight at 56 weeks and a significantly higher proportion of patients received greater than 5%, 10%, or 15% weight loss with combination therapy compared to placebo.[22] The studies also found significant reductions in waist circumference, fasting triglycerides, and fasting glucose in the intervention groups. Common adverse effects seen in this and other studies were paresthesia, dry mouth, constipation, dysgeusia, and insomnia.[23] There were few serious adverse events, notably nephrolithiasis in the high-dose phentermine/topiramate group.[22] As with the possible side effects and adverse effects, it is critical for prescribers to be aware of certain contraindications of phentermine/topiramate including pregnancy, breastfeeding, coronary artery disease, uncontrolled hypertension, cardiac arrhythmias, hyperthyroidism, glaucoma, MAO inhibitor use, and it is not recommended for patients on selective serotonin reuptake inhibitors.[19]

Phentermine and phentermine/topiramate have been studied as adjunct therapy for weight loss for bariatric surgery and have been shown to be viable options for weight loss in patients with WR or weight loss plateau after bariatric surgery. In a retrospective study of patients who had undergone Roux-en-Y gastric bypass (RYGB) or laparoscopic adjustable gastric banding (LAGB), patients on phentermine lost 6.45 kg (12.8% excess weight loss [EWL]) and those on phentermine/topiramate lost 3.81 kg (12.9% EWL) at 90 days postsurgery, but this study was limited by short-term follow-up period.[24] An open label trial of patients with BMI of 50 or greater who had planned to undergo laparoscopic sleeve gastrectomy (LSG) were prescribed phentermine/topiramate 7.5/46 to 15/92 mg or no therapy for at least 3 months preoperatively and 2 years postoperatively, and the study found that the combination therapy (phentermine/topiramate + LSG) group lost over twice as much weight compared to controls in the preoperative period (28.1 kg vs 12.3 kg) and lost 11.2% more of initial weight than controls 2 years after surgery[25] (**Fig. 1**). Also, a higher proportion of patients in the phentermine/topiramate plus LSG group achieved a BMI of less than 40 kg/m^2 than LSG alone after 2 years of treatment, favoring adjunct therapy for longer term weight loss after LSG.

Topiramate alone was shown to be effective in at least 2 studies of inadequate weight loss after bariatric surgery. In a cohort of patients who had underdone RYGB or sleeve gastrectomy who received medication after surgery for inadequate weight loss or WR, topiramate was the only medication that demonstrated a

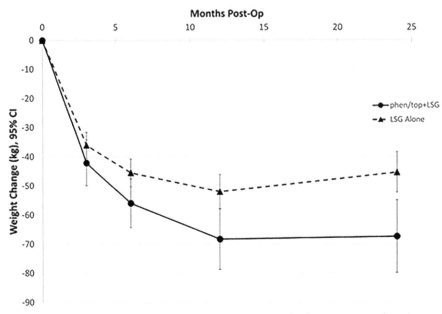

Fig. 1. Change in weight after LSG for those treated with phentermine and topiramate extended release (phen/top) + LSG versus LSG alone. (*From* Ard JD, Beavers DP, Hale E, Miller G, McNatt S, Fernandez A. Use of phentermine-topiramate extended release in combination with sleeve gastrectomy in patients with BMI 50 kg/m2 or more. Surg Obes Relat Dis. 2019;15(7):1039-1043. https://doi.org/10.1016/j.soard.2019.04.017.)

statistically significant response for weight loss, where patients were twice as likely to lose at least 10% of their weight compared to those not on topiramate.[26] A small, prospective study of patients with binge eating and inadequate weight loss after AGB were prescribed topiramate for 3 months (doses from 12.5 to 50 mg per day) found there was a mean increase in excess weight from 20.4% to 34.1%,[27] suggesting that topiramate may be a useful adjunct therapy in this patient population.

Naltrexone/Bupropion

Naltrexone and bupropion are both FDA approved as monotherapies for indications other than weight loss but were approved by the FDA as combination therapy for long-term weight management in patients with obesity in 2014.[28] Naltrexone is an opioid antagonist that is FDA approved for alcohol and opioid dependence and inhibits the autoinhibition of anorexigenic neurons in the hypothalamus.[12] Bupropion is a dopamine/norepinephrine reuptake inhibitor used to treat depression and to aid in smoking cessation. Bupropion is thought to stimulate the secretion of anorexigenic α-melanocyte stimulating hormone (αMSH) from pro-opiomelanocortin (POMC)-producing hypothalamic cells; however, it may also induce secretion of endogenous opioid products of POMC that may inhibit αMSH secretion.[28] Naltrexone alone has little efficacy for weight management; however, it is thought to counteract the autoinhibitory actions of the endogenous opioids stimulated by bupropion.[28]

The approval for combination therapy was based on a number of randomized trials that demonstrated its efficacy for weight loss. Contrave Obesity Research I was a randomized, double-blind, placebo-controlled phase 3 trial that compared naltrexone 32 mg plus bupropion 360 mg to naltrexone 16 mg plus bupropion 360 mg to placebo and found a statistically significant difference in weight loss compared to placebo after 56 weeks. The placebo group lost only 1.3%, while the lower dose naltrexone group lost a mean of 5.0% body weight and the higher dose lost 6.1% of body weight[29] (**Fig. 2**). Subsequent trials (COR-II, COR-BMOD, and COR-DM) also demonstrated statistically significant and clinically meaningful weight loss after 1 year of treatment, compared to placebo, with an average weight loss across the studies of 11 to 22 lbs (5–9 kg).[30] Some reported adverse effects include dry mouth, irritability, GI symptoms (nausea, vomiting, diarrhea, and constipation), dizziness, hypertension, seizures, and insomnia.[19] Similarly to phentermine/topiramate, there are a number of contraindications that providers need to be aware of to ensure patient safety, including pregnancy, breastfeeding, uncontrolled hypertension, seizure disorders, bipolar disorder, anorexia nervosa or bulimia, chronic opioid use, undergoing abrupt discontinuation of alcohol of anticonvulsant drugs and MAO inhibitor use.[19]

While the efficacy of combination therapy has been studied as pharmacotherapy, to date, there are no studies of the individual efficacies of naltrexone, bupropion, or combination therapy in the postbariatric surgery population.[12] Randomized controlled trials of obesity pharmacotherapy often exclude patients with a history of bariatric surgery as a control. Given the proposed mechanism of naltrexone/bupropion for weight loss as a mediator of appetite in the hypothalamus, perhaps, it would be useful adjunct therapy for patients experiencing WR, inadequate weight loss, or weight loss plateau due to dietary indiscretion after bariatric or endoscopic bariatric surgery.

Liraglutide

The development of glucagon-like peptide type 1 (GLP-1) agonists has dramatically changed the landscape of weight loss pharmacotherapy. Liraglutide, a GLP-1 agonist with 97% homology for human GLP-1,[8] given as a once daily subcutaneous injection, was approved by the FDA for the treatment of type 2 diabetes in 2013 and for weight loss at a higher dose in 2014.[31] GLP-1 is an incretin hormone that has effects on blood

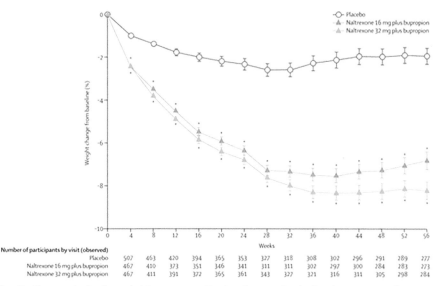

Fig. 2. Change in body weight among patients who received placebo versus naltrexone 16 mg plus bupropion or naltrexone 32 mg plus bupropion. (*Reprinted with permission from* Elsevier. The Lancet, August 2010, 376 (9741), 595-605.)

glucose as well as weight loss, as it stimulates the release of insulin from pancreatic beta cells after eating, suppresses glucagon secretion, and slows gastric emptying.[32]

Liraglutide at the highest dose, 3.0 mg daily, which was approved for weight loss under the brand name Saxenda (Novo Nordisk A/S, DK-2880 Bagsvaerd, Denmark), has been shown to result in clinically meaningful weight loss in overweight and obese patients across numerous studies. A large, randomized, controlled trial of over 3500 patients with a BMI greater than 30 or 27 with comorbidities and without type 2 diabetes found a mean weight loss of 8.4 kg in the liraglutide group compared to 2.8 kg in the placebo group (difference of −5.6 kg, $P<.001$) and 33.1% of the liraglutide group compared to 10.6% of the placebo group lost at least 10% of their body weight after 56 weeks of treatment[33] (**Fig. 3**). Greater reduction in hemoglobin A1c, fasting glucose and fasting insulin levels were noted in the liraglutide compared to the placebo group. Another randomized trial of patients with overweight or obesity receiving liraglutide 3.0 mg daily versus placebo found that patients lost an additional 6.2% of their body weight with liraglutide compared to 0.2% with placebo after 56 weeks of treatment after an initial run in period with a low-calorie diet.[34] The Liraglutide Effect and Action in Diabetes trials compared liraglutide to other oral antidiabetic drug therapies for type 2 diabetes and showed that liraglutide was associated with improvement in beta-cell function as well as weight reduction across all the trials, which included more than 4000 patients across 40 countries. The most common adverse effects were GI, mainly nausea.[35] Contraindications include a personal or family history of medullary thyroid carcinoma or in patients with multiple endocrine neoplasia syndrome type 2 (MEN2).[36]

While liraglutide alone has shown efficacy for weight loss, it has also been demonstrated as a useful adjunct to bariatric surgeries[37–39] and more recently for endoscopic bariatric surgeries. The first placebo controlled trial of adjunctive GLP-1 agonist therapy in patients with diabetes after bariatric surgery found a statistically significant mean weight change from baseline to week 26 for patients receiving liraglutide 1.8 mg daily compared to placebo.[40] There was also a statistically significant reduction in hemoglobin A1c between the groups, favoring liraglutide. A retrospective study of patients with prior bariatric surgery who experienced weight recidivism (>10% WR from lowest postsurgical weight), inadequate weight loss (<20% weight loss from initial assessment or presurgical weight), and weight loss plateau (patient desired further weight loss) found that those who had been on high-dose liraglutide had a median weight loss of 7.1% at 16 weeks and 9.7% at 28 weeks of therapy[41] (**Fig. 4**). A subgroup analysis supported the concept of "early responders" and "early

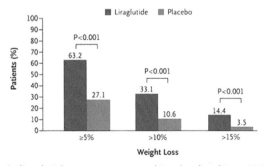

Fig. 3. Weight loss in liraglutide groups compared to placebo. (*From* Pi-Sunyer X, Astrup A, Fujioka K, et al. A Randomized, Controlled Trial of 3.0 mg of Liraglutide in Weight Management. N Engl J Med. 2015;373(1):11-22. https://doi.org/10.1056/NEJMoa1411892.)

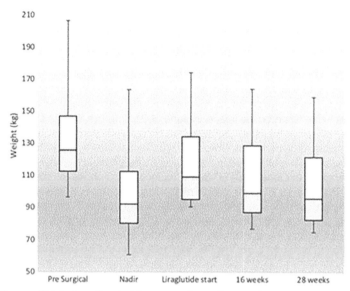

Fig. 4. Efficacy of high-dose liraglutide as an adjunct for weight loss in patients with prior bariatric surgery. (*From* Ye P, Modi R, Cawsey S, Sharma AM. Efficacy of High-Dose Liraglutide as an Adjunct for Weight Loss in Patients with Prior Bariatric Surgery. Obes Surg. 2018;28(11):3553-3558. https://doi.org/10.1007/s11695-018-3393-7.)

nonresponders," which is a cutoff of 5% weight loss at 16 weeks to predict a clinically significant weight loss at 28 weeks. This cut off has been used in the nonsurgical population to predict superior weight loss and glycemic parameters at 160 weeks after therapy.[42] A pooled data study from the SCALE Obesity and Prediabetes and SCALE diabetes trials of liraglutide found that weight loss 4% or greater at 16 weeks best predicted 5% or greater weight loss after 56 weeks.[43] This cutoff may prove useful for not only predicting long-term outcomes in pharmacotherapy alone but may also be informative for the timing and use of adjunctive pharmacotherapy with bariatric procedures.

GLP-1 agonists such as liraglutide have variably been shown to be an effective adjunctive therapy for weight loss among patients who have undergone endoscopic bariatric interventions. Endoscopic bariatric procedures, such as ESG and IGB, face the same challenges of WR and inadequate weight loss as surgical bariatric procedures. In a retrospective study, 26 matched patients who underwent ESG were offered liraglutide 5 months after ESG, and a statistically significant TBWL was found after 7 months of treatment (1 year after ESG) compared to patients who refused treatment (24.72% vs 20.51%, $P < .001$).[44] While liraglutide plus ESG showed promising results, a study of liraglutide after IGB found that combination therapy did not decrease the risk of WR 6 months after balloon removal.[31] This study of 108 patients who received IGB alone versus IGB plus liraglutide 1 month after IGB insertion found higher mean weight loss after combination therapy. However, after adjusting for covariates, the IGB group alone had higher mean body weight loss at time of IGB removal and higher odds of treatment success 6 months after IGB removal. Of note, significantly more patients in the IGB alone group tolerated the therapy for 6 months (54 vs 46% $P = .038$), but there were otherwise no significant differences between the groups regarding GI symptoms, pain, early IGB removal or migration, or small bowel obstruction (SBO). Liraglutide was discontinued 1 month after IGB removal. Although this study did not find decreased WR with combination therapy, perhaps, the timing of the initiation and termination of liraglutide could have yielded different results.

Semaglutide

Semaglutide, a newer GLP-1 agonist, is given as a weekly subcutaneous injection for both diabetes and weight management. It was FDA approved for type 2 diabetes in 2017 and for chronic weight management in adults with obesity or overweight with at least one weight-related condition in June 2021.[45] In the SUSTAIN 1 to 7 trials of semaglutide efficacy and safety, semaglutide consistently demonstrated a greater degree and sustained glycemic control and weight loss versus comparators,[46] which led to further investigation of its role in weight loss. The phase 3 Semaglutide Treatment Effect in People with Obesity (STEP) program included 5 phase 3 trials that evaluated the safety and efficacy of semaglutide at 2.4 mg subcutaneously weekly in patients with overweight or obesity, with or without weight-related complications.[47] The STEP 1 trial enrolled 1961 adults with obesity or overweight with a weight-related coexisting condition without diabetes and found that the mean change in body weight from baseline to week 68 was −14.9% and 15.3 kg in the semaglutide 2.4 mg group compared with −2.4% and 2.6 kg in the placebo group.[48] The STEP 2 trial similarly found a significant weight loss in the semaglutide 2.4 mg group compared to placebo among patients with diabetes and at 68 weeks, the estimated change in mean body-weight from baseline was −9.6% with semaglutide versus −3.4% with placebo.[49] Weight loss in the semaglutide group was −16.0% from baseline compared to −5.7% for placebo in the STEP 3 trial, which compared semaglutide 2.4 mg to placebo in adults with overweight or obesity (without diabetes), both combined with intensive behavioral therapy and initial low-calorie diet in adults with overweight or obesity.[50] Compared to liraglutide, semaglutide has shown to be a more effective weight loss agent in multiple studies.[51] Similar to liraglutide, the most common side effects of semaglutide were nausea and diarrhea; however, more participants in the semaglutide group than placebo group discontinued the treatment due to GI side effects.[48] The contraindications to prescribing semaglutide are common to GLP-1 agonists, including family or personal history of medullary thyroid cancer or MEN2.

Semaglutide also has an oral formulation, Rybelsus (Novo Nordisk A/S, DK-2880 Bagsvaerd, Denmark), which was approved by the FDA for the treatment of type 2 diabetes in 2019.[52] It is available in 3, 7, and 14 mg daily doses, with the 3 mg dosage intended for treatment initiation and not for glycemic control.[53] The PIONEER phase III clinical trial program included 10 studies of patients with type 2 diabetes and compared oral semaglutide to placebo and other glycemic control agents. The trials found that oral semaglutide resulted in effective glycemic control, reductions in body weight, and reductions in systolic blood pressure. They found low risk of hypoglycemia and the most common adverse events were mild-to-moderate GI effects, most frequently nausea and diarrhea,[52] similar to the injectable formulation of GLP agonists. The PIONEER I trial found a mean reduction in body weight of −2.3 kg at 26 weeks with oral semaglutide 14 mg daily compared to placebo.[54] Compared to both liraglutide 1.8 mg SC daily and to placebo, oral semaglutide 14 mg daily was found to be superior in decreasing body weight at week 26 (−4.4 kg) in semaglutide group.[55]

Of note, the oral formulation of semaglutide helps to address the challenge that some patients express a preference for noninjectable therapy. Studies have reported avoidance of injections of glucose-lowering agents, such as insulin, due to concerns about injection burden, interference with daily activities and injection pain.[56] In general, the oral route of medications improves patient compliance and is a more physiologic means of delivering certain molecules to liver and intestinal targets (such as GLP-1 agonists).[57] However, ensuring sufficient systemic exposure of peptide-based drugs via oral administration is challenged by the acidic environment and proteolytic enzymes in the stomach, as well as limited permeability of peptides and proteins through the GI epithelium.[58] A study of oral semaglutide in the fed compared to fasting state found that the administration of semaglutide in the fasting state with water and at least 30 minute postdose fasting results in clinically relevant semaglutide exposure.[59] Oral semaglutide, taken appropriately, therefore, provides an effective option for patients who wish to avoid injectable weight loss therapies.

The delivery methods and absorption of GLP-1 agonists are important considerations not only in patient adherence and efficacy of therapy for weight loss pharmacotherapy alone but also in their use as adjunct therapy for weight loss interventions such as bariatric and endoscopic bariatric surgeries. Semaglutide has been extensively studied as an adjunct therapy for bariatric surgery patients who have WR or weight loss plateau after surgery. A Swiss study reviewed patients who had experienced WR after surgery who received 6 months of GLP-1 agonist therapy with either semaglutide or liraglutide. Patients who had a mean WR of 15.1%, and who received semaglutide (1.0 mg subcutaneous [SC] weekly or 14 mg PO daily) for at least 6 months had TBWL of 15% or greater loss by nearly one-quarter of patients. Combined with results from a liraglutide group, the authors concluded that two-thirds of WR after bariatric surgery can be safely lost with GLP-1 agonist therapy.[51] Another study of patients with WR or insufficient weight loss found statistically significant weight loss during semaglutide treatment with a mean of −10.3 kg at 6 months[60] (**Fig. 5**). The mean time from surgery to initiation of semaglutide was 64.7 months with no difference between RYGB or sleeve gastrectomy (SG). The timing of the initiation of adjunct pharmacotherapy is an important factor in determining how to optimize the use of obesity drugs, such as semaglutide, for weight loss recidivism after bariatric surgery. Of note, the patients in those studies received a maximum dose of semaglutide 1.0 mg

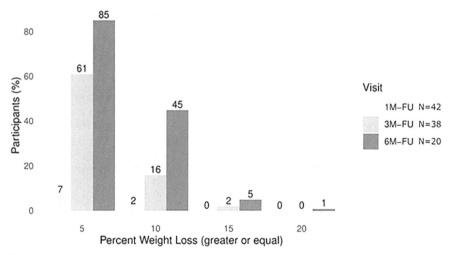

Fig. 5. Percentages of patients who reached weight loss of at least 5%, 10%, 15%, and 20%, respectively, following adjunct treatment with semaglutide once weekly for 1, 3, and 6 months. FU, follow-up; N, number of individuals. (*From* Lautenbach A, Wernecke M, Huber TB, et al. The Potential of Semaglutide Once-Weekly in Patients Without Type 2 Diabetes with Weight Regain or Insufficient Weight Loss After Bariatric Surgery-a Retrospective Analysis. Obes Surg. 2022;32(10):3280-3288. https://doi.org/10.1007/s11695-022-06211-9.)

SC weekly, as it had not yet been approved for obesity at the time. Perhaps, the higher dose of semaglutide that is now approved for weight loss, 2.4 mg weekly, would yield even greater weight loss results in this patient population.

Tirzepatide

Tirzepatide is the first dual gastric inhibitory peptide (GIP) and GLP-1 coagonist approved for the treatment of type 2 diabetes in the United States.[61] GIP is also an incretin hormone that, like GLP-1, provides glucose-dependent insulin secretion from pancreatic β cells. Both GIP and GLP-1 are both thought to play a role in appetite and satiety.[62] The safety profile is comparable to the other GLP-1 agonists, with the most common adverse effects being a dose-dependent increase in mild-to-moderate and transient GI events, such as nausea, diarrhea, and vomiting,[63] and rare fatal adverse effects, such as severe hypoglycemia, acute pancreatitis, cholelithiasis, or cholecystitis.[64] The SURPASS 1 to 5 trials among patients with type 2 diabetes demonstrated that tirzepatide at doses of 5 to 15 mg per week for 40 weeks not only significantly reduces hemoglobin A1c but also reduces weight by 5.4 to 11.7 kg and 20.7% to 68.4% of patients lost more than 10% of their baseline body weight.[61] Compared to semaglutide 1 mg SC weekly, tirzepatide at 5, 10, or 15 mg doses resulted in greater weight loss (−1.9, −3.6, and −5.5 kg, respectively) after 40 weeks of treatment.[65] The SURMOUNT-1 trial of tirzepatide among patients with obesity who did not have diabetes demonstrated an average of 15%, 19.5%, and 20.9% weight loss over 72 weeks with tirzepatide 5, 10, and 15 mg, respectively, versus 3.1% in the placebo group. In this trial, more than 35% of participants in the highest dose tirzepatide group had more than 25% weight reduction.[66] For comparison, bariatric surgery has been shown to result in estimated weight reduction up to 30% at 1 year after surgery.[67] **Fig. 6** shows a comparison between lifestyle, GLP-1 agonists (liraglutide, semaglutide, and tirzepatide), endoscopic interventions, and surgery after 12 months. Tirzepatide is expected to be approved for weight loss in the near future. It will be a valuable addition to available weight loss pharmacotherapies and may be an effective adjunct therapy for surgical and endoscopic weight loss interventions.

DISCUSSION
Weight Loss Pharmacotherapies Under Investigation

Retatrutide

A phase 2 study of a once-weekly injectable triple agonist, Retatrutide (Eli Lilly and Company, Indianapolis, IN, USA), was published in August 2023, and it showed substantial weight loss in adults with obesity. Retatrutide is an agonist at the GIP, GLP-1, and glucagon receptors. Glucagon receptor agonism is thought to decrease food intake, promote lipolysis, and weight loss.[68] In the phase 2 trial, 83% of the participants in the highest dose group (12 mg weekly) had achieved more than 15% weight loss, compared to 2% in the placebo group.[69] The side effect profile was comparable to those of GLP-1 agonists and GIP/GLP-1 agonists. It is currently undergoing phase III trials for use in obesity.

Orforglipron

Orforglipron is a nonpeptide GLP-1 receptor agonist that was recently developed and studied in a phase 2 trial of weight loss in adults with obesity. After 36 weeks, patients who received orforglipron lost up to a mean of 14.7% body weight compared to 2.3% in the placebo group. Weight reduction of at least 10% was seen in at least 46% of participants in the intervention group during the study period.[70] Adverse events were similar to those with injectable GLP-1 receptor agonists. Orforglipron may be

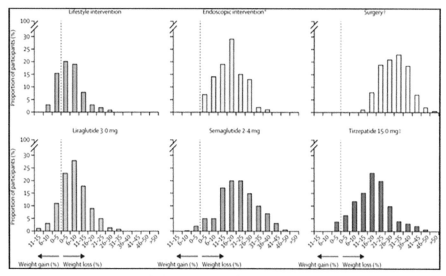

Fig. 6. Heterogeneity in weight loss response after approximately 12 months with several therapeutic approaches currently available. *For endoscopic intervention, mean results for intragastric balloon and endoscopic gastroplasty are shown for which data were available. †For surgery, mean results for sleeve gastrectomy and Roux-en-Y gastric bypass have been given as they account for 95% of all bariatric surgeries worldwide. ‡For tirzepatide, since published data reached only 25% weight loss or more, the proportion of participants obtaining higher weight losses has been presumptively assigned following the unimodal distribution observed for other anti-obesity medications. (*Reprinted with permission from Elsevier. The Lancet, April 2023, 401 (10382), 1116-1130.*)

a promising future option for effective weight loss among patients who are not amenable to injectable weight loss pharmacotherapy.

Timing of Adding Pharmacotherapy to Bariatric Interventions

Our multidisciplinary group at the Margaret Corbin (Manhattan) Campus of the VA New York Harbor Healthcare System initiated care for veterans with obesity and excess weight complications in 2017, and since this time, it has integrated obesity pharmacotherapy with bariatric endoscopy into a combined therapy. In our initial 1 year follow-up cohort study, we observed that weight loss outcomes were significantly greater in the combined cohort compared to only bariatric endoscopy. In comparison, all weight loss parameters were significantly greater in the combined therapy cohort at 12 months compared to obesity pharmacotherapy. This difference, specifically percent change in BMI and percent excess weight loss (% EWL), was sustained at 24 months. In a cohort of 58 patients who underwent outpatient IGBs or ESG and had at least 12 months of follow-up data, 43% of patients were also trialed on obesity pharmacotherapy with phentermine-topiramate, bupropion naltrexone, liraglutide, or semaglutide. At 1 year follow-up post-EBT, there was no difference in TBWL, change in BMI, or EWL between IGB and ESG cohorts. By year 3, EWL was significantly greater in ESG patients at 40.4 ± 31.6% compared to IGB patients at 17.4 ± 19.8% (*P* = .025). These promising longitudinal results suggest that the combination of obesity pharmacotherapy and bariatric endoscopy results in greater sustained weight loss than each modality alone and address the chronic nature of obesity and weight management requiring multimodal therapies.

Optimal timing for pharmacotherapy initiation with bariatric intervention (both surgical and endoscopic) remains unclear. In a prospective study of 1000 consecutive patients undergoing ESG, the greatest rate of weight loss was observed within the first 6 months following ESG. Average percent total body weight loss (% TWL) at 1, 3, 6, 9, 12, and 18 month follow-up was $8.9 \pm 2.9\%$, $10.5 \pm 4.5\%$, $13.7 \pm 6.8\%$, $15.2 \pm 8.3\%$, $15.0 \pm 7.7\%$, and $14.8 \pm 8.5\%$, respectively, with a plateau in weight loss observed at 9 months postprocedure.[71] Obesity medications could be considered during this deceleration in weight loss following ESG prior to any WR. This finding is corroborated by a study by Badurdeen and colleagues,[44] where patients post-ESG who opted to take liraglutide at 5 months postprocedure had superior weight loss compared to those who underwent ESG alone.

It has previously been posited that GLP-1 agonist initiation at the onset of endoscopic bariatric intervention may increase side effects like nausea and abdominal pain. However, in a recent study of 58 patients randomized to either semaglutide versus placebo just 1 month after ESG, those in the semaglutide cohort had approximately 7% higher TBWL in comparison to the placebo group with no serious side effects.[72] Limited data exist on the efficacy of medications prior to bariatric intervention, though one study examining the effect of preoperative orlistat prior to gastric bypass found that there was no additional difference in weight loss.[73]

A qualitative study of 16 patients examining weight loss patterns after gastric bypass described patterns that may help inform the optimal timing of pharmacotherapy (**Fig. 7**). In the "honeymoon" period immediately after surgery and continuing for 6 to 12 months, weight loss was significant and rapid. This was followed by a weight "stabilization" period, followed by a "work begins" period when patients needed to implement cognitive and behavioral effort to maintain weight loss.

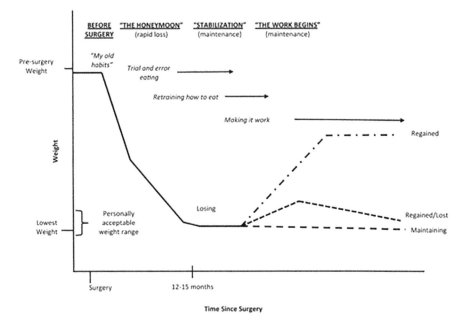

Fig. 7. Gastric bypass patients' postsurgery weight outcome trajectories and dietary management phases. (*From* Lynch A. "When the honeymoon is over, the real work begins:" Gastric bypass patients' weight loss trajectories and dietary change experiences. Soc Sci Med. 2016;151:241-249. https://doi.org/10.1016/j.socscimed.2015.12.024.)

Participants who regained weight reported a return to prior dietary habits including lack of portion control, snacking, and emotional eating.[74] Pharmacotherapies that specifically decrease appetite, such as GLP-1 agonists, phentermine/topiramate and naltrexone/bupropion, may play a role in ameliorating these habits to prevent WR in the months to years following bariatric surgery. Further studies are needed to determine the optimal timing of combining pharmacotherapy to bariatric interventions to maximize weight loss and tolerability.

SUMMARY

In conclusion, there are a number of safe and effective options for the pharmaco-therapy of obesity. New and improved weight loss drugs continue to emerge and a number of new multiagonist and multihormonal therapies are currently in the pipeline, and we hope that it will be approved for obesity in the near future. Understanding the individual mechanisms, tolerability, and efficacy of each of these weight loss drugs is essential to inform how they may best be used not only as monotherapy but also how they may be powerful adjuncts to endoscopic and surgical bariatric procedures. As discussed, some studies have already demonstrated the utility of the combination of bariatric surgery and pharmacotherapy for optimizing weight loss. With the increased use of less invasive bariatric procedures, such as endoscopic surgeries, more studies are needed to evaluate the role of weight loss drugs as adjunct therapy with such procedures. The optimal timing of adjunct obesity pharmacotherapy also re-quires further investigation in order to help provide patients with the most efficacious, tolerable, and long-lasting weight loss achievable.

CLINICS CARE POINTS

- Multihormonal agonists such as tirzepatide, and retatrutide are currently being evaluated for their efficacy in weight loss management comparable to weight loss procedures.
- The use and timing of obesity pharmacotherapy with surgical and endoscopic interventions requires further investigation.

DISCLOSURE

J.O. Alemán is a consultant for Novo Nordisk and clinical advisory board member for Intellihealth. The authors declare that they have no relevant or material financial inter-ests that relate to the data described in this study.

FUNDING

Doris Duke Charitable Foundation (JOA), American Heart Association 17-SFRN33490004 (JOA), NIH K08 DK117064 (JOA), NIH NHLBI P01 HL 160470-01A1 (JOA).

REFERENCES

1. Adult obesity prevalence maps. in: center for disease control and prevention. na-tional center for chronic disease prevention and health promotion, division of nutrition, physical activity, and obesity. 2023. Available at: https://www.cdc.gov/obesity/data/prevalence-maps.html. [Accessed 27 September 2022].

2. Powell-Wiley TM, Poirier P, Burke LE, et al. Obesity and cardiovascular disease: a scientific statement from the American Heart Association. Circulation 2021; 143(21):e984–1010.
3. King LK, March L, Anandacoomarasamy A. Obesity & osteoarthritis. Indian J Med Res 2013;138(2):185–93.
4. Pati S, Irfan W, Jameel A, et al. Obesity and cancer: a current overview of epidemiology, pathogenesis, outcomes, and management. Cancers 2023;15(2):485. Published 2023 Jan 12.
5. Mertens IL, Van Gaal LF. Overweight, obesity, and blood pressure: the effects of modest weight reduction. Obes Res 2000;8(3):270–8.
6. Wing RR. The challenge of defining the optimal lifestyle weight loss intervention for real-world settings. JAMA 2022;328(22):2213–4.
7. Dombrowski SU, Knittle K, Avenell A, et al. Long term maintenance of weight loss with non-surgical interventions in obese adults: systematic review and meta-analyses of randomised controlled trials. BMJ 2014;348:g2646. Published 2014 May 14.
8. Bray GA, Frühbeck G, Ryan DH, et al. Management of obesity. Lancet 2016; 387(10031):1947–56.
9. Jensterle M, Rizzo M, Haluzík M, et al. Efficacy of GLP-1 RA approved for weight management in patients with or without diabetes: a narrative review. Adv Ther 2022;39(6):2452–67.
10. Dave N, Dawod E, Simmons OL. Endobariatrics: a still underutilized weight loss tool. Curr Treat Options Gastroenterol 2023;21(2):172–84.
11. Popov VB, Ou A, Schulman AR, et al. The impact of intragastric balloons on obesity-related co-morbidities: a systematic review and meta-analysis. Am J Gastroenterol 2017;112(3):429–39.
12. Lucas E, Simmons O, Tchang B, et al. Pharmacologic management of weight regain following bariatric surgery. Front Endocrinol 2023;13:1043595. Published 2023 Jan 9.
13. Sjöström L, Rissanen A, Andersen T, et al. Randomised placebo-controlled trial of orlistat for weight loss and prevention of weight regain in obese patients. European Multicentre Orlistat Study Group. Lancet 1998;352(9123):167–72.
14. Torgerson JS, Hauptman J, Boldrin MN, et al. XENical in the prevention of diabetes in obese subjects (XENDOS) study: a randomized study of orlistat as an adjunct to lifestyle changes for the prevention of type 2 diabetes in obese patients. Diabetes Care 2004;27(1):155–61 [published correction appears in Diabetes Care. 2004 Mar;27(3):856].
15. Jain SS, Ramanand SJ, Ramanand JB, et al. Evaluation of efficacy and safety of orlistat in obese patients. Indian J Endocrinol Metab 2011;15(2):99–104.
16. Zoss I, Piec G, Horber FF. Impact of orlistat therapy on weight reduction in morbidly obese patients after implantation of the Swedish adjustable gastric band. Obes Surg 2002;12(1):113–7.
17. Filippatos TD, Derdemezis CS, Gazi IF, et al. Orlistat-associated adverse effects and drug interactions: a critical review. Drug Saf 2008;31(1):53–65.
18. Müller TD, Blüher M, Tschöp MH, et al. Anti-obesity drug discovery: advances and challenges. Nat Rev Drug Discov 2022;21(3):201–23.
19. Perdomo CM, Cohen RV, Sumithran P, et al. Contemporary medical, device, and surgical therapies for obesity in adults. Lancet 2023;401(10382):1116–30.
20. Herrero AI, Del Olmo N, González-Escalada JR, et al. Two new actions of topiramate: inhibition of depolarizing GABA(A)-mediated responses and activation of a potassium conductance. Neuropharmacology 2002;42(2):210–20.

21. Lonneman DJ Jr, Rey JA, McKee BD. Phentermine/topiramate extended-release capsules (qsymia) for weight loss. P T 2013;38(8):446–52.

22. Smith SM, Meyer M, Trinkley KE. Phentermine/topiramate for the treatment of obesity. Ann Pharmacother 2013;47(3):340–9.

23. Allison DB, Gadde KM, Garvey WT, et al. Controlled-release phentermine/topiramate in severely obese adults: a randomized controlled trial (EQUIP). Obesity 2012;20(2):330–42.

24. Schwartz J, Chaudhry UI, Suzo A, et al. Pharmacotherapy in conjunction with a diet and exercise program for the treatment of weight recidivism or weight loss plateau post-bariatric surgery: a retrospective review. Obes Surg 2016;26(2): 452–8 [published correction appears in Obes Surg. 2016 Mar;26(3):706. Chaudhry, Umer I; Tychonievich, Kirsten; and Durkin, Nicholas [Added]].

25. Ard JD, Beavers DP, Hale E, et al. Use of phentermine-topiramate extended release in combination with sleeve gastrectomy in patients with BMI 50 kg/m2 or more. Surg Obes Relat Dis 2019;15(7):1039–43.

26. Stanford FC, Alfaris N, Gomez G, et al. The utility of weight loss medications after bariatric surgery for weight regain or inadequate weight loss: a multi-center study. Surg Obes Relat Dis 2017;13(3):491–500.

27. Zilberstein B, Pajecki D, Garcia de Brito AC, et al. Topiramate after adjustable gastric banding in patients with binge eating and difficulty losing weight. Obes Surg 2004;14(6):802–5.

28. Yanovski SZ, Yanovski JA. Naltrexone extended-release plus bupropion extended-release for treatment of obesity. JAMA 2015;313(12):1213–4.

29. Greenway FL, Fujioka K, Plodkowski RA, et al. Effect of naltrexone plus bupropion on weight loss in overweight and obese adults (COR-I): a multicentre, randomised, double-blind, placebo-controlled, phase 3 trial. Lancet 2010;376(9741): 595–605 [published correction appears in Lancet. 2010 Aug 21;376(9741):594] [published correction appears in Lancet. 2010 Oct 23;376(9750):1392].

30. Apovian CM. Naltrexone/bupropion for the treatment of obesity and obesity with type 2 diabetes. Future Cardiol 2016;12(2):129–38.

31. Mosli MM, Elyas M. Does combining liraglutide with intragastric balloon insertion improve sustained weight reduction? Saudi J Gastroenterol 2017;23(2):117–22 [published correction appears in Saudi J Gastroenterol. 2017 May-Jun;23 (3):211].

32. Ladenheim EE. Liraglutide and obesity: a review of the data so far. Drug Des Devel Ther 2015;9:1867–75. Published 2015 Mar 30.

33. Pi-Sunyer X, Astrup A, Fujioka K, et al. A randomized, controlled trial of 3.0 mg of liraglutide in weight management. N Engl J Med 2015;373(1):11–22.

34. Wadden TA, Hollander P, Klein S, et al. Weight maintenance and additional weight loss with liraglutide after low-calorie-diet-induced weight loss: the SCALE Maintenance randomized study. Int J Obes 2013;37(11):1443–51 [published correction appears in Int J Obes (Lond). 2013 Nov;37(11):1514] [published correction appears in Int J Obes (Lond). 2015 Jan;39(1):187].

35. Blonde L, Russell-Jones D. The safety and efficacy of liraglutide with or without oral antidiabetic drug therapy in type 2 diabetes: an overview of the LEAD 1-5 studies. Diabetes Obes Metab 2009;11(Suppl 3):26–34.

36. Victoza (liraglutide) injection prescribing information. Food and Drug Administration. 2019. Available at: https://www.accessdata.fda.gov/drugsatfda_docs/label/2019/022341s031lbl.pdf. [Accessed 27 September 2023].

37. Pajecki D, Halpern A, Cercato C, et al. Short-term use of liraglutide in the management of patients with weight regain after bariatric surgery. Rev Col Bras Cir 2013;40(3):191–5.

38. Creange C, Lin E, Ren-Fielding C, et al. A5163 - use of liraglutide for weight loss in patients with prior bariatric surgery. Surg Obes Relat Dis 2016;12(7, Supplement):S157.

39. Gorgojo-Martínez JJ, Feo-Ortega G, Serrano-Moreno C. Effectiveness and tolerability of liraglutide in patients with type 2 diabetes mellitus and obesity after bariatric surgery. Surg Obes Relat Dis 2016;12(10):1856–63.

40. Miras AD, Pérez-Pevida B, Aldhwayan M, et al. Adjunctive liraglutide treatment in patients with persistent or recurrent type 2 diabetes after metabolic surgery (GRAVITAS): a randomised, double-blind, placebo-controlled trial. Lancet Diabetes Endocrinol 2019;7(7):549–59.

41. Rye P, Modi R, Cawsey S, et al. Efficacy of high-dose liraglutide as an adjunct for weight loss in patients with prior bariatric surgery. Obes Surg 2018;28(11):3553–8.

42. Proietto J, Lau DCW, Fujioka K, et al. Early weight loss responders to liraglutide 3.0mg had greater weight loss, regression to normoglycaemia, and reduced T2D development at 3 years vs early non-responders: SCALE obesity and prediabetes. Obes Res Clin Pract 2019;13(1):55–6.

43. Fujioka K, O'Neil PM, Davies M, et al. Early weight loss with liraglutide 3.0 mg predicts 1-year weight loss and is associated with improvements in clinical markers. Obesity 2016;24(11):2278–88.

44. Badurdeen D, Hoff AC, Hedjoudje A, et al. Endoscopic sleeve gastroplasty plus liraglutide versus endoscopic sleeve gastroplasty alone for weight loss. Gastrointest Endosc 2021;93(6):1316–24.e1.

45. FDA approves new drug treatment for chronic weight management, first since 2014. 2021. Available at: https://www.fda.gov/news-events/press-announcements/fda-approves-new-drug-treatment-chronic-weight-management-first-2014. [Accessed 27 September 2023].

46. Aroda VR, Ahmann A, Cariou B, et al. Comparative efficacy, safety, and cardiovascular outcomes with once-weekly subcutaneous semaglutide in the treatment of type 2 diabetes: Insights from the SUSTAIN 1-7 trials. Diabetes Metab 2019;45(5):409–18.

47. Kushner RF, Calanna S, Davies M, et al. Semaglutide 2.4 mg for the treatment of obesity: key elements of the STEP trials 1 to 5. Obesity 2020;28(6):1050–61.

48. Wilding JPH, Batterham RL, Calanna S, et al. Once-weekly semaglutide in adults with overweight or obesity. N Engl J Med 2021;384(11):989–1002.

49. Davies M, Færch L, Jeppesen OK, et al. Semaglutide 2·4 mg once a week in adults with overweight or obesity, and type 2 diabetes (STEP 2): a randomised, double-blind, double-dummy, placebo-controlled, phase 3 trial. Lancet 2021;397(10278):971–84.

50. Wadden TA, Bailey TS, Billings LK, et al. Effect of subcutaneous semaglutide vs placebo as an adjunct to intensive behavioral therapy on body weight in adults with overweight or obesity: the STEP 3 randomized clinical trial. JAMA 2021;325(14):1403–13.

51. Jensen AB, Renström F, Aczél S, et al. Efficacy of the glucagon-like peptide-1 receptor agonists liraglutide and semaglutide for the treatment of weight regain after bariatric surgery: a retrospective observational study. Obes Surg 2023;33(4):1017–25.

52. Andersen A, Knop FK, Vilsøll T. A pharmacological and clinical overview of oral semaglutide for the treatment of type 2 diabetes. Drugs 2021;81(9):1003–30.
53. Rybelsus® Semaglutide tablets, Prescribing information. Novo Nordisk. 2023. Available at: https://www.novo-pi.com/rybelsus.pdf. [Accessed 27 September 2023].
54. Aroda VR, Rosenstock J, Terauchi Y, et al. PIONEER 1: randomized clinical trial of the efficacy and safety of oral semaglutide monotherapy in comparison with placebo in patients with type 2 diabetes. Diabetes Care 2019;42(9):1724–32.
55. Pratley R, Amod A, Hoff ST, et al. Oral semaglutide versus subcutaneous liraglutide and placebo in type 2 diabetes (PIONEER 4): a randomised, double-blind, phase 3a trial. Lancet 2019;394(10192):39–50 [published correction appears in Lancet. 2019 Jul 6;394(10192):e1].
56. Peyrot M, Rubin RR, Kruger DF, et al. Correlates of insulin injection omission. Diabetes Care 2010;33(2):240–5.
57. Maher S, Brayden DJ. Overcoming poor permeability: translating permeation enhancers for oral peptide delivery. Drug Discov Today Technol 2012;9(2):e113–9.
58. Bruno BJ, Miller GD, Lim CS. Basics and recent advances in peptide and protein drug delivery. Ther Deliv 2013;4(11):1443–67.
59. Bækdal TA, Breitschaft A, Donsmark M, et al. Effect of various dosing conditions on the pharmacokinetics of oral semaglutide, a human glucagon-like peptide-1 analogue in a tablet formulation. Diabetes Ther 2021;12(7):1915–27.
60. Lautenbach A, Wernecke M, Huber TB, et al. The potential of semaglutide once-weekly in patients without type 2 diabetes with weight regain or insufficient weight loss after bariatric surgery-a retrospective analysis. Obes Surg 2022;32(10):3280–8.
61. Nauck MA, D'Alessio DA. Tirzepatide, a dual GIP/GLP-1 receptor co-agonist for the treatment of type 2 diabetes with unmatched effectiveness regrading glycaemic control and body weight reduction. Cardiovasc Diabetol 2022;21(1):169. Published 2022 Sep 1.
62. Seino Y, Fukushima M, Yabe D. GIP and GLP-1, the two incretin hormones: Similarities and differences. J Diabetes Investig 2010;1(1–2):8–23.
63. Rosenstock J, Wysham C, Frías JP, et al. Efficacy and safety of a novel dual GIP and GLP-1 receptor agonist tirzepatide in patients with type 2 diabetes (SURPASS-1): a double-blind, randomised, phase 3 trial [published correction appears in Lancet. 2021 Jul 17;398(10296):212]. Lancet 2021;398(10295):143–55.
64. Mishra R, Raj R, Elshimy G, et al. Adverse events related to tirzepatide. J Endocr Soc 2023;7(4):bvad016. Published 2023 Jan 26.
65. Frías JP, Davies MJ, Rosenstock J, et al. Tirzepatide versus semaglutide once weekly in patients with type 2 diabetes. N Engl J Med 2021;385(6):503–15.
66. Jastreboff AM, Aronne LJ, Ahmad NN, et al. Tirzepatide once weekly for the treatment of obesity. N Engl J Med 2022;387(3):205–16.
67. Maciejewski ML, Arterburn DE, Van Scoyoc L, et al. Bariatric surgery and long-term durability of weight loss. JAMA Surg 2016;151(11):1046–55.
68. Day JW, Ottaway N, Patterson JT, et al. A new glucagon and GLP-1 co-agonist eliminates obesity in rodents. Nat Chem Biol 2009;5(10):749–57.
69. Jastreboff AM, Kaplan LM, Frías JP, et al. Triple-hormone-receptor agonist retatrutide for obesity - a phase 2 trial. N Engl J Med 2023;389(6):514–26.
70. Wharton S, Blevins T, Connery L, et al. Daily oral glp-1 receptor agonist orforglipron for adults with obesity. N Engl J Med 2023;389(10):877–88.

71. Alqahtani A, Al-Darwish A, Mahmoud AE, et al. Short-term outcomes of endo-scopic sleeve gastroplasty in 1000 consecutive patients. Gastrointest Endosc 2019;89(6):1132–8.

72. Carolina Hoff A, Barrichello S, Badurdeen D, et al. "Semaglutide in association to endoscopic sleeve gastroplasty: taking endoscopic batriatric procedures out-comes to the next level". Gastrointest Endosc 2021;93(6):AB6–7.

73. Lo H-C, Hsu S-C. Effectiveness of a preoperative orlistat-based weight manage-ment plan and its impact on the results of oneanastomosis gastric bypass: A retrospective study. PLoS One 2023;18(7):e0289006.

74. Lynch A. "When the honeymoon is over, the real work begins:" Gastric bypass pa-tients' weight loss trajectories and dietary change experiences. Soc Sci Med 2016;151:241–9.

Bariatric Surgery
Current Trends and Newer Surgeries

Ruben D. Salas-Parra, MD[a], Caroline Smolkin, MD[a],
Sarah Choksi, MD[b], Aurora Dawn Pryor, MD, MBA[c,d],*

KEYWORDS

- Bariatric surgery • Sleeve gastrectomy • Roux-en-Y gastric bypass
- Single anastomosis duodeno–ileal bypass • Duodenal switch

KEY POINTS

- Bariatric surgery remains a safe and highly effect treatment for obesity and related metabolic conditions.
- Bariatric procedures have continued to evolve with sleeve gastrectomy and Roux-en-Y gastric bypass still being commonly employed.
- Revisional surgery is gaining in popularity and includes many nuances in surgical technique.
- Novel procedures are being developed, which may employ a combination of surgical and endoscopic approaches.

INTRODUCTION

The prevalence of obesity is on the rise, leading to a significant increase in metabolic and bariatric surgery around the world. Metabolic and bariatric surgery consists of procedures that are gastric specific or reliant on intestinal bypass either alone or in combination for the treatment of obesity. Although we have seen substantial evolution in procedures, Roux-en-Y gastric bypass (RYGB) and sleeve gastrectomy are the most commonly performed bariatric operations, with newer techniques gaining recent popularity, most notably single anastomosis duodeno–ileal bypass with sleeve gastrectomy (SADI-S) and one anastomosis gastric bypass (OAGB) (**Fig. 1**).

Long-term data confirm the safety and efficacy of these surgeries, supporting procedure adoption. Recent guidelines recommend bariatric surgery in individuals with

a Department of Surgery, Long Island Jewish Medical Center and North Shore University Hospital, Northwell, New Hyde Park, NY, USA; b Department of Surgery, Lenox Hill Hospital, Northwell Health, New York, NY, USA; c Long Island Jewish Medical Center, Northwell Health; d Donald and Barbara Zucker School of Medicine at Hofstra/Northwell, 240-05 76th Avenue, Suite B-241, New Hyde Park, NY 11040, USA
* Corresponding author.
E-mail address: apryor@icloud.com
Twitter: @AuroraPryor (A.D.P.)

Gastrointest Endoscopy Clin N Am 34 (2024) 609–626
https://doi.org/10.1016/j.giec.2024.06.005
1052-5157/24/© 2024 Elsevier Inc. All rights reserved, including those for text and data mining, AI training, and similar technologies.

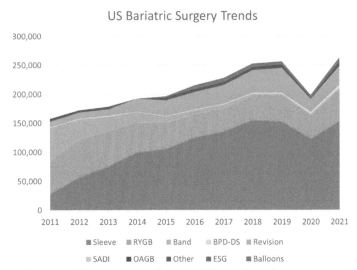

Fig. 1. United States (US) bariatric procedure trends in number of cases per year. Procedures included are sleeve gastrectomy (sleeve), Roux-en-Y Gastric Bypass (RYGB), Laparoscopic adjustable gastric banding (band), Biliopancreatic Diversion with Duodenal Switch (BPD-DS), Revision following primary bariatric surgery (revision), Single Anastomosis Duodeno-ileostomy (SADI), One Anastomosis Gastric Bypass (OAGB), other surgical procedures (Other), Endoscopic Sleeve Gastroplasty (ESG) and Intragastric Balloons (Balloons). (Estimate of Bariatric Surgery Numbers, 2011-2022. https://asmbs.org/resources/estimate-of-bariatric-surgery-numbers/, accessed 1/3/2024.)

body mass index (BMI) greater than 35 kg per m^2, irrespective of their comorbidities, or BMI greater than 30 kg per m^2 in individuals with type 2 diabetes or have not achieved significant weight loss or improvement of comorbidities with non-surgical methods. Also, older individuals who stand to benefit from metabolic and bariatric surgery should not be longer restricted by an upper age limit.[1]

HISTORY OF BARIATRIC SURGERY

In the literature, it is recognized that the first weight loss surgery was performed by Dr A.J. Kremen, who initially translated his animal experiment to the first jejunal-ileal bypass (JIB) in humans on April 9, 1954. The JIB is performed by joining the proximal small intestine and the distal ileum, thereby bypassing a large segment of small bowel using an open right mid abdomen transverse incision.[2,3]

With time, the Jejunoileal bypass and its modifications during the next decades were abandoned due to serious complications. These complications included severe diarrhea and electrolyte abnormalities, vitamin, protein, and mineral deficiencies, blind loop syndrome with associated bacterial overgrowth in the defunctionalized limb and most significantly liver dysfunction, which ranged from mild to cirrhosis and liver failure. These high severity morbidities significantly impacted patients' quality of life.[2]

Later, with the decline of the Jejunoileal bypass, gastric-based surgeries were developed, with the initial restrictive technique described by Mason creating a small proximal reservoir with a band reinforcing the outlet of the stomach–the vertical banded gastroplasty. These procedures led to significant weight loss but with the downside of weight regain due to the loss of the restriction offered initially with dilation of the pouch and connecting channel and associated staple line dehiscence.[2,4]

Dr Mason continued his innovation with the creation of the gastric bypass, diving the stomach horizontally and connecting a loop gastrojejunostomy to the proximal gastric pouch, originally described in 1968.[5] This technique was then modified by adjusting the size and shape of the gastric pouch for an adequate volume restriction as proposed by Alder and Terry at the end of 1970's and later modified by Griffen, decreasing the bile reflux and the tension on the loop by doing a Roux-en-Y gastrojejunostomy.[6] The RYGB is the first procedure to stand the test of time and it was successfully performed laparoscopically by Wittgrove in the 1990's, reporting the initial large series of 500 patients.[7]

To create a less invasive procedure without altering the gastrointestinal (GI) tract continuity, in 1978 the initial attempts at a non-adjustable gastric band were reported by Wilkinson and Peloso.[2] The initial experiences were unsuccessful due to complications including band slippage, gastric prolapse, strictures, and erosions.[2] Later developments led to an adjustable silicone gastric band connected to a subcutaneous port to allow fluid to be added to the band and produce restriction.[2] The concept of "metabolic surgery" where the surgical intervention performed on a normal organ to achieve a potential health benefit due to its biologic results was published by Kremen and Varco in 1978, which later was further proven by Purnell and colleagues where the association between gastric bypass and diabetes resolution was demonstrated long-term.[3,8]

All the techniques were continuously modified to improve their outcomes, but it was the development of laparoscopic surgery in the 1990s that led to rapid expansion in bariatric surgery. Laparoscopic adjustable gastric banding (LAGB) and RYGB were the first widespread procedures.[7,9] The LAGB underwent many modifications and soon rose to its peak in popularity in 2008 with 42% of total bariatric procedures being LAGB, but the popularity of the procedure declined in the later years (see **Fig. 1**). Band failure is attributed to long-term complications related to the band (pouch dilation, erosions, slippage, and intolerance), weight gain or poor weight loss, reflux, and reoperations as high as 50%. Alongside this, more effective and highly safe procedures such as sleeve gastrectomy, described as follows, were developed.[2,4,10,11]

Biliopancreatic diversion was described by Scopanario in 1976. This procedure combines a horizontal gastrectomy with an intestinal bypass. Duodenal switch (DS) was first performed by Hess and Hess in 1988 as a modification of this procedure, incorporating a vertically sleeved stomach with a duodenal bypass with very short common channel with their 9 years outcomes reported in 1998.[12] Gagner and Pomp proposed separating the DS into an initial gastric sleeve followed by a staged intestinal bypass.[13] The majority of patients undergoing Biliopancreatic Diversion with Duodenal Switch (BPD-DS) did well with the initial sleeve alone, leading to the most popular bariatric surgical procedure today.[14]

Gastric bypass was modified to a single anastomosis approach with Rutledge's 1997 mini gastric bypass.[15] This technique involved the formation of a long-sleeved gastric pouch from the lesser curvature of the stomach extending proximally toward the angle of His. A gastrojejunostomy was created antecolic, 3 to 5 cm wide, and 180 to 220 cm from the ligament of Treitz. Over the years this technique has been modified into the modern OAGB. The length of the loop may vary based on patients BMI and risk factors—250 cm in super obese, 180 to 200 cm in elderly or vegetarians, and 150 cm in patients with type II diabetes.[15,16] The most current technique was proposed by Carbajo and Caballero in 2002 in which a side-to-side anastomosis between the gastric pouch and jejunum is formed about 250 to 350 cm from the ligament of Treitz to prevent gastroesophageal (GE) bile reflux.[17] Single anastomosis modification of the duodenal switch has also gained popularity. It is a newer technique, initially described by Sanchez-Pernaute. This procedure typically involves a sleeve gastrectomy with a SADI-S with the distal common channel typically of 200 to 350 cm.

Multiple authors have reported their series of laparoscopic gastric bypass, which achieved comparable outcomes to the open approach in terms of anastomotic leak, complications, and sustained weight loss in the 10 years after the first laparoscopic bypass. However, the marked improvements in patient outcomes were driven quality programs, which led to marked advancement in techniques, outcomes, and reduced complications. According to the American Society for Metabolic and Bariatric Surgery (ASMBS), sleeve gastrectomy was the most common procedure in 2021 (over 152000 cases). Primary RYGB is the second most common bariatric surgery performed, with over 56000 cases in 2021.[18] This trend has been consistently seen since at least 2015. Before 2015, the sleeve and RYGB were performed almost equally, and the gastric band was performed as often as the RYGB. As of the writing of this article, the gastric band is being minimally performed with only approximately 1000 cases in 2021 (see **Fig. 1**).[18]

Trends in bariatric surgery in the United States (US) over the last 10 years are depicted in **Fig. 1**.

BACKGROUND
Laparoscopic Adjustable Gastric Band

The adjustable gastric band works by restriction, achieving weight loss by limiting intake of calories. Two main techniques have been described in the literature: the perigastric and the pars-flaccida techniques. While both are effective for weight loss, the perigastric technique has been associated with higher complication rates.[19] (**Fig. 2**).

Studies demonstrate a long-term excess weight loss ranging from 33% to 60% and a total weight loss (%) (%TWL) at 1 year of 23.73%; however, long-term complications

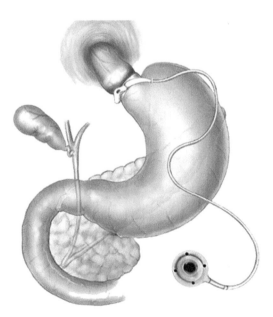

Fig. 2. Laparoscopic adjustable gastric banding (LAGB). (*Reprinted with permission from Elsevier. The Lancet Gastroenterology & Hepatology, 2021; 6(3):238-251.*)

have led to more gastric band removals than placements.[11,20-22] Complications of a LAGB include reflux, esophageal dysmotility, slipped band, band erosion, and band obstruction.[23] A slipped band, or gastric prolapse, is seen when the lower stomach herniates superiorly through the device. The band slip can be anterior or posterior depending on which portion of the stomach herniates through the band. The patient with slippage usually presents with dysphagia, vomiting, regurgitation, and food intolerance. Diagnosis can be made by plain abdominal radiograph or upper GI series. The band is normally oriented diagonally from the 2 to 8 o'clock position and points toward the left shoulder while a slipped band will appear more horizontal and point toward the left hip. The first step is to deflate the band to alleviate the symptoms. If symptoms persist, urgent surgery is warranted. Treatment options include removal of the band, repositioning of the band, and conversion to another bariatric procedure such as sleeve gastrectomy or RYGB. Failure to diagnose and treat a slipped band may lead to gastric ischemia. Band erosion usually presents with port site infection, abdominal pain, or failure of appetite suppression. Endoscopy can be used to confirm the diagnosis and potentially for band removal. Treatment involves removal of the band and possibly repairs of the stomach wall with drainage. Band obstruction is secondary to an over filled band, which leads to gastric pouch and esophageal dilation. Treatment is deflation or removal of the band.

While laparoscopic adjustable gastric banding was once a popular procedure, it has lost its popularity with newer literature showing high long-term reoperation rates and fewer efficacies than newer procedures.[23-25] Surgeons are moving away from this procedure given its requirement for close follow-up, low patient compliance, and high reoperation rates. Sleeve gastrectomy, in contrast, is gaining popularity given its effectiveness for weight loss, low complication rates, and technical ease of operation.[24,26]

Sleeve Gastrectomy

Sleeve Gastrectomy (SG) is a restrictive and metabolic weight loss procedure that is typically performed laparoscopically or robotically. In a study from 2013, sleeve gastrectomy was the most common bariatric procedure performed in the USA and Canada.[10] (**Fig. 3**). Sleeve is a partial gastrectomy performed vertically, preserving the lesser curvature of the stomach to make a tubular organ.

SG can lead to excess weight loss up to 70% in year one, which is maintained up to at least 3 years, and a %TWL of 29.5% and 27% at 1 and 5 years, respectively.[27-32] SG also helps reduce rates of diabetes, hypertension, hyperlipidemia, and sleep apnea similar to RYBG.[30,32,33]

Since cancer is also another condition associated with obesity, it is important to note that metabolic and bariatric surgery has shown reduction of the risk of obesity-related cancers (GI and hepatobiliary, genitourinary, and gynecologic). Another important benefit of bariatric surgery is to work as a bridge for severely obese patients requiring other surgical treatments for abdominal wall hernias, transplants, or arthroplasty. Also, life expectancy after bariatric surgery is increased, with some studies reporting up to an additional 6 years of longevity.[1]

Intraoperatively and early postoperatively, bleeding and staple line leaks are the most common complications.[32] Staple line leakage occurs in about 1% to 3% of patients and bleeding occurs in less than 1% of patients.[34,35] These patients are also prone to mesenteric or portal venous thrombosis in the early post-operative period. Longer term, the most common vitamin deficiencies after SG include vitamin B12, iron, calcium, and vitamin D.[36] However, studies show that patients experience fewer nutrient deficiencies after SG compared to RYGB.[28] Strictures in the distal sleeve

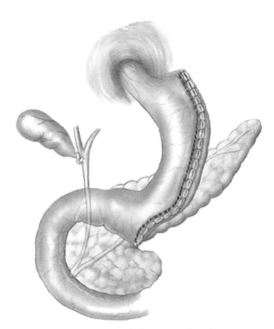

Fig. 3. Laparoscopic sleeve gastrectomy (SG). (*Reprinted with permission from* Elsevier. The Lancet Gastroenterology & Hepatology, 2021; 6(3):238-251.)

occur in about 4% of SG patients and present with inability to tolerate oral intake, nausea, and vomiting, which can be diagnosed by upper GI series or endoscopy, with subsequent therapeutic endoscopic dilation.[37]

Sleeve patients may develop GE reflux disease or some esophageal dysmotility. A high incidence of Barrett's esophagus has also been described.[38] Given the technical ease, low complication rate and high weight loss, sleeve gastrectomy continues to be a safe and popular option for bariatric surgery.

Roux-en-Y Gastric Bypass

RYGB is an option for bariatric surgery in individuals with higher BMI and potentially with obesity-related comorbidities. The technique may vary by surgeon; however, the steps include a creation of a gastric pouch of 20 to 30 cc in volume (primarily involving the lesser curve of the stomach), creation of a 50 to 150 cm biliopancreatic limb, jejunojejunostomy creation, and creation of a 75 to 150 cm Roux limb with gastrojejunostomy. RYGB is typically performed laparoscopically or robotically.[39] (**Fig. 4**).

When compared to SG, few studies have reported better weight loss outcomes with the RYGB, while others have suggested only minor weight loss differences in the long-term.[40,41] Studies have shown similar trends between RYGB and SG in changes in weight loss percentage and percent excess weight loss from baseline up to 3 years post-surgery.[40] RYGB mean excess weight loss (EWL) has been documented as 59.1 plus minus 20.3%, with some anticipated weight regain following the initial nadir and %TWL at 1 year of 31.9% and at 5 years of 28.1%.[31,41]

In a meta-analysis conducted with 20 studies from 2013 to 2023 by Kim and colleagues, RYGB and SG were found to have superior weight loss outcomes compared to medical therapy. RYGB was found to have the most effect on maintaining weight loss over SG, gastric banding, and medical therapy. For type 2 diabetic patients, the STAMPEDE randomized control trial by Schauer and colleagues showed that

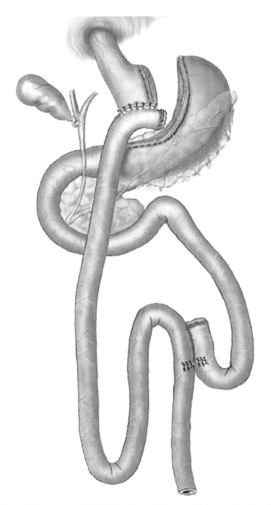

Fig. 4. Roux-en-Y gastric bypass (RYGB). (*Reprinted with permission from* Elsevier. The Lancet Gastroenterology & Hepatology, 2021; 6(3):238-251.)

bariatric surgery with medical therapy was more effective than medical therapy alone in reducing hyperglycemia.[42] Multiple other studies have also shown the benefit of bariatric surgery in the remission of type 2 diabetes.[43,44] The results for resolution of hyperlipidemia are not as straight forward.[45] However, there are studies that show that hyperlipidemia may fully resolve with RYGB.[46,47] Hypertension also had improvement after RYGB and SG in the short- and long-term.[45,46]

Early post-operative complications after RYGB include bleeding, leak, and obstruction. Post-operative bleeding is reported with a rate of 0.9% to 4.4%, with rates decreasing more recently with advancements to surgical technique. Bleeding is either intraluminal or extraluminal, with intraluminal bleeding occurring 3x more often than extraluminal. If bleeding is present, it is often at an anastomosis site and may be managed endoscopically if the bleeding does not resolve with conservative management.[48] Longer term complications include small bowel obstruction secondary to an internal hernia, gastrojejunal anastomosis stenosis, gastrogastric fistula, and marginal ulcer.[37] There are 3 potential spaces for internal herniation: (1) mesenteric defect at the enteroenterostomy (most common); (2) retro alimentary limb space between Roux limb, transverse mesocolon, and the retroperitoneum (Peterson's space); and (3) mesocolon window created in the mesentery of the transverse colon in retrocolic techniques through which the Roux limb [afferent limb of jejunum] will pass toward the gastric pouch".[49,50] A meta-analysis, which included over 31000 patients, showed the incidence rate of internal hernia was 1% to 3%.[50] A randomized clinical trial found that closure of the mesenteric defects in laparoscopic RYGB reduced the risk of small bowel obstruction (14.9% vs 7.8%).[51] Marginal ulcers are seen in 16% of post-RYGB patients, often within 1 year post-operatively. They may be related to technical factors or to patient factors such as diabetes, smoking, alcohol use, and steroid or nonsteroidal anti-inflammatory use. Endoscopy should be first line for diagnosis, and proton pump inhibitors should be first line treatment.[52] Surgical revision may be required.

Biliopancreatic Diversion with Duodenal Switch or Single Anastomosis Duodenal Ileal Bypass-Sleeve

The duodenal switch is depicted in **Fig. 5**.This procedure combines the SG with significant intestinal bypass. The BPD-DS consist in 3 primary components: a longitudinal gastrectomy, providing decreased gastric acid production, maintaining normal gastric emptying, and encouraging caloric restriction; then a 250 to 350 cm total alimentary limb to decrease absorption of calories; and lastly, a common channel measuring 100 to 125 cm in length decreasing protein and fat absorption by mixing the food with the biliopancreatic juices.[53] In terms of weight loss, at 1 year can offer a 43.22 %TWL.[54] DS has the greatest resolution of diabetes (>90% in patient with oral medications for type 2 diabetes) and weight loss effectiveness with a %TWL at 1 year of 40%, but despite these benefits, is not commonly performed worldwide.[6,55] Complications after this type of operations are related to the sleeve (staple leak, strictures), or related to its anastomosis (anastomotic leak, stenosis), but due to its malabsorptive mechanism, the BPD-DS is associated with micronutrient deficiencies (primarily fat-soluble vitamins, iron, and zinc), requiring need for extra supplementation and long-term follow.[53,56]

More recently, there has been increasing interest in a modification of this procedure that omits the ileo-ileal anastomosis. Most commonly called the SADI or SADI-S, SADI is technically easier to perform than traditional DS, with an enhanced safety profile and relatively equivalent short-term outcomes. It consists of a sleeve gastrectomy over a 50 to 60 Fr Bougie, with a duodenoileostomy 250 to 350 cm from the ileocecal valve.[6] (**Fig. 6**). Some studies have shown comparable outcomes of remission of comorbidities with significant percentage of excess weight loss around 80% to 89% and %TWL at 1 year of 42% and at 5 years of 38%.[57] Postoperative complications have been lower in comparison to BPD-DS.[58] Longer term, there is some evidence that weight loss maintenance may be better with traditional DS. Nowadays, these procedures are also options for conversion for inadequate weight loss or weight regain after sleeve.[59,60]

One Anastomosis Gastric Bypass

In 2018, the International Federation for the Surgery of Obesity and Metabolic Disorders published the OAGB as the third most performed primary surgical bariatric procedure with a rate of 4.8%.[61] This procedure combines a long lesser curvature based gastric pouch with a loop gastrojejunostomy and shorter common channel (**Fig. 7**) reducing the long-term risk internal hernia reduction since no mesenteric defects were created.[62] According to the ASMBS, approximately 1149 OAGB were performed in 2021 in the US.[18]

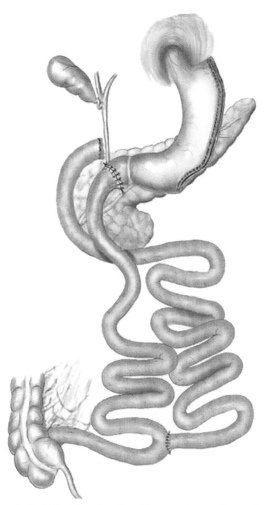

Fig. 5. Duodenal switch (DS). (*Reprinted with permission from* Elsevier. The Lancet Gastroenterology & Hepatology, 2021; 6(3):238-251.)

The weight loss after OAGB is reported as %TWL of 26.6 plus minus 5.9% and 20.9 plus minus 9.3% at 1 year and 5 years, respectively, and other studies as 68.6% to 85% excess weight lost at greater than or equal to 5-year follow-up, closer to DS than RYGB.[63–67] Randomized control studies have shown the excess weight loss to be comparable and with no significant difference between OAGB versus RYGB, as well as OAGB versus SG.[67–69]

The studies that have assessed short- and long-term outcomes have noted comparable complication rates to more prevalent bariatric procedures.[67] Early complication rates are reported as between 3.5% and 7.5%.[65,67] Some of these complications included reoperation for intra-abdominal bleeding, leaks, or small bowel obstruction.[65] A prospective, randomized trial of 80 patients reported that the OAGB produces similar results when compared to the RYGB when comparing late complications, EWL, BMI, quality of life improvement, and comorbidity improvement. This study also noted that OAGB had shorter operative times.[66]

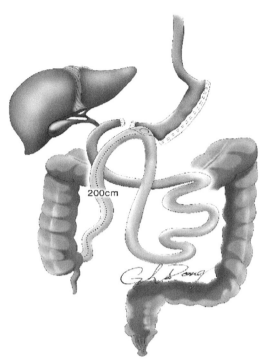

Fig. 6. Single anastomosis duodeno-ileal bypass with sleeve gastrectomy (SADI-S). (Anjian Wu et al., Single-anastomosis duodeno-ileal bypass with sleeve gastrectomy (SADI-S) as a revisional surgery, Surgery for Obesity and Related Diseases, 14 (11), 2018, 1686-1690, https://doi.org/10.1016/j.soard.2018.08.008.)

The limited popularity as OAGB as a mainstay choice in US bariatric surgery is attributed to the side effect of biliary reflux secondary to the creation of the loop gastrojejunostomy.[62] Rates of biliary reflux have been reported as between 0.9% and 4% of patients and concern of biliary reflux centers around the potential for stomach and esophageal malignancy.[62,64,65] Revision with a Braun enteroenterostomy or with Roux-en-Y conversion can address this complication. Modern techniques with angulation of the biliopancreatic limb may minimize reflux. The technical ease and favorable complication profile of this procedure are leading to an increase in its adoption.

Newer Techniques

With the interest in metabolic procedures, there has been much innovation in recent years and a long list of alternative procedures has been proposed.[6] Some of these procedures have been modified to accommodate lower risk anastomoses or potentially combined endoscopic or surgical approaches. Two of these techniques are depicted in **Fig. 8** the Single Anastomosis Sleeve Ileostomy and the SADI with duodenal bipartitioning. Although early outcomes of these procedures seem favorable, longer follow-up is needed. These procedures are also promising as potential targets for magnetic GI anastomoses.

PRE-OPERATIVE OR PRE-PROCEDURE PLANNING

Bariatric surgery requires a comprehensive preoperative work-up, which consists of a multidisciplinary team (primary care provider, nutritionist, psychologist/psychiatrist,

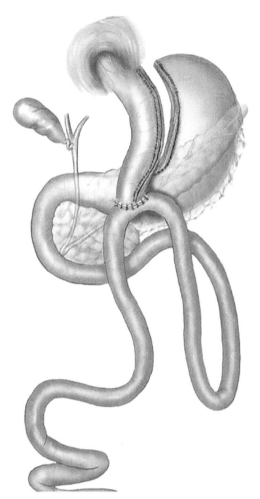

Fig. 7. One anastomosis gastric bypass (OAGB). (*Reprinted with permission from* Elsevier. The Lancet Gastroenterology & Hepatology, 2021; 6(3):238-251.)

nurse, medical subspecialties, and bariatric surgeon). This team facilitates long-term lifestyle modifications essential for a successful completion of the bariatric surgery program. A psychosocial assessment is required and aim to identify and address psychiatric disorders or substance abuse before surgery, and to assess ability to cope with the changes in lifestyle, body image, and stressors that would affect the long-term effects of surgery.[1] Medical and nutritional assessments are required as well preoperatively with the goal of to optimize potential tolerance of surgery and to educate and assess macro and micronutrients deficiencies, as well as food choice guidance.

Enhanced recovery pathways recommend preoperative and postoperative nutrition screening as essential, focusing on providing protein rather than calories, promoting feeding until late in the preoperative period and restarting diet early postoperatively. Oral nutrition supplements should be considered for all patients.[70] Some other patients will require additional evaluations depending on the risk factors or comorbidities.

In evaluating a patient for bariatric surgery, further assessments are determined by medical history, physical examination, laboratory testing, or preoperative medical

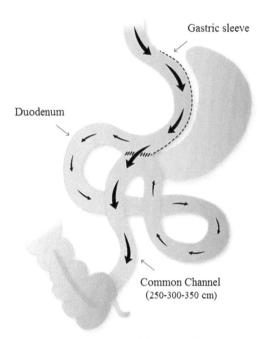

Fig. 8. Bipartitioning procedure. If anastomosis is to the distal sleeve, the procedure is called Single anastomosis sleeve ileostomy (SASI). Is the anastomosis is to the duodenum, this represents transit bipartitioning after sleeve. (Najmeddine Attia et al., The single anastomosis sleeve ileal (SASI) bypass: A review of the current literature on outcomes and statistical results, Obesity Medicine, 27, 2021, 100370, https://doi.org/10.1016/j.obmed.2021.100370.)

assessments. Completion of sleep apnea screening with STOP-BANG with further testing based on screening results is recommended due to the high prevalence of obstructive sleep apnea in obese patients. Patients with preoperative reflux or dysphagia may benefit from upper endoscopy, upper gastrointestinal series, manometry, or esophageal pH study before surgery.[71] Cancer screening should follow age-appropriate recommendations.

Medically supervised weight loss programs are not clinically indicated, but education regarding post-operative diet and exercise programs is essential. Patients should also be able to demonstrate an understanding of these programs prior to surgery. Female patients are encouraged to avoid pregnancy for 18 months until weight loss has stabilized to avoid nutrient deficiencies.

PERIOPERATIVE MANAGEMENT

In 2021, an evidence-based guideline for the perioperative care of patients undergoing bariatric surgery was published by the Enhanced Recovery After Surgery Society.[72] These guidelines advocate that a pre-operative liquid diet can be used to shrink liver volume. In addition, bowel preparation may have a benefit on post-operative constipation, but is not yet universally applied.[73] A multimodal approach to PONV prophylaxis should be adopted based on a high level of evidence and strong recommendations suggesting total intravenous anesthesia with Propofol, avoidance of volatile anesthetics and fluid overload, and minimization of intra- and postoperative opioids.[72] Perioperative venous thromboembolism (VTE) prophylaxis is recommended for every bariatric surgical patient in addition to early ambulation, mechanical thromboprophylaxis, and adequate hydration.[74] In high risk patients, there are insufficient high-quality data to support administration of post-discharge chemoprophylaxis to meaningfully decrease the risk of VTE events in these patients. Although no clear consensus exists on the choice, dosing, and duration of chemoprophylaxis after bariatric surgery, high-risk SG patients may benefit given the risk and severity of VTE events in this group.[74]

PROCEDURAL APPROACH

The field of bariatric surgery is constantly shifting, particularly with the increasing availability of robotic surgery. In the case of robotic SG, no significant differences have been found in complications, length of stay, or blood loss, but robotic surgery is associated with longer operative time and increased cost.[75] An MBSAQIP database study reported the outcomes of bariatric surgery (RYGB) when comparing robotic versus laparoscopic approaches between the years 2015 and 2019, only 16.6% of RYGB cases were done robotically.[76] Robotic cases were found to have longer operative times; however, were shown to reduce infectious complications and transfusion requirements.[76,77] A similar study using 2015 to 2016 data compared laparoscopic versus robotic-assisted cases and found that the robotic-assisted RYGB cohort was older and had a slightly lower BMI. However, patients undergoing robotic-assisted RYGB had a higher prevalence of pre-operative comorbidities, including hypertension, hyperlipidemia, obstructive sleep apnea, and so forth.[77] Post-operatively, the robotic-assisted group demonstrated higher rates of readmission but similarly lower rates of transfusions, superficial surgical site infections, and aggregate wound infections.[77] The results were the same in both unmatched and matched comparisons.

RECOVERY & REHABILITATION

After bariatric surgery, the patients are usually sent home 1 to 2 days after surgery, but some have advocated for same day discharge, with success rates of same day discharge reported as 63% to 100% after sleeve and RYGB in a systematic review and meta-analysis.[78]

Patients typically are encouraged to ambulate early in the postoperative care unit. No drains or catheters are usually left, which allow the patient easier mobilization. Following recovery from anesthesia, patients start a liquid diet, consuming 1 to 2 ounces every 15 minutes, with the quantity increasing as tolerated. Additionally, the incorporation of protein-containing liquid diet (with a minimum of 60 g/day) is recommended. Several studies have demonstrated early feeding with protein containing liquid diet is safe, and effective in enhanced recovery pathways and associated with shorter length of stay for patients.[79] Subsequently, diet advancement occurs over time. Under the guidance of the nutritionist, the bariatric diet progresses through bariatric phases. Phase I involves a full liquid diet and very thin puree for 2 to 3 weeks, followed by Phase II, consisting of a soft and semi-solid diet for the subsequent 1 to 2 months. Finally, Phase III encourages the maintenance of a regular diet. A regimen of life-long vitamin and mineral supplementation and nutritional biochemical monitoring is necessary.[72]

SUMMARY

Many procedures have been trialed for metabolic and bariatric surgery. All these techniques employ modification of the stomach or small intestine. Currently the most popular procedures are RYGB and SG, but newer procedures continue to be developed. With modern techniques, most patients experience sustained weight loss of at least 60% of their excess weight and resolution of many weight-related co-morbidities. Although these procedures have an excellent safety profile, physicians caring for these patients should be aware; however, of their altered anatomy and potential for post-operative complications and the need for long-term follow-up.

CLINICS CARE POINTS

- Use established criteria for patient selection based on the current ASMBS guidelines for metabolic and bariatric surgery. Selecting patients without a thorough assessment of psychological health or comorbid conditions, could negatively impact surgery outcomes and patient adherence.
- Ensure that patients receive information about the risk, benefits, and expected outcomes of the surgery, since inadequate information, can lead to unrealistic expectations or dissatisfaction with the outcomes of the surgery.
- Preoperative multidisciplinary approach and counseling is crucial as postoperative structured follow-up schedule.

DISCLOSURE

Dr A.D. Pryor receives honoraria for speaking from Gore, Medtronic and Stryker. She has research support from Allurion.

REFERENCES

1. Eisenberg D, Shikora SA, Aarts E, et al. 2022 American Society for Metabolic and Bariatric Surgery (ASMBS) and International Federation for the Surgery of Obesity and Metabolic Disorders (IFSO): Indications for Metabolic and Bariatric Surgery. Surg Obes Relat Dis 2022;18(12):1345–56.
2. Baker MT. The history and evolution of bariatric surgical procedures. Surg Clin North Am 2011;91(6):1181–1201, viii.
3. Samczuk P, Ciborowski M, Kretowski A. Application of Metabolomics to Study Effects of Bariatric Surgery. J Diabetes Res 2018;2018:6270875.
4. Sundbom M. Laparoscopic revolution in bariatric surgery. World J Gastroenterol 2014;20(41):15135–43.
5. Mason EE, Ito C. Gastric bypass in obesity. Surg Clin North Am 1967;47(6):1345–51.
6. Bhandari M, Fobi MAL, Buchwald JN. Standardization of Bariatric Metabolic Procedures: World Consensus Meeting Statement. Obes Surg 2019;29(Suppl 4):309–45.
7. Wittgrove AC, Clark GW. Laparoscopic gastric bypass, Roux-en-Y- 500 patients: technique and results, with 3-60 month follow-up. Obes Surg 2000;10(3):233–9.
8. Purnell JQ, Dewey EN, Laferrère B, et al. Diabetes Remission Status During Seven-year Follow-up of the Longitudinal Assessment of Bariatric Surgery Study. J Clin Endocrinol Metab 2021;106(3):774–88.
9. Belachew M, Legrand M, Vincent V, et al. Laparoscopic adjustable gastric banding. World J Surg 1998;22(9):955–63.
10. Angrisani L, Santonicola A, Iovino P, et al. Bariatric Surgery Worldwide 2013. Obes Surg 2015;25.

11. Ugale S, Vennapusa A, Katakwar A, et al. Laparoscopic bariatric surgery-current trends and controversies. Annals of Laparoscopic and Endoscopic Surgery 2017;2(10).
12. Hess DS, Hess DW. Biliopancreatic diversion with a duodenal switch. Obes Surg 1998;8(3):267–82.
13. Marceau P, Hould FS, Simard S, et al. Biliopancreatic diversion with duodenal switch. World J Surg 1998;22(9):947–54.
14. Marceau P, Biron S, Bourque RA, et al. Biliopancreatic Diversion with a New Type of Gastrectomy. Obes Surg 1993;3(1):29–35.
15. Salgaonkar H, Sharples A, Marimuthu K, et al. One Anastomosis Gastric Bypass (OAGB). In: Lomanto D, Chen WT-L, Fuentes MB, editors. Mastering endo-laparoscopic and thoracoscopic surgery: ELSA manual. Singapore: Springer Nature Singapore; 2023. p. 297–304.
16. Bindal V, Bhatia P, Dudeja U, et al. Review of contemporary role of robotics in bariatric surgery. J Minimal Access Surg 2015;11(1):16–21.
17. Cal P ea. Totally robotic single anastomosis gastric bypass is safe and feasible compared to laparoscopic approach. SAGES 2017 Annual Meeting 2017. Houston, TX.
18. Estimate of Bariatric Surgery Numbers, 2011-2021. ASMBS 2021. Available at: https://asmbs.org/resources/estimate-of-bariatric-surgery-numbers.
19. O'Brien PE, Dixon JB, Laurie C, et al. A prospective randomized trial of placement of the laparoscopic adjustable gastric band: comparison of the perigastric and pars flaccida pathways. Obes Surg 2005;15(6):820–6.
20. Carvalho Silveira F, Maranga G, Mitchell F, et al. First-year weight loss following gastric band surgery predicts long-term outcomes. ANZ J Surg 2021;91(11):2443–6.
21. Furbetta N, Cervelli R, Furbetta F. Laparoscopic adjustable gastric banding, the past, the present and the future. Ann Transl Med 2020;8(Suppl 1):S4.
22. Seeras K, Acho RJ, Prakash S. Laparoscopic gastric band placement. [Updated 2023 Jan 19]. In: StatPearls [Internet]. Treasure Island (FL): StatPearls Publishing; 2024.
23. Eid I, Birch DW, Sharma AM, et al. Complications associated with adjustable gastric banding for morbid obesity: a surgeon's guides. Can J Surg 2011;54(1):61–6.
24. Li L, Yu H, Liang J, et al. Meta-analysis of the effectiveness of laparoscopic adjustable gastric banding versus laparoscopic sleeve gastrectomy for obesity. Medicine (Baltimore) 2019;98(9):e14735.
25. DeMaria EJ, Sugerman HJ, Meador JG, et al. High failure rate after laparoscopic adjustable silicone gastric banding for treatment of morbid obesity. Ann Surg 2001;233(6):809–18.
26. Carlin AM, Zeni TM, English WJ, et al. The comparative effectiveness of sleeve gastrectomy, gastric bypass, and adjustable gastric banding procedures for the treatment of morbid obesity. Ann Surg 2013;257(5):791–7.
27. Diamantis T, Apostolou KG, Alexandrou A, et al. Review of long-term weight loss results after laparoscopic sleeve gastrectomy. Surg Obes Relat Dis 2014;10(1):177–83.
28. Gehrer S, Kern B, Peters T, et al. Fewer nutrient deficiencies after laparoscopic sleeve gastrectomy (LSG) than after laparoscopic Roux-Y-gastric bypass (LRYGB)-a prospective study. Obes Surg 2010;20(4):447–53.
29. Ruban A, Stoenchev K, Ashrafian H, et al. Current treatments for obesity. Clin Med (Lond) 2019;19(3):205–12.

30. Seeras K, Sankararaman S, Lopez PP. Sleeve gastrectomy. [Updated 2023 Jan23]. In: StatPearls [Internet]. Treasure Island (FL): StatPearls Publishing; 2024.

31. van Rijswijk AS, van Olst N, Schats W, et al. What Is Weight Loss After Bariatric Surgery Expressed in Percentage Total Weight Loss (%TWL)? A Systematic Review. Obes Surg 2021;31(8):3833–47.

32. Kheirvari M, Dadkhah Nikroo N, Jaafarinejad H, et al. The advantages and disadvantages of sleeve gastrectomy; clinical laboratory to bedside review. Heliyon 2020;6(2):e03496.

33. Peterli R, Wölnerhanssen BK, Peters T, et al. Effect of Laparoscopic Sleeve Gastrectomy vs Laparoscopic Roux-en-Y Gastric Bypass on Weight Loss in Patients With Morbid Obesity: The SM-BOSS Randomized Clinical Trial. JAMA 2018; 319(3):255–65.

34. Abou Rached A, Basile M, El Masri H. Gastric leaks post sleeve gastrectomy: review of its prevention and management. World J Gastroenterol 2014;20(38): 13904–10.

35. Zafar SN, Felton J, Miller K, et al. Staple Line Treatment and Bleeding After Laparoscopic Sleeve Gastrectomy. JSLS 2018;22(4). e2018.00056.

36. Sarker A, Meek CL, Park A. Biochemical consequences of bariatric surgery for extreme clinical obesity. Ann Clin Biochem 2016;53(Pt 1):21–31.

37. Larsen M, Kozarek R. Therapeutic endoscopy for the treatment of post-bariatric surgery complications. World J Gastroenterol 2022;28(2):199–215.

38. Bevilacqua LA, Obeid NR, Yang J, et al. Incidence of GERD, esophagitis, Barrett's esophagus, and esophageal adenocarcinoma after bariatric surgery. Surg Obes Relat Dis 2020;16(11):1828–36.

39. Wittgrove AC, Clark GW, Tremblay LJ. Laparoscopic Gastric Bypass, Roux-en-Y: Preliminary Report of Five Cases. Obes Surg 1994;4(4):353–7.

40. Alfadda AA, Al-Naami MY, Masood A, et al. Long-term weight outcomes after bariatric surgery: a single center saudi arabian cohort experience. J Clin Med 2021; 10(21):4922.

41. Pucci A, Batterham RL. Mechanisms underlying the weight loss effects of RYGB and SG: similar, yet different. J Endocrinol Invest 2019;42(2):117–28.

42. Schauer PR, Bhatt DL, Kirwan JP, et al. Bariatric Surgery versus Intensive Medical Therapy for Diabetes - 5-Year Outcomes. N Engl J Med 2017;376(7):641–51.

43. Dixon JB, le Roux CW, Rubino F, et al. Bariatric surgery for type 2 diabetes. Lancet 2012;379(9833):2300–11.

44. Maggard-Gibbons M, Maglione M, Livhits M, et al. Bariatric surgery for weight loss and glycemic control in nonmorbidly obese adults with diabetes: a systematic review. JAMA 2013;309(21):2250–61.

45. Kim JC, Kim MG, Park JK, et al. Outcomes and Adverse Events After Bariatric Surgery: An Updated Systematic Review and Meta-analysis, 2013-2023. J Metab Bariatr Surg 2023;12(2):76–88.

46. Ricci C, Gaeta M, Rausa E, et al. Long-term effects of bariatric surgery on type II diabetes, hypertension and hyperlipidemia: a meta-analysis and meta-regression study with 5-year follow-up. Obes Surg 2015;25(3):397–405.

47. Spivak H, Sakran N, Dicker D, et al. Different effects of bariatric surgical procedures on dyslipidemia: a registry-based analysis. Surg Obes Relat Dis 2017;13(7): 1189–94.

48. Odovic M, Clerc D, Demartines N, et al. Early Bleeding After Laparoscopic Roux-en-Y Gastric Bypass: Incidence, Risk Factors, and Management — a 21-Year Experience. Obes Surg 2022;32(10):3232–8.

49. Altieri MS, Rogers A, Afaneh C, et al. Bariatric emergencies for the general surgeon. Surg Obes Relat Dis 2023;19(5):421–33.

50. Geubbels N, Lijftogt N, Fiocco M, et al. Meta-analysis of internal herniation after gastric bypass surgery. Br J Surg 2015;102(5):451–60.

51. Stenberg E, Ottosson J, Magnuson A, et al. Long-term safety and efficacy of closure of mesenteric defects in laparoscopic gastric bypass surgery: a randomized clinical trial. JAMA Surgery 2023;158(7):709–17.

52. Tian Y, Rogers AM. Marginal Ulcer: Diagnosis and Treatment. In: Docimo Jr S, Pauli EM, editors. Clinical algorithms in general surgery : a practical guide. Cham: Springer International Publishing; 2019. p. 827–9.

53. Biertho L, Lebel S, Marceau S, et al. Biliopancreatic diversion with duodenal switch: surgical technique and perioperative care. Surg Clin North Am 2016; 96(4):815–26.

54. Wang L, Zhang Z, Wang Z, et al. First study on the outcomes of biliopancreatic diversion with duodenal switch in Chinese patients with obesity. Front Surg 2022;9:934434.

55. Roslin M, Sabrudin S, Pearlstein S, et al. Conversion and revisional surgery: duodenal switch. In: Reavis KM, Barrett AM, Kroh MD, editors. The SAGES manual of bariatric surgery. Cham: Springer International Publishing; 2018. p. 521–33.

56. Sorribas M, Casajoana A, Sobrino L, et al. Experience in biliopancreatic diversion with duodenal switch: results at 2, 5 and 10 years. Cir Esp 2021.

57. Sánchez-Pernaute A, Herrera MÁR, Ferré NP, et al. Long-term results of single-anastomosis duodeno-ileal bypass with sleeve gastrectomy (SADI-S). Obes Surg 2022;32(3):682–9.

58. Esparham A, Roohi S, Ahmadyar S, et al. The Efficacy and Safety of Laparoscopic Single-Anastomosis Duodeno-ileostomy with Sleeve Gastrectomy (SADI-S) in Mid- and Long-Term Follow-Up: a Systematic Review. Obes Surg 2023; 33(12):4070–9.

59. Spivak H, Giorgi M, Luhrs A. Conversion of gastric sleeve to Roux-en-Y gastric bypass and biliopancreatic diversion/duodenal switch: safe and viable options. Surg Obes Relat Dis 2023;19(2):131–5.

60. Lee Y, Ellenbogen Y, Doumouras AG, et al. Single- or double-anastomosis duodenal switch versus Roux-en-Y gastric bypass as a revisional procedure for sleeve gastrectomy: A systematic review and meta-analysis. Surg Obes Relat Dis 2019;15(4):556–66.

61. Angrisani L, Santonicola A, Iovino P, et al. IFSO Worldwide Survey 2016: Primary, Endoluminal, and Revisional Procedures. Obes Surg 2018;28(12):3783–94.

62. Aleman R, Lo Menzo E, Szomstein S, et al. Efficiency and risks of one-anastomosis gastric bypass. Ann Transl Med 2020;8(Suppl 1):S7.

63. Kermansaravi M, Karami R, Valizadeh R, et al. Five-year outcomes of one anastomosis gastric bypass as conversional surgery following sleeve gastrectomy for weight loss failure. Sci Rep 2022;12(1):10304.

64. Bruzzi M, Rau C, Voron T, et al. Single anastomosis or mini-gastric bypass: long-term results and quality of life after a 5-year follow-up. Surg Obes Relat Dis 2015; 11(2):321–6.

65. Carbajo MA, Luque-de-León E, Jiménez JM, et al. Laparoscopic One-Anastomosis Gastric Bypass: Technique, Results, and Long-Term Follow-Up in 1200 Patients. Obes Surg 2017;27(5):1153–67.

66. Lee W-J, Yu P-J, Wang W, et al. Laparoscopic Roux-en-Y versus mini-gastric bypass for the treatment of morbid obesity: a prospective randomized controlled clinical trial. Annals of Surgery 2005;242(1):20–8.
67. Parikh M, Eisenberg D, Johnson J, et al. American Society for Metabolic and Bariatric Surgery review of the literature on one-anastomosis gastric bypass. Surg Obes Relat Dis 2018;14(8):1088–92.
68. Lee W-J, Ser K-H, Lee Y-C, et al. Laparoscopic Roux-en-Y Vs. Mini-gastric Bypass for the Treatment of Morbid Obesity: a 10-Year Experience. Obes Surg 2012;22(12):1827–34.
69. Seetharamaiah S, Tantia O, Goyal G, et al. LSG vs OAGB—1 Year Follow-up Data—a Randomized Control Trial. Obes Surg 2017;27(4):948–54.
70. Wischmeyer PE, Carli F, Evans DC, et al. American society for enhanced recovery and perioperative quality initiative joint consensus statement on nutrition screening and therapy within a surgical enhanced recovery pathway. Anesth Analg 2018;126(6):1883–95.
71. Lim R.B., Bariatric surgery for management of obesity: Indications and preoperative preparation. In: D. Jones & W. Chen Editors. UpToDate, Wolters Kluwer; the Netherlands. 2024.
72. Stenberg E, Dos Reis Falcão LF, O'Kane M, et al. Guidelines for Perioperative Care in Bariatric Surgery: Enhanced Recovery After Surgery (ERAS) Society Recommendations: A 2021 Update. World J Surg 2022;46(4):729–51.
73. Sethi I, Lam K, Sanicola C, et al. Efficacy of Bowel Regimen in Decreasing Postoperative Constipation in Bariatric Surgery Patients. In: Obesity surgery. 2024.
74. Aminian A, Vosburg RW, Altieri MS, et al. The American Society for Metabolic and Bariatric Surgery (ASMBS) updated position statement on perioperative venous thromboembolism prophylaxis in bariatric surgery. Surg Obes Relat Dis 2022; 18(2):165–74.
75. Elli E, Gonzalez-Heredia R, Sarvepalli S, et al. Laparoscopic and robotic sleeve gastrectomy: short- and long-term results. Obes Surg 2015;25(6):967–74.
76. Wesley Vosburg R, Haque O, Roth E. Robotic vs. Laparoscopic Metabolic and Bariatric Surgery, Outcomes over 5 Years in Nearly 800,000 Patients. Obes Surg 2022;32(7):2341–8.
77. Acevedo E, Mazzei M, Zhao H, et al. Outcomes in conventional laparoscopic versus robotic-assisted primary bariatric surgery: a retrospective, case–controlled study of the MBSAQIP database. Surg Endosc 2020;34(3):1353–65.
78. Vanetta C, Dreifuss NH, Angeramo CA, et al. Outcomes of same-day discharge sleeve gastrectomy and Roux-en-Y gastric bypass: a systematic review and meta-analysis. Surg Obes Relat Dis 2023;19(3):238–49.
79. Bevilacqua LA, Obeid NR, Spaniolas K, et al. Early postoperative diet after bariatric surgery: impact on length of stay and 30-day events. Surg Endosc 2019; 33(8):2475–8.

Managing the Bariatric Surgery Patient
Presurgery and Postsurgery Considerations

Sujani Yadlapati, MD[a], Sergio A. Sánchez-Luna, MD, ABOM-D[b],
Mark A. Gromski, MD[a], Ramzi Mulki, MD[b],*

KEYWORDS

• Obesity • Bariatric surgery • Preoperative assessment • Postoperative care

KEY POINTS

• The preoperative assessment for bariatric surgery is a comprehensive and meticulous process.
• Gastroenterologists assume a pivotal role in evaluating the gastrointestinal health of patients through procedures such as esophagogastroduodenoscopy, manometry, and pH/impedance testing before surgery.
• Postoperative care includes the management of potential complications like bleeding, leaks, and infections, coupled with optimizing recovery through adept pain management and wound care.
• Providing essential nutritional support to prevent deficiencies is integral, while ongoing guidance on behavioral and lifestyle changes, including dietary adjustments and exercise regimens, constitutes a cornerstone for long-term success.

INTRODUCTION

The prevalence of obesity continues to escalate, despite its association with a myriad of medical conditions. Body mass index (BMI) allows for anthropometric classification of individuals into discrete groupings. BMI considers weight in kilograms (kg) and height in meters (m) (kg/m^2).[1] While BMI is not a perfect measure for assessing the severity of obesity, a BMI of 18.5 kg/m^2 to 25 kg/m^2 is considered normal. A BMI of 30 kg/m^2 or more is considered obese (with 3 distinct grades within this BMI range).[1,2] Per the World Health Organization, roughly 650 million adults in the world are considered obese.[3] Numerous studies have highlighted an association between obesity and

[a] Department of Gastroenterology and Hepatology, Indiana University Health, Indiana University School of Medicine, 550 University Boulevard, Indianapolis, IN 46202, USA;
[b] Department of Gastroenterology and Hepatology, University of Alabama, Heersink School of Medicine, 1720 university Boulevard, Birmingham, AL 35294, USA
* Corresponding author. Department of Gastroentrology and Hepatology, Univesity of Alabama, 1720 university Blvd, Birmingham, Alabama 35294.
E-mail address: ramzi.mulki@gmail.com

Gastrointest Endoscopy Clin N Am 34 (2024) 627–638
https://doi.org/10.1016/j.giec.2024.04.002
1052-5157/24/Published by Elsevier Inc.

decreased life expectancy.[4] Comorbidities associated with obesity include metabolic, cardiovascular, respiratory, musculoskeletal, and neurologic conditions. Medical and behavioral therapies for weight loss may be ineffective for many patients with obesity. Bariatric surgery has gained importance as a sustainable alternative to address morbid obesity and associated comorbidities. Individuals undergoing bariatric surgery exhibit enduring weight loss and improvement in obesity-related comorbidities.[5]

Bariatric surgery utilizes techniques that can be restrictive, malabsorptive, or a combination of both. Malabsorptive methods, such as jejunoileal bypass and biliopancreatic bypass, are rarely performed at present. Restrictive procedures include vertical sleeve gastrectomy (VSG), laparoscopic adjustable gastric banding (LAGB), and vertical banded gastroplasty.[1] Roux-en-Y gastric bypass (RYGB) is considered both a restrictive and malabsorptive procedure. Obese patients often have several comorbidities and are, therefore, at increased risk of anesthesia-related complications while undergoing any surgery. Preoperative assessment and postoperative care play a critical role in ensuring optimal outcomes following surgery. Preoperative assessment includes appropriate patient selection, psychosocial evaluation, nutritional analysis, and behavioral/medical counseling. Postoperative assessment includes immediate perioperative care, diet transition, nutritional needs management, and handling of complications associated with bariatric surgery. This article focuses on the preoperative and postoperative management strategies required to achieve successful and durable outcomes in bariatric surgery patients. Medical and endoscopic management of obesity, the selection of a bariatric surgery procedure, and intraoperative care is beyond the scope of this article. However, these aspects typically involve a comprehensive multidisciplinary evaluation, consideration of patient preferences, and adherence to institutional protocols.

INDICATIONS AND CONTRAINDICATIONS FOR BARIATRIC SURGERY

Determining suitable candidates for bariatric surgery relies on specific BMI criteria and associated comorbidities (**Table 1**). This criterion was originally defined by the National Institutes of Health Consensus Development Panel and later modified by the International Federation for the Surgery of Obesity and Metabolic Disorders and the American Society for Metabolic and Bariatric Surgery.[6,7] Criteria for weight loss surgery include a BMI of 40 kg/m2 or more or a BMI greater than 35 kg/m2 with obesity-associated comorbidities. Surgery should be contemplated for individuals who cannot achieve lasting weight loss or experience improvement in comorbidities solely through lifestyle modifications and lifestyle interventions. A supervised weight loss program involving exercise and lifestyle modifications is recommended before surgery. The willingness of a patient to comply with such a regimen often reflects the commitment required to adhere to postoperative nutritional restrictions.[8,9] Bariatric surgery is contraindicated in those with a history of substance abuse, alcoholism, underlying eating disorders, pregnant patients, as well as those with severe coagulopathies. Identifying patients who are unlikely to adhere to follow-up appointments, sustain lifestyle changes, and comply with medical advice following bariatric surgery is crucial. Additionally, severe cardiovascular disease is a contraindication due to increased anesthesia-related risks.

ROLE OF A GASTROENTEROLOGIST IN MANAGING THE BARIATRIC SURGERY PATIENT

Gastroenterologists play a crucial role in caring for bariatric surgery patients. Obese patients are more likely to experience numerous gastrointestinal (GI) and hepatobiliary

Table 1
World Health Organization classification of obesity and indications/contraindications for bariatric surgery

Classification	Body Mass Index (kg/m²)
Underweight	<18.5
Normal weight	18.5–24.9
Overweight	25–29.9
Obese	30 or above
Class I obesity (obese)	30.0–34.9
Class II obesity (morbid obesity)	35.0–39.9
Class III obesity (super obesity)	40 or more

Indications for bariatric surgery
- BMI over 40 kg/m²
- BMI over 35 kg/m² with obesity-related metabolic or major systemic disorders
  ○ Type 2 diabetes mellitus
  ○ Hypertension
  ○ Hyperlipidemia
  ○ Obstructive sleep apnea
  ○ Cardiomyopathy related to obesity
  ○ Severe osteoarthritis

Contraindications for bariatric surgery
- Major depression or psychiatric disorders
- Eating disorders
- Pregnancy
- Active malignancy
- Severe coagulopathies
- Drug or alcohol abuse
- Evidence of medical noncompliance

conditions like gastroesophageal reflux disease (GERD), Barrett's esophagus (BE), metabolic dysfunction–associated fatty liver disease and an increased risk of cancers such as pancreatic cancer, esophageal adenocarcinoma, and gallbladder cancer, among others.[10] Historically, gastroenterologists focused on pre-bariatric and post-bariatric surgery assessments. Now, their role includes medical and endoscopic approaches to obesity management as well. This article excludes details on medical and endoscopic obesity management. A preoperative esophagogastroduodenoscopy (EGD) is frequently performed for patients considering weight loss surgery to evaluate anatomy, assess for hiatal hernia, and rule out *Helicobacter pylori* infection, peptic ulcer disease, reflux esophagitis, BE, or pathologic lesions in the upperGI tract.[11] It is important to keep in mind that this is often done irrespective of symptoms, since pathologic findings may influence the choice of surgery and it is often difficult to assess an excluded stomach once patients undergo RYGB.[11,12] For instance, a large hiatal hernia may complicate surgery, potentially necessitating concurrent or prior repair. Notably, the presence of BE is a contraindication for VSG, as this procedure could exacerbate GERD and contribute to BE progression.[13] Recent studies, including a meta-analysis, underscore the importance of vigilance after VSG, revealing a 13% annual risk of esophagitis and suggesting consideration for BE screening even in asymptomatic patients.[14] As per the Bariatric Outcomes Longitudinal Database, a registry documenting bariatric surgeries at centers of excellence, RYGB proved to be more effective in addressing GERD when compared to alternative weight loss procedures.[15] *H pylori* infection, if detected, should be treated prior to bariatric surgery to prevent complications like peptic ulcers or anastomotic ulcers. Some patients may need a presurgical assessment of GI motility. LAGB patients may face postoperative challenges like dysphagia or pseudo-achalasia, highlighting the need for thorough preoperative evaluation.

Postoperative complications like anastomotic leaks, depending on chronicity, can be addressed using different therapeutic modalities such as overstitch, covered metal stents, and X-tack among others. Postsurgical bleeding, whether immediate or delayed, can be approached with endoscopic therapy. Anastomotic strictures may require endoscopic dilation or stenting. Nutritional deficiencies and complications are discussed later in the article. Apart from conducting preoperative and postoperative assessments, gastroenterologists are taking on a more prominent role in the management of bariatric surgery patients, as medical and endoluminal therapies play an expanding role in obesity management.

PREOPERATIVE CONSIDERATIONS IN THE BARIATRIC SURGERY PATIENT

A detailed medical history and physical examination should be performed during the initial visit. Initial laboratory assessment includes a metabolic panel, complete blood count, hemoglobin A1C (HBA1C), lipid panel, as well as measurements of vitamin B12, folic acid, vitamin D, and iron levels. Evaluating albumin and prealbumin levels provides insights into overall nutritional status. The importance of preoperative nutritional deficiencies varies based on the risk of malabsorption specific to the planned procedure.[16] Individuals considering weight loss surgery should undergo a preoperative assessment for underlying endocrinopathies. For long-standing or medically refractory diabetes, an endocrinologist's involvement is mandatory.[17] To reduce the intraoperative and postoperative risks in diabetic patients, certain criteria should be satisfied, including a HBA1C level between 6.5% and 7%.[16,18]

Patients with obesity face increased anesthesia-related risks, often compounded by respiratory conditions like obstructive sleep apnea (OSA) or hypoventilation syndrome of obesity, which may be known or undiagnosed.[19–21] In such instances, it is recommended to seek advice from a pulmonologist. Preoperative weight loss is the recommended strategy for addressing obesity hypoventilation syndrome. Despite the implementation of these risk reduction measures, it is common for patients undergoing weight loss surgery to require postoperative admission to the intensive care unit, and counseling regarding this possibility is crucial.[19] Lastly, to decrease the cardiopulmonary intraoperative anesthesia risk, some patients may be candidates to "bridge" therapy with bariatric and metabolic endoscopy modalities such as intragastric balloon placement to achieve weight loss and improve certain metabolic parameters that could decrease the risks.

It is also important to screen these patients for major mental health disorders, severe depression, and eating disorders. Patients with a history of alcohol dependence should undergo formal rehabilitation prior to being considered for bariatric surgery. Preoperative eating behavior and postoperative dietary adherence have been identified as factors influencing weight loss after gastric bypass surgery. Delving deeper into the specific dietary patterns associated with successful weight loss could guide the development of personalized dietary recommendations for bariatric surgery patients. Understanding the impact of cultural and socioeconomic factors on dietary habits presurgery and postsurgery could aid in the development of more inclusive nutritional guidelines.

Expectations should be set regarding weight loss after surgery. Typically, individuals undergoing sleeve gastrectomy (SG) aim to lose around 60 to 65% of excess body weight within a 2-year timeframe, while those undergoing RYGB should anticipate a weight loss in the range of 70 to 75% of excess body weight over the same period. Furthermore, discussions with patients should encompass strategies for maintaining weight loss after surgery. A supervised weight loss program should be recommended for best outcomes. This program should include guidance for dietary and exercise planning. Clearly defined weight loss objectives should be monitored consistently throughout each visit in the preoperative phase. Individuals with obesity considering weight loss surgery should be educated about the potential for excess skin and tissue following significant weight loss. The transformations in the body after substantial weight loss may pose mental and emotional challenges, impacting overall well-being. Consulting with a plastic surgeon to explore medical and surgical interventions for improving the overall body image after weight loss can assist in tackling these challenges.[22] It is crucial to recommend smoking cessation at least 6 weeks prior to the surgery and to maintain abstinence in the postoperative period.[16] Smoking substantially increases the likelihood of numerous intraoperative and postoperative complications, including hindered wound healing, thromboembolic and cardiovascular events, and the onset of marginal ulcers. Additionally, patients should be educated about postponing pregnancy for minimum of 12 to 18 months after surgery. Nutritional deficiencies that may arise after bariatric surgery pose risks to both the patient and a potential fetus if pregnancy occurs in this time.

POSTOPERATIVE CONSIDERATIONS IN THE BARIATRIC SURGERY PATIENT
Short-Term Postoperative Care

While the weight loss surgical procedure itself is pivotal, the period following surgery is equally crucial in determining long-term outcomes. Laparoscopic bariatric procedures are typically linked to swift recovery, shorter hospital stays, and a lower incidence of postoperative pain and complications. Inpatient postoperative care for the first 24 hours focuses on pain control, symptomatic management of nausea or vomiting, intravenous fluids therapy, pulmonary hygiene, and early ambulation. Obesity increases the work of breathing and prolongs the risk of postoperative atelectasis. Minimally invasive surgical techniques, opioid-sparing analgesia, and continuous positive airway pressure/bilevel positive airway pressure use can mitigate cardiopulmonary risks in OSA patients undergoing bariatric surgery. All patients undergoing bariatric surgery should be placed on a venous thromboembolism prevention regimen. Early ambulation within 4 to 6 hours after surgery should be encouraged. Patients who have an anastomotic leak, bleeding, or obstruction in the early postoperative period should immediately return to the operating room for surgical revision or undergo diagnostic and therapeutic upper endoscopy.

Following bariatric surgery, the initiation of oral intake starts with a clear liquid diet within the initial 24 hours, dependent on water tolerance and the absence of clinical concerns such as a staple line or anastomotic leak.[23] After successfully tolerating a low-fat, full-liquid diet and demonstrating the ability to ambulate, patients are released with protein supplements, vitamins, and a gradual shift in food consistency. Generally, protein intake of 60 to 80 g/day or 1.0 to 1.5 g/kg of ideal body weight is suggested for individuals undergoing SG, adjustable gastric band, and RYGB. In the early postoperative period, thiamine deficiency is at risk due to small nutrient reserves, rapid weight loss, poor nutritional intake, and nonadherence with supplements. Signs of Wernicke encephalopathy include neuropathy, myopathy, and encephalopathy. Thiamine deficiency requires immediate supplementation. In the initial stages following bariatric surgery, patients rely on stored adipose tissue to meet their energy requirements.

Consequently, the dietary focus in the early postoperative period is centered on fulfilling essential nutrient needs and ensuring proper hydration. As weight stabilizes and most energy needs are derived from dietary sources, the nutritional guidelines for macronutrients align with those recommended for the general population.

Nutritional Deficiencies After Surgery

Common vitamin deficiencies after bariatric surgery include iron, folate, vitamin B12, vitamin D, zinc, copper, and selenium (**Table 2**). Procedures involving malabsorption increase the risk of deficiencies in vitamins A, E, and K.[24,25] Patients must consistently follow lifelong vitamin and mineral supplementation and periodic biochemical monitoring customized to the surgical procedure. Iron deficiency results from bypassing the duodenum and proximal jejunum. Concerning vitamin B12, it is usually absorbed in the terminal ileum after binding with intrinsic factor (IF). IF is secreted by the parietal cells of the gastric antrum. The exclusion of the gastric antrum during RYGB disrupts the timely interaction of IF and B12, leading to inadequate absorption in the terminal ileum and subsequent deficiency. The treatment for deficiencies of both iron and B12 includes oral supplementation and injectable or intravenous routes if needed.[26,27]

Complications Associated with Bariatric Surgery

Complications after bariatric surgery are both medical and surgical in nature (**Box 1**).[28,29] The management of complications involves early detection and medical, endoscopic, or surgical therapy.

Gastroesophageal reflux disease/Barrett's esophagus

For cases involving VSG, it is imperative to appropriately address common concerns such as GERD. Nevertheless, there is presently inadequate evidence to endorse the routine utilization of proton pump inhibitors (PPIs) following VSG, despite findings of reflux-related complications in certain studies.[30,31]

Postsurgery dysphagia

Usually underrecognized, postsurgical dysphagia occurs in up to 10% of patients undergoing an SG or an RYGB.[32] This has a time-dependent relationship and can present as post-obesity surgery esophageal dysfunction or achalasia. The diagnosis requires upper endoscopy and high-resolution manometry, and its treatment can involve Botox injection, dilation, laparoscopic Heller myotomy, and per-oral endoscopic myotomy.

Dumping syndrome

This occurs due to swift passage of undigested food into the small bowel, leading to GI and vasomotor symptoms. Two types of dumping syndromes have been described. Early dumping occurs within 30 minutes of meal intake, whereas delayed dumping happens up to 3 hours after food intake. A Danish survey involving 1429 gastric bypass patients revealed that 9.4% experienced moderate to severe symptoms of early dumping, while 6.6% reported hypoglycemic symptoms. The overall prevalence of 1 or both types of symptoms was 12.6% (95% confidence interval 10.9–14.4). Individuals under the age of 35 or with a BMI below 25 kg/m^2 were more prone to display symptoms in contrast to their older or higher BMI counterparts.[33] It's worth noting that dumping may contribute to weight loss by influencing changes in a patient's eating habits. Patients with dumping syndrome experience abdominal pain, diarrhea, nausea, and later hypoglycemia. Symptoms are typically managed by avoiding foods with simple sugars and consuming diet rich in protein, fiber, and complex carbohydrates. Refractory dumping syndrome can also be treated endoscopically by transoral outlet reduction (TORe) in selected individuals after a multidisciplinary discussion.[34]

Table 2
Micronutrient deficiencies in bariatric surgery patients

Nutrient	Symptoms	Recommended Daily Allowance	Recommended Supplement	Recommended Supplementation
Vitamin B12	Fatigue, weakness, neuropathy, macrocytic anemia	2.4 mcg	Vitamin B12 supplements (sublingual or intramuscular)	350–1000 mcg/day or 1000mcg IM or SQ monthly.
Iron	Fatigue, dyspnea, pica, pale skin, microcytic anemia	8–18 mg per day (higher requirements for women in menstruating age group)	Iron supplements (ferrous sulfate, ferrous fumarate)	150–300 mg up to 3 times a day.
Calcium	Bone pain, muscle cramps, weakness	1000–1200 mg	Calcium citrate supplements	1200–2400 mg/day (divided doses)
Vitamin D	Bone pain, muscle weakness, increased fractures	600–800 IU (maintain 25(OH)D level of >30 ng/mL)	Vitamin D supplements (D2 or D3)	3000 IU D3 daily
Folate (B9)	Fatigue, macrocytic anemia, pancytopenia	400 mcg	Folate supplements (folic acid or methyl folate)	400–1000 mcg/day. (Maximum dose should be no more than 1 mg/day)
Thiamine (B1)	Fatigue, confusion, ataxia, Wernicke-Korsakoff syndrome, beriberi	1.5 mg	Thiamine supplements (thiamine mononitrate)	50–100 mg/day
Zinc	Impaired wound healing, increased infections	8–11 mg	Zinc supplements (zinc sulfate, zinc gluconate)	100%–200% of RDA
Copper	Microcytic anemia, Ataxia, Neutropenia	900 mcg	Copper supplements (copper gluconate)	1–2 mg/day orally (100%–200% RDA)
Vitamin A	Night blindness, dry skin, loss of taste	700–900 mcg or 2300–3000 IU	Vitamin A supplements (retinyl palmitate)	10,000–25,000 IU daily orally until improved. Several doses of 50,000–100,000 IU IM if corneal changes

Abbreviations: IM, intramuscular; IU, international units; RDA, recommended daily allowance; SQ, subcutaneous.

Box 1
Complications associated with bariatric surgery

Early complications
- Anastomotic dehiscence/leak (1%–3%)—Leaks or fistulas can potentially cause infection, abscess formation, or peritonitis.
- PE/DVT (<1%)
- Gastrointestinal bleeding (<2%)
- Wound infections
- Cardiovascular complications

Late complications
- *Nutritional deficiencies*—Deficiencies in vitamin B12, iron, calcium, vitamin D, and folate can lead to long-term medical problems such as malnutrition and failure to thrive.
- *GERD/BE*—It occurs more frequently with sleeve gastrectomy. It is treated with acid suppression therapy and conversion to RYGB if reflux is poorly controlled with medical therapy
- *Psychological and behavioral issues*—Changes in eating habits, body image, and relationships may contribute to mental health challenges, including depression, anxiety, and eating disorders.
- *Dumping syndrome*—It is the rapid emptying of the stomach contents into the small bowel. Patients present with nausea, sweating, weakness, and diarrhea.
- *Bowel obstruction*—It is caused by adhesions, hernias, or strictures.
- *Stricture*—This is formation at the surgical site.
- *Marginal ulcers*—These are seen at the site of surgical anastomosis.
- *Gallstones*—These occur because of rapid weight loss. It can ultimately result in acute cholecystitis or choledocholithiasis.
- *Weight gain*—It is multifactorial and difficult to treat. Endoscopic options are preferred over surgical revision.

Abbreviations: BE, Barrett's esophagus; DVT, deep vein thrombosis; GERD, gastroesophageal reflux disease; PE, pulmonary embolism; RYGB, Roux-en-Y gastric bypass.

Marginal ulceration

Marginal ulcers occur in approximately 25% of individuals undergoing RYGB. Patients present with abdominal pain and nausea. If ulcers fail to heal, they may lead to complications such asGI bleeding or perforation. Risk factors for marginal ulcers involve the use of tobacco and nonsteroidal anti-inflammatory drugs. Marginal ulcers can be treated using open-capsule PPIs and sucralfate. Smoking cessation is important in the overall management of this condition. Endoscopic treatment usually involves the removal of staples and sutures since they cause a foreign body reaction that may impair the proper healing of these ulcers and oversewing in refractory cases.

Cholelithiasis

Mechanisms for cholelithiasis include changes in bile composition after bariatric surgery and increased gallstone formation after rapid weight loss. Cholecystectomy, though not recommended prophylactically, may be performed at the time of RYGB; however, if the gallbladder is not removed, patients are started on ursodeoxycholic acid (ursodiol) 300 mg orally twice a day for 6 months to prevent gallstone formation.

Stenosis

Post-SG, there is a potential risk of gastric outlet obstruction, which may manifest as symptoms such as dysphagia or vomiting. It can happen in up to 4% of patients. Post-SG strictures are usually present at the gastroesophageal junction and incisura angularis. Diagnosis typically involves an EGD and endoscopic dilation with or without stenting, and, in severe cases, tunneled stricturotomy. In instances where endoscopic measures prove ineffective, surgical revision may be considered as an alternative. Gastrojejunal anastomotic stricture is a known complication in patients undergoing RYGB. They are usually associated with marginal ulceration, and thus, they have the same medical treatment. Nonetheless, endoscopic treatment is still the mainstay of treatment with endoscopic balloon dilation and stenting being the most common treatment approaches.

Depression
Patients can experience mood changes and increased depression after RYGB. Emotional aspects of food loss should be addressed, and antidepressants or behavioral therapies may be recommended.

Anastomotic or staple line leaks
Leaks often present in the immediate postoperative period and are associated with sepsis, need for repeat intervention, and intensive care unit stay. Patients often develop signs of peritonitis and systemic inflammatory response syndrome. When suspected, immediate operative intervention should be pursued. Image-guided drainage, antibiotics, and initiation of parenteral nutrition are typically required. Endoscopic stenting across the leaking staple line or endoscopic closure of fistulae defects may be needed.

Internal hernias
Internal herniation is a relatively uncommon complication occurring in 1% to 3% of individuals undergoing bariatric surgery, particularly those opting for RYGB. Patients often present with symptoms like abdominal pain, nausea, and vomiting, sometimes indicative of bowel obstruction. Early detection is crucial, and diagnostic tools such as an upper GI series and a computed tomography scan play a key role. The standard treatment approach involves laparoscopic exploration to locate and reduce the hernia, accompanied by the closure of the defect. In around 5% of cases, bowel resection may be necessary to address the herniation effectively.

Weight gain
This can be seen in both post-SG and RYGB patients, and its cause is usually multifactorial. Though its approach is beyond the scope of this article, recent advancements in bariatric and metabolic endoscopic (endoscopic re-suturing of SG, TORe in RYGB, among other techniques) are safer alternatives than surgical revision and thus preferred. Nevertheless, ruling out a gastro-gastric fistula is mandatory in RYGB patients presenting with weight regain.

Failure to thrive/malnutrition
Though the exact prevalence of this complication is not well known, patients with a history of malabsorptive surgical procedures can be more prone to these conditions in the setting of prolonged illnesses such as a cancer diagnosis. Enteral and parenteral support are often needed in this setting.

SUMMARY

The preoperative assessment for bariatric surgery is a comprehensive and meticulous process. Establishing criteria for surgery and considering contraindications form the foundation of this evaluative phase. The evaluation also addresses cardiorespiratory status, airway intricacies, and specific factors relevant to obese patients. Gastroenterologists assume a pivotal role in evaluating the GI health of patients through procedures such as EGD, manometry, and pH/impedance testing before surgery. Additionally, a gastroenterologist is involved in assessing the integrity of surgical anastomosis and addressing complications such as ulceration, bleeding, or alterations in bowel habits. Simultaneously, they contribute to providing nutritional guidance and addressing long-term issues. Postoperative care includes the management of potential complications like bleeding, leaks, and infections, coupled with optimizing recovery through adept pain management and wound care. Providing essential nutritional support to prevent deficiencies is integral, while ongoing guidance on behavioral and lifestyle changes, including dietary adjustments and exercise regimens, constitutes a cornerstone for long-term success. In summary, the success of bariatric treatment hinges on meticulous preoperative assessment and diligent postoperative care. The collaborative efforts of specialists within the interdisciplinary team underscore the significance of a holistic approach for achieving optimal outcomes in bariatric surgery.

CLINICS CARE POINTS

- Bariatric surgery necessitates a meticulous approach encompassing both preoperative assessments and postoperative care to ensure optimal outcomes. Existing evidence highlights the significance of a multidisciplinary team, emphasizing collaboration among specialists to conduct thorough preoperative evaluations, including cardiorespiratory and gastrointestinal assessments.

- Encouraging preoperative weight loss, providing nutritional supplementation, and offering behavioral counseling are crucial to enhancing patient readiness and promoting long-term success.

- Regular follow-up post-surgery is essential for monitoring weight loss, nutritional status, and psychological well-being, facilitating early intervention and complication management.

- Clinical pitfalls underscore the risks associated with inadequate preoperative assessments, neglecting nutritional needs, and overlooking mental health considerations. Failing to provide comprehensive support, including behavioral counseling and structured follow-up care, may lead to poor adherence to dietary and lifestyle changes, increasing the likelihood of complications and weight regain. Addressing these pitfalls through thorough assessments, multidisciplinary collaboration, and ongoing support can mitigate risks, improve patient outcomes, and enhance the effectiveness of bariatric surgery as a treatment for obesity.

REFERENCES

1. Mayoral LP, Andrade GM, Mayoral EP, et al. Obesity subtypes, related biomarkers & heterogeneity. Indian J Med Res 2020;151(1):11–21.
2. Benalcazar DA, Cascella M. Obesity surgery preoperative assessment and preparation. In: StatPearls. Treasure Island (FL): StatPearls Publishing; 2023. Available at: https://www.ncbi.nlm.nih.gov/books/NBK546667/?report=classic.
3. World Health Organization. Fact sheet: Obesity and overweight. Available at: https://www.who.int/en/news-room/fact-sheets/detail/obesity-and-overweight. [Accessed 12 March 2020].
4. Shafiee G, Qorbani M, Heshmat R, et al. Socioeconomic inequality in cardiometabolic risk factors in a nationally representative sample of Iranian adolescents using an Oaxaca-Blinder decomposition method: the CASPIAN-III study. J Diabetes Metab Disord 2019;18(1):145–53.
5. Smelt HJM, Pouwels S, Smulders JF, et al. Patient adherence to multivitamin supplementation after bariatric surgery: a narrative review. J Nutr Sci 2020;9:e46.

6. NIH conference. Gastrointestinal surgery for severe obesity. Consensus Development Conference Panel. Ann Intern Med 1991;115(12):956–61.

7. Eisenberg D, Shikora SA, Aarts E, et al. 2022 American Society for Metabolic and Bariatric Surgery (ASMBS) and International Federation for the Surgery of Obesity and Metabolic Disorders (IFSO): Indications for Metabolic and Bariatric Surgery. Surg Obes Relat Dis 2022;18(12):1345–56.

8. Thorell A, MacCormick AD, Awad S, et al. Guidelines for Perioperative Care in Bariatric Surgery: Enhanced Recovery After Surgery (ERAS) Society Recommendations. World J Surg 2016;40(9):2065–83.

9. Desogus D, Menon V, Singhal R, et al. An Examination of Who Is Eligible and Who Is Receiving Bariatric Surgery in England: Secondary Analysis of the Health Survey for England Dataset. Obes Surg 2019;29(10):3246–51.

10. Nam SY. Obesity-Related Digestive Diseases and Their Pathophysiology. Gut Liver 2017;11(3):323–34.

11. Moulla Y, Lyros O, Mehdorn M, et al. Preoperative Upper-GI Endoscopy Prior to Bariatric Surgery: Essential or Optional? Obes Surg 2020;30(6):2076–84.

12. Wolter S, Duprée A, Miro J, et al. Upper Gastrointestinal Endoscopy prior to Bariatric Surgery-Mandatory or Expendable? An Analysis of 801 Cases. Obes Surg 2017;27(8):1938–43.

13. Davrieux CF, Palermo M, Nedelcu M, et al. Reflux After Sleeve Gastrectomy: An Update. J Laparoendosc Adv Surg Tech 2021;31(9):978–82.

14. Qumseya BJ, Qumsiyeh Y, Ponniah SA, et al. Barrett's esophagus after sleeve gastrectomy: a systematic review and meta-analysis. Gastrointest Endosc 2021;93(2):343–52.e2.

15. Pallati PK, Shaligram A, Shostrom VK, et al. Improvement in gastroesophageal reflux disease symptoms after various bariatric procedures: review of the Bariatric Outcomes Longitudinal Database. Surg Obes Relat Dis 2014;10(3):502–7.

16. Mechanick JI, Youdim A, Jones DB, et al. Clinical practice guidelines for the perioperative nutritional, metabolic, and nonsurgical support of the bariatric surgery patient–2013 update: cosponsored by American Association of Clinical Endocrinologists, the Obesity Society, and American Society for Metabolic & Bariatric Surgery. Surg Obes Relat Dis 2013;9(2):159–91.

17. Swoboda L, Held J. Impaired wound healing in diabetes. J Wound Care 2022; 31(10):882–5.

18. Handelsman Y, Bloomgarden ZT, Grunberger G, et al. American association of clinical endocrinologists and american college of endocrinology - clinical practice guidelines for developing a diabetes mellitus comprehensive care plan - 2015. Endocr Pract 2015;21(Suppl 1):1–87.

19. Rasmussen JJ, Fuller WD, Ali MR. Sleep apnea syndrome is significantly underdiagnosed in bariatric surgical patients. Surg Obes Relat Dis 2012;8(5):569–73.

20. Fritscher LG, Mottin CC, Canani S, et al. Obesity and obstructive sleep apnea-hypopnea syndrome: the impact of bariatric surgery. Obes Surg 2007; 17(1):95–9.

21. Stefura T, Droś J, Kacprzyk A, et al. Influence of Preoperative Weight Loss on Outcomes of Bariatric Surgery for Patients Under the Enhanced Recovery After Surgery Protocol. Obes Surg 2019;29(4):1134–41.

22. Gunnarson GL, Frøyen JK, Sandbu R, et al. Plastic surgery after bariatric surgery. Tidsskr Nor Laegeforen 2015;135(11):1044–9.

23. Kassir R, Debs T, Blanc P, et al. Complications of bariatric surgery: Presentation and emergency management. Int J Surg 2016;27:77–81.

24. Shoar S, Poliakin L, Rubenstein R, et al. Single Anastomosis Duodeno-Ileal Switch (SADIS): A Systematic Review of Efficacy and Safety. Obes Surg 2018;28(1): 104–13.
25. Homan J, Betzel B, Aarts EO, et al. Vitamin and Mineral Deficiencies After Biliopancreatic Diversion and Biliopancreatic Diversion with Duodenal Switch–the Rule Rather than the Exception. Obes Surg 2015;25(9):1626–32.
26. Ziegler O, Sirveaux MA, Brunaud L, et al. Medical follow up after bariatric surgery: nutritional and drug issues. General recommendations for the prevention and treatment of nutritional deficiencies. Diabetes Metab 2009;35(6 Pt 2):544–57.
27. Poitou Bernert C, Ciangura C, Coupaye M, et al. Nutritional deficiency after gastric bypass: diagnosis, prevention and treatment. Diabetes Metab 2007; 33(1):13–24.
28. Daigle CR, Brethauer SA, Tu C, et al. Which postoperative complications matter most after bariatric surgery? Prioritizing quality improvement efforts to improve national outcomes. Surg Obes Relat Dis 2018;14(5):652–7.
29. Wolfe BM, Kvach E, Eckel RH. Treatment of Obesity: Weight Loss and Bariatric Surgery. Circ Res 2016;118(11):1844–55.
30. Sebastianelli L, Benois M, Vanbiervliet G, et al. Systematic Endoscopy 5 Years After Sleeve Gastrectomy Results in a High Rate of Barrett's Esophagus: Results of a Multicenter Study. Obes Surg 2019;29(5):1462–9.
31. Mandeville Y, Van Looveren R, Vancoillie PJ, et al. Moderating the Enthusiasm of Sleeve Gastrectomy: Up to Fifty Percent of Reflux Symptoms After Ten Years in a Consecutive Series of One Hundred Laparoscopic Sleeve Gastrectomies. Obes Surg 2017;27(7):1797–803.
32. Miller AT, Matar R, Abu Dayyeh BK, et al. Postobesity Surgery Esophageal Dysfunction: A Combined Cross-Sectional Prevalence Study and Retrospective Analysis. Am J Gastroenterol 2020;115(10):1669–80.
33. Nielsen JB, Pedersen AM, Gribsholt SB, et al. Prevalence, severity, and predictors of symptoms of dumping and hypoglycemia after Roux-en-Y gastric bypass. Surg Obes Relat Dis 2016;12(8):1562–8.
34. Vargas EJ, Abu Dayyeh BK, Storm AC, et al. Endoscopic management of dumping syndrome after Roux-en-Y gastric bypass: a large international series and proposed management strategy. Gastrointest Endosc 2020;92(1):91–6.

Endoscopic Management of Weight Regain After Bariatric Surgery

Daniel Szvarca, MD[a,b], Pichamol Jirapinyo, MD, MPH[a,b],*

KEYWORDS

- Bariatric surgery • Roux-en-Y gastric bypass (RYGB) • Sleeve gastrectomy (SG)
- Weight regain • Weight recurrence • Transoral outlet reduction (TORe)
- Restorative obesity surgery endoluminal • Argon plasma coagulation (APC)

KEY POINTS

- Metabolic and bariatric surgery is an effective treatment for patients with obesity and obesity-related comorbidities; however, postoperative weight regain, that is, recurrent weight gain, is prevalent.
- Roux-en-Y gastric bypass (RYGB) and sleeve gastrectomy (SG) are the most commonly performed bariatric surgeries worldwide and can be revised endoscopically for patients experiencing weight regain.
- Transoral outlet reduction is an endoscopic revisional procedure for patients with weight regain after RYGB with level I evidence. The procedure focuses on reducing the size of the gastrojejunal anastomosis and/or pouch.
- Sleeve-in-sleeve is an endoscopic revisional procedure for patients with weight regain after SG. The procedure focuses on reducing the width and/or length of the sleeve body.

INTRODUCTION

Metabolic and bariatric surgery (MBS) is the most effective treatment for patients with obesity and obesity-related comorbidities.[1,2] Over the past decade, the most commonly performed MBSs are Roux-en-Y gastric bypass (RYGB) and sleeve gastrectomy (SG), which are associated with approximately 32% and 23% total weight loss (TWL) at 1 year, respectively.[3,4] Although these interventions are effective, weight regain is not uncommon.[1] Of note, the newer term for weight regain is recurrent weight gain. Throughout the remainder of this article, the authors use the traditional terminology of "weight regain."

[a] Division of Gastroenterology, Hepatology and Endoscopy, Brigham and Women's Hospital, 75 Francis Street, Boston, MA 02115, USA; [b] Harvard Medical School, 25 Shattuck Street, Boston, MA 02115, USA
* Corresponding author. Division of Gastroenterology, Hepatology and Endoscopy, Brigham and Women's Hospital, 75 Francis Street, Boston, MA 02115.
E-mail address: pjirapinyo@bwh.harvard.edu

Gastrointest Endoscopy Clin N Am 34 (2024) 639–654
https://doi.org/10.1016/j.giec.2024.04.007
1052-5157/24/© 2024 Elsevier Inc. All rights reserved.

NATURE OF THE PROBLEM

Due to a lack of consensus on the definition of weight regain, the prevalence of weight regain after MBS has a wide, estimated range from 9% to 91%.[5] A large, observational study of 4047 patients found that the amount of weight loss after RYGB was maximal at 1 to 2 years with patients regaining an average of 30% of their initial lost weight by 10 years.[4] With regard to SG, a systematic review showed the prevalence of weight regain ranging from 5.7% at 2 years to 75.6% at 6 years.[6] Overall, it is estimated that, in the long-term, patients typically regain about 30% of their maximum lost weight, with approximately 30% of them regaining nearly all of their lost weight within 10 to 12 years following MBS.[7]

Weight regain after MBS is complex. Patient factors include medical, genetic, dietary, psychological, and behavioral components, while anatomic factors include gastrojejunal anastomosis (GJA) diameter, gastric pouch size, and surgical complications such as gastro-gastric fistulas (GGFs).[8–10] Therefore, the management of weight regain requires a comprehensive, yet individualized approach.

Recent advancements in anti-obesity medications (AOMs), especially glucagon-like peptide-1 receptor agonists, have shown promise in the treatment of weight regain after MBS.[11] Although promising, these AOMs are sometimes difficult for patients to tolerate and are often expensive.[12] On the other hand, surgical revisions and/or conversions of MBS are effective; however, they are technically challenging and are associated with significant morbidity compared to the index procedure.[13] Therefore, endoscopic interventions have recently emerged as minimally invasive, safe, and effective treatment options for patients who experience weight regain after MBS.[2,14] This review will outline the endoscopic techniques used to treat weight regain, specifically after RYGB and SG, and their clinical outcomes.

ANATOMY
Roux-en-Y Gastric Bypass

During RYGB, the surgeon first creates a small gastric pouch (20–30 mL) in the proximal stomach and separates it from the remnant stomach. The biliopancreatic limb (~ 50 cm) is then created, consisting of the duodenum and proximal jejunum, which remain contiguous with the remnant stomach. A Roux limb is measured 75 to 150 cm from the jejunal division point and is then connected to the distal end of the biliopancreatic limb at the jejunojejunostomy. Finally, the proximal end of the Roux limb is brought up to the pouch and a side-to-side gastrojejunostomy is created. The cumulative effect of the procedure results in both reduced gastric volume and altered nutrient flow from exclusion of the proximal small bowel leading to weight loss (**Fig. 1**).[15]

Sleeve Gastrectomy

During SG, the surgeon uses a tissue stapler to resect along the greater curvature of the stomach from around 5 cm proximal to the pylorus up to the Angle of His (**Fig. 2**).[16] This resection reduces the gastric volume by approximately 70% and induces rapid gastric emptying and hormonal changes, which lead to weight loss.

PRE-ENDOSCOPIC REVISIONAL PROCEDURE PLANNING

Prior to considering endoscopic revision of MBS, a thorough evaluation of the patient's medical and surgical history, weight loss history, and weight loss goals is necessary. Patients are evaluated by a bariatric multidisciplinary team including bariatric surgeons, bariatric endoscopists, obesity medicine specialists, psychologists,

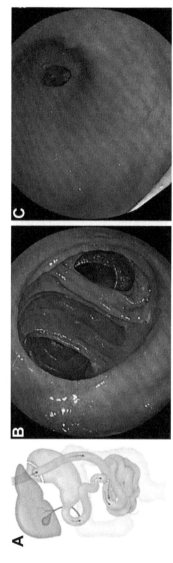

Fig. 1. (A) RYGB anatomy, (B) endoscopic view of dilated GJA, and (C) endoscopic view of gastric pouch. (*From* Jirapinyo P, Thompson CC. Obesity Primer for the Practicing Gastroenterologist. Am J Gastroenterol. 2021 May 1;116(5):918 to 934. with permission (A)).

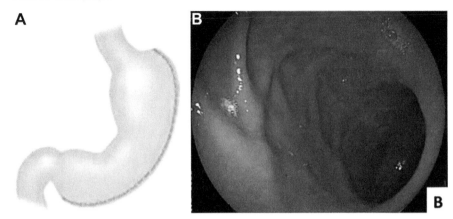

Fig. 2. (*A*) SG anatomy and (*B*) endoscopic view of SG anatomy. (*From* Jirapinyo P, Thompson CC. Obesity Primer for the Practicing Gastroenterologist. Am J Gastroenterol. 2021 May 1;116(5):918 to 934. with permission (A)).

dieticians, and exercise physiologists. A comprehensive review of treatment options for weight regain is then discussed including behavioral, pharmacologic, surgical, and endoscopic approaches.

For patients considering an endoscopic revision of MBS, they are scheduled for an esophagogastroduodenoscopy to assess anatomy and identify any structural abnormalities that may contribute to weight regain. Depending on the findings, patients may require further radiographic evaluation prior to the revisional procedure.

Patients are also recommended to discuss with their primary care physician to ensure that their medications can be converted to a liquid or crushable form after the revisional procedure.

PREP AND PATIENT POSITIONING

On the day prior to the procedure, patients are encouraged to take a bowel preparation to minimize constipation while on a liquid diet after the procedure. At 8 hours prior to the procedure, patients start a clear liquid-only diet. A carbohydrate-loading beverage is also encouraged the night before and at 3 hours prior to the procedure to help reduce postoperative nausea and vomiting. At 2 hours prior to the procedure, patients stop all intake by mouth.

In the preoperative area, patients are given a scopolamine patch, intravenous dexamethasone, and intravenous ondansetron to minimize postoperative nausea and vomiting. Additionally, they are placed on pneumatic compression devices and given a dose of subcutaneous heparin to minimize the risks of post-procedural deep vein thrombosis and pulmonary embolism.

Patient positioning during the procedure depends on the type of revisional procedure and device, but usually involves either a left lateral or supine position. Similarly, depending on the procedure, intravenous antibiotics may be administered interprocedurally, and most cases are performed under general anesthesia with all cases utilizing carbon dioxide insufflation.

PROCEDURAL APPROACH
Endoscopic Treatments of Weight Regain Following RYGB

Overview
There are several factors that contribute to weight regain following RYGB. From an anatomic standpoint, dilation of the GJA, presence of a GGF, and dilation of the gastric

pouch have been shown to be associated with weight regain.[9,10] Although traditionally, surgical revisions have been performed to treat weight regain, revisional surgeries are complex and carry an increased morbidity compared to the index MBS.[13] Therefore, over the past decades, less invasive, endoscopic approaches to treat weight regain following RYGB have been increasingly performed with good efficacy and safety profiles.[17]

Transoral outlet reduction

Transoral outlet reduction (TORe) is an endoscopic approach for the management of weight regain following RYGB with level I evidence.[18] In 2013, Thompson and colleagues[19] reported the result of a prospective, multicenter, randomized, blinded, sham-control trial (RESTORe) demonstrating that patients who underwent TORe had significantly greater weight loss than those who underwent a sham procedure (3.5% vs 0.4% TWL at 6 months, respectively; $P = .021$). In this trial, a partial thickness suturing device was used, which has now been shown to be inferior to full-thickness suturing devices.[20] Currently, there are two endoscopic, full-thickness tissue approximation devices used for TORe: (1) the Overstitch endoscopic suturing device (Boston Scientific, Marlborough, MA, USA; **Fig. 3**A), which recently received Food and Drug Administration (FDA) marketing de novo authorization for endoscopic sleeve gastroplasty as well as TORe and (2) the Incisionless Operating Platform (IOP) endoscopic plication device (USGI Medical, San Clemente, CA, USA; **Fig. 3**B [21]), which is FDA-cleared for tissue approximation. Of note, in general, suturing refers to when the tissue is approximated in a mucosa-to-mucosa manner, while plication refers to when the tissue is approximated in a serosa-to-serosa manner.

Suturing-TORe

The suturing-TORe (S-TORe) procedure is performed using the Overstitch endoscopic suturing device (Boston Scientific). The device consists of a curved needle driver, an anchor exchange catheter, and an operating handle that attaches near the endoscopic working channels (**Fig. 3**C). Sutures are loaded onto the anchor exchange and passed back and forth between the needle driver and anchor exchange catheter to place stitches. A tissue helix may also be used to grasp and pull the tissue into the Overstitch device. Over the last decade, there have been several advancements in TORe procedures, encompassing various aspects such as suture patterns and tissue

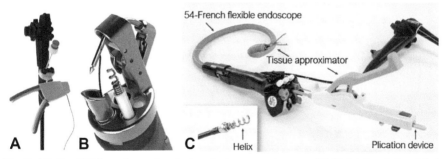

Fig. 3. (A) OverStitch endoscopic suturing device on endoscope. (B) Distal tip of OverStitch device with needle, helix, and working channel for anchor exchange catheter. (C) IOP endoscopic plication device. (*With permission from* Apollo Endosurgery, Inc, Austin, Texas. (A) Jirapinyo P, de Moura DTH, Thompson CC. Sleeve in sleeve: endoscopic revision for weight regain after sleeve gastrectomy. VideoGIE. 2019 Aug 13;4(10):454 to 457 (B)).

preparation techniques, all of which have continued to improve weight loss outcomes.[22,23]

In 2013, Jirapinyo and colleagues[24] reported the use of the first-generation Overstitch device used to reduce GJA diameter and treat weight regain. Shortly afterward, the second-generation Overstitch device enabled endoscopists to place multiple stitches with a single suture allowing for several suture patterns, including running and purse-string, in addition to the interrupted pattern.[25] In 2018, Schulman and colleagues[22] demonstrated that the pursestring TORe technique was superior to the original interrupted TORe suture pattern with the efficacy of 8.6% versus 6.4% TWL at 12 months, respectively (*P* = .02; **Fig. 4**). From a tissue preparation standpoint, a meta-analysis showed that performing argon plasma coagulation (APC) circumferentially around the GJA prior to suturing the anastomosis resulted in greater weight loss compared to suturing alone (24.2% vs 11.7% excess weight loss, respectively; *P*<.001).[2] Most recently, the combination of modified endoscopic submucosal dissection (ESD) performed around the GJA, followed by APC and pursestring suturing of the GJA has been shown to be safe and effective. Subsequently, in our practice, ESD-TORe is now the first-line treatment for patients with RYGB with weight regain and a dilated GJA.

STEPS OF THE PROCEDURE (S-TORe)

1. First, a diagnostic endoscopy is performed to evaluate the RYGB anatomy, measure anatomic landmarks, and assess for any contraindications (eg, marginal ulceration) (**Fig. 5**).
2. Approximately 60 mL of simethicone is then deployed in the distal Roux limb to minimize abdominal bloating after the procedure.
3. For APC-TORe, a straight-fire APC catheter is used to perform APC (forced APC, flow 0.8 L/min and power of 70 W) approximately 1 cm around the GJA. Then, proceed to step 8.
4. For ESD-TORe, a cap is placed at the tip of the gastroscope. A solution of hetastarch mixed with methylene blue and epinephrine is then injected into the submucosal layer of the GJA using an injection needle.
5. An electrosurgical knife is used to make a circumferential mucosal incision approximately 1 cm from the anastomotic rim. Subsequently, the same knife is

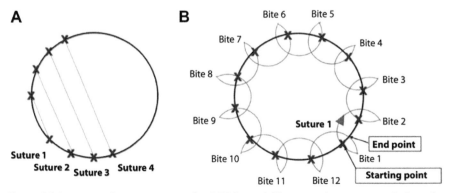

Fig. 4. (*A*) Interrupted suture pattern for S-TORe and (*B*) pursestring suture technique for S-TORe. (*From:* Jirapinyo P, Kumar N, AlSamman MA, Thompson CC. Five-year outcomes of transoral outlet reduction for the treatment of weight regain after Roux-en-Y gastric bypass. Gastrointest Endosc. 2020 May;91(5):1067–1073).

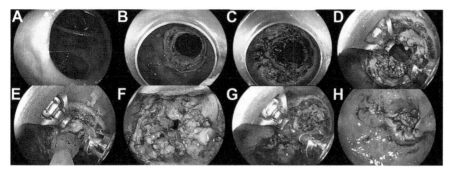

Fig. 5. (*A*) Dilated GJA, (*B*) GJA after modified-ESD, (*C*) GJA after APC, (*D*) pursestring suturing around the GJA, (*E*) cinching around CRE balloon, (*F*) GJA after cinching, (*G*) reinforcement interrupted suture in the distal pouch, and (*H*) GJA immediately after ESD-TORe.

used to trim and expose the submucosal/muscular layer circumferentially around the GJA.

6. Any exposed foreign body materials such as surgical staples or prior sutures should be removed to prevent a bent needle during the suturing step and to optimize tissue healing after the procedure.

7. APC (forced APC, flow 0.8 L/min and power of 70 W) is then used to ablate the inner and outer rims of the exposed submucosal/muscular bed. This step helps minimize bleeding during the suturing step and further defines the borders of the submucosal/muscular bed.

8. The gastroscope is exchanged to a double channel endoscope, which is attached to the Overstitch suturing device. The suturing device is then used to place 12 to 14 stitches with a single suture in a pursestring suture pattern around the GJA. Of note, our practice is to place the first stitch through the ablated area (for APC-TORe) or exposed submucosal/muscular layer (for ESD-TORe) at the 5 o'clock position and then subsequent stitches approximately 5 mm apart in a counterclockwise manner.

9. Once a full pursestring is performed around the GJA, the last stitch is intentionally crossed with the first stitch to lock the suture. The tissue anchor is dropped, which becomes a T-tag to secure one end of the suture.

10. The other end of the suture is loaded onto the cinching device, which is passed down the working channel of the double channel endoscope. A hydrostatic dilation balloon (CRE balloon dilator; Boston Scientific, Marlborough, MA) is passed down through the second channel of the double channel endoscope. The CRE balloon is placed through the GJA and inflated to 6 to 8 mm. The suture is tightened and cinched over the inflated balloon to size the final anastomotic diameter. The suture is then cut.

11. The final step is to place an interrupted suture pattern in the distal pouch proximal to the GJA to reinforce the pursestring suture. Additionally, if the pouch is long (usually >5 cm), pouch reduction may be performed using a running suture pattern.

Outcomes

S-TORe has now become the most commonly performed endoscopic revisional procedure for patients with weight regain after RYGB. In 2017, Jirapinyo and colleagues[25] reported the efficacy of pursestring TORe on 252 patients with weight regain after RYGB to be 9.6% and 8.4% TWL at 6 and 12 months, respectively. There were two serious adverse events (SAEs; 0.8%) including gastrointestinal bleeding and GJA stenosis, which were treated endoscopically.

Within S-TORe, modified ESD-TORe has been shown to be superior to APC-TORe. Specifically, in Jirapinyo and colleagues,[26] 15 patients with ESD-TORe were matched 1:3 to 45 patients with APC-TORe based on baseline GJA and pouch sizes. At 12 months, the ESD-TORe group experienced 12.1% TWL compared to 7.5% in the APC-TORe group ($P = .04$). Additionally, 83.3% of the ESD-TORe group experienced 5% or greater TWL compared to 56.1% in the APC-TORe group.

Regarding durability, Jirapinyo and colleagues[17] in 2020 reported that of a cohort of 331 patients with RYGB who underwent TORe, the mean TWL was 8.8% at 5 years postprocedure. Moreover, the 5 year efficacy of TORe has been demonstrated to be similar to surgical RYGB revision (11.5% [TORe] vs 13.1% [surgical] TWL; $P = .67$), but with significantly fewer adverse events (AEs; 6.5% vs 29%; $P = .043$).[27]

Lastly, with the emerging role of AOMs, the combination therapy of medical and endoscopic approaches for treating weight regain has gained popularity. Recently, a study of 145 patients with RYGB treated with both AOMs (most commonly topiramate, phentermine, and liraglutide) along with TORe, found that combination therapy is more effective than either AOMs or TORe alone.[28] Specifically, combination therapy was associated with 15.2% versus 6.8% TWL for AOMs alone ($P<.0001$) and 8.7% for TORe alone ($P<.0001$) at 12 months. SAE rates were similar for combination therapy (2.1%), AOM alone (4.7%), and TORe alone (0.6%) ($P>.05$). Combination therapy also yielded similar 12 month weight loss compared to surgical revision with a lower SAE rate.

Plication-TORe

The plication-TORe (P-TORe) procedure, also known as restorative obesity surgery endoluminal, utilizes the IOP plication device (USGI Medical) to invert the stomach with tissue anchor placement achieving serosa-to-serosa apposition and reducing the size of the GJA and/or pouch (**Fig. 6**). The device consists of 4 components: the transport-R (a 54F flexible endoscope with 4 working channels), the 16 mm G-Prox (for grasping and approximating tissue), the G-Lix (a helix for pulling tissue into the jaws of the G-Prox), and the G-Cath (for deploying tissue anchors) (see **Fig. 3**).[29]

STEPS OF THE PROCEDURE (P-TORe)

1. First, a diagnostic endoscopy is performed to evaluate the RYGB anatomy, measure anatomic landmarks, and assess for contraindications to the procedure (eg, marginal ulceration). Of note, given the size of the IOP system, the pouch should be at least 3 cm in length (see **Fig. 6**).
2. Approximately 60 mL of simethicone is then deployed in the distal Roux limb to minimize abdominal bloating after the procedure.
3. APC (setting: forced APC, flow 0.8 L/min and power of 70 W) is performed on the mucosal rim on the gastric side of the GJA. Of note, APC prior to P-TORe is performed to a narrow width of approximately 5 mm, in contrast to 10 mm or greater for S-TORe.
4. The gastroscope is then exchanged for the IOP plication system with an ultraslim gastroscope.
5. Plications are placed around the GJA a few millimeters outside the ablated area to allow for plication of more compliant tissue. To place each plication, the G-Lix is

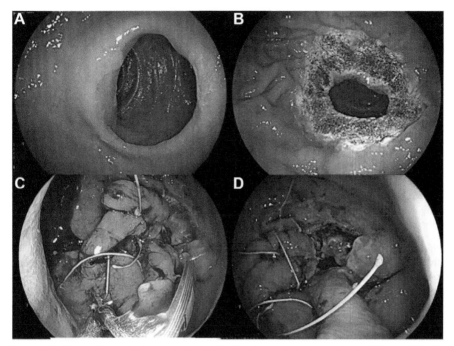

Fig. 6. (A) Dilated GJA, (B) GJA after APC, (C) plications placed around the GJA, and (D) GJA after P-TORe.

used to pull tissue into the G-Prox. The needle from the G-Cath is then passed through the tissue and a pair of snowshoe tissue anchors are deployed on both sides of the tissue prior to cinching. The suture is then cut and released.[30]

6. These steps are repeated until the GJA diameter is reduced to approximately 8 to 10 mm in diameter. Subsequently, additional plications are placed in the pouch to reduce its length.

Outcomes

In 2010, Horgan and colleagues[30] reported an outcome of a multicenter registry study including 116 patients who underwent P-TORe with the average TWL of 4.2% at 12 months. Since then, there have been advancements to the IOP device, and most recently, Jirapinyo and colleagues[29] showed that P-TORe with APC around the GJA prior to plication resulted in 9.5% TWL at 12 months. There were no reported SAEs. The GJA stenotic rate was 9.9%, all of which were treated endoscopically.

Argon Plasma Coagulation

APC emits argon gas which is ionized by an electrical current leading to coagulation of the mucosal surface (**Fig. 7**). APC can be applied circumferentially around the GJA to decrease its diameter and compliance over several sessions and ultimately induce weight loss. The settings for APC reported in the literature vary from 45 to 80 W. The procedure can be performed under moderate sedation and patients go home on the same day. The procedure is then repeated every 3 months until the GJA size is reduced to approximately 8 to 10 mm or until the ideal body weight is achieved.

Outcomes

An 8 center study including 558 patients who underwent serial APC for weight regain demonstrated a 6.9% to 10.4% TWL at 12 months.[31] The AE rate was 5.4% with the 3 most common including GJA stenosis (2.7%), GJA ulcers (0.9%), and vomiting (0.9%). All were treated conservatively or endoscopically.

Another study demonstrated that high-dose (70–80 W) APC was superior to low-dose (45–55 W) APC for the treatment of weight regain. Specifically, a single-center study including 217 patients who underwent 411 APC sessions showed that the 12 month TWL was 9.7% in the high-dose APC group versus 5.1% in the low-dose APC group (P = .008), with no significant difference in the GJA stenosis rate.[32]

Additionally, a more recent randomized, controlled trial of 40 patients showed that serial APC was comparable to S-TORe (8.3% TWL in the APC group vs 7.5% in the S-TORe group at 12 months; P = .71).[33] However, it is important to note that in this study, S-TORe was performed using the figure-of-eight suture pattern which is inferior to the pursestring suture pattern.

Other techniques

Other techniques for endoscopic treatment of weight regain following RYGB include cryoablation, sclerotherapy, and over-the-scope clips (OTSCs; Ovesco Endoscopy AG; Tubingen, Germany). Cryoablation utilizes a balloon to ablate the mucosal layer of the dilated GJA and pouch with the goal of inducing fibrosis and reducing their size. Sclerotherapy involves the injection of a sclerosing agent (classically sodium morrhuate) around the dilated GJA to decrease its compliance and diameter. OTSCs are made of Nitinol and have multiple therapeutic applications including the treatment of weight regain after RYGB as a way to reduce the size of the GJA and pouch.

Outcomes

With cryoablation, a retrospective study of 22 patients with RYGB demonstrated that at 8 weeks following treatment, the GJA diameter was reduced from a mean of 24.1 to 17.1 mm and the pouch size was reduced from a mean of 5.0 to 3.9 cm.[34] The average TWL was 8.1% at 8 weeks and the AE rate was 13.6% including 2 gastric ulcers treated with proton-pump inhibitors and one GJA stenosis treated endoscopically. For sclerotherapy, a retrospective analysis of 231 patients with RYGB with weight regain who underwent 575 sclerotherapy sessions demonstrated a mean weight loss of 10 lbs at 12 months, representing 18% of the weight regained from the nadir post-RYGB weight and 4.4% TWL from the pre-sclerotherapy weight.[35] The most common AEs included transient diastolic blood pressure increases 64 (15%), gastro-intestinal bleeding which was treated endoscopically 14 (2.4%), and small, incidental ulcerations on repeat endoscopy 6 (1%). Regarding OTSC, a retrospective study including 94 patients who underwent 2 OTSC placements (one on each side of the

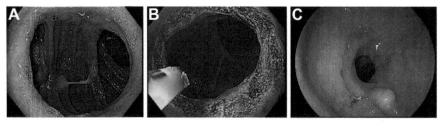

Fig. 7. (*A*) Dilated GJA, (*B*) GJA after first APC session, and (*C*) GJA after 3 APC sessions.

GJA) demonstrated that this technique could reduce the GJA size by 80%.[36] The mean body mass index decreased from 32.8 kg/m^2 prior to the revisional procedure to 27.4 kg/m^2 at 1 year postprocedure. Five patients reported postprocedural dysphagia requiring endoscopic evaluation with 2 patients requiring endoscopic dilation of the GJA.

Endoscopic Treatment of Weight Regain Following Sleeve Gastrectomy

Overview
Although SG is an effective surgical treatment for obesity, weight regain is common.[6] Traditionally, weight regain following SG is treated with surgical re-sleeve or conversion to RYGB.[37,38] Although surgical revision is effective and sometimes needed for reflux management, it is associated with higher morbidity compared to the index surgery.[13,14] Therefore, over the recent years, endoscopic revisional procedures of SG, also known as sleeve-in-sleeve (SIS), have been increasingly performed for the management of weight regain after SG as a less-invasive alternative.

Similar to endoscopic revision of RYGB, endoscopic revision of SG can be performed via a suturing or plication technique. For the suturing approach, the Overstitch suturing device (Boston Scientific) is utilized to place several running and interrupted suture patterns along the greater curvature of the sleeve body to reduce its width. For the plication approach, the IOP plication system (USGI Medical) is utilized to place plications in a belt-and-suspenders pattern to reduce the width and length of the dilated sleeve.

STEPS OF THE PROCEDURE (SUTURING TECHNIQUE)

1. A diagnostic endoscopy is performed to evaluate the sleeve anatomy, measure anatomic landmarks, and assess for any contraindications to endoscopic revision of SG, such as an ulceration or stenosis (**Fig. 8**).
2. Approximately 60 mL of simethicone is then deployed in the distal duodenum to minimize abdominal bloating after the procedure.
3. The gastroscope is exchanged to a double channel endoscope, which is attached to the Overstitch suturing device.
4. Using the suturing device, a running suture is placed starting at the anterior wall of the incisura and then moving down along the greater curvature and posterior wall to reduce the diameter of the sleeve body.
5. Once the running suture is completed, the needle is dropped, which becomes a T-tag. The other end of the suture is loaded onto the cinching device, which is then advanced through the working channel of the double channel endoscope. Constant tension is applied to tighten the suture and a cinch is deployed to secure and cut the suture.
6. In our practice, the next suture is used to place an interrupted suture pattern adjacent to the first suture. This reinforces the running suture and further narrows the width of the sleeve.
7. Subsequently, a running suture alternating with an interrupted suture is placed proximally to the previous sutures along the greater curvature, with the final suture being placed at the proximal sleeve body sparing the fundic remnant.

STEPS OF THE PROCEDURE (PLICATION TECHNIQUE)

1. A diagnostic endoscopy is performed to evaluate the sleeve anatomy, measure anatomic landmarks, and assess for any contraindications to endoscopic revision of SG, such as an ulceration or stenosis (**Fig. 9**).

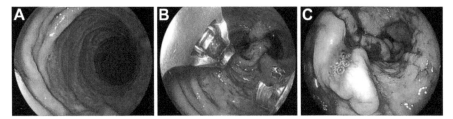

Fig. 8. (A) Dilated SG, (B) sleeve body being narrowed using running and interrupted sutures, and (C) sleeve body immediately after suturing SIS.

2. Approximately 60 mL of simethicone is then deployed in the distal duodenum to minimize abdominal bloating after the procedure.
3. The gastroscope is then exchanged for the IOP plication system with an ultraslim gastroscope.
4. Distal belt plications are placed at the incisura to reduce the width of the dilated sleeve.
5. Next, two rows of suspender plications are placed in parallel to the greater curvature to shorten the length of the sleeve.
6. Finally, proximal belt plications are placed at the junction between the sleeve body and fundic remnant to further reduce the width at the proximal sleeve.

Outcomes

In 2020, a multicenter study of 82 patients who underwent endoscopic revision of SG via suturing technique demonstrated an average of 13.2% TWL at 6 months and 15.7% at 12 months.[39] One patient had stenosis of the gastroesophageal junction treated with endoscopic dilation. Using the IOP device to perform SIS has also been shown to be a feasible approach with 8% TWL at 3 months.[21] Additionally, plication SIS has also been compared to the surgical options of re-sleeve and conversion to RYGB. In this study including 18 patients (9 SIS and 9 surgical revisions), there was no difference in TWL at 6 and 12 months (9.75% vs 10.53% and 9.75% vs 9.87%, respectively; $P>.05$). However, patients who underwent endoscopic SIS had a shorter length of hospital stay and fewer AEs, although the later did not reach statistical significance potentially due to a small sample size.[40]

RECOVERY AND REHABILITATION

Most revisional procedures can be performed as outpatient procedures. To minimize postprocedural nausea and vomiting, in addition to preprocedural antiemetics, we

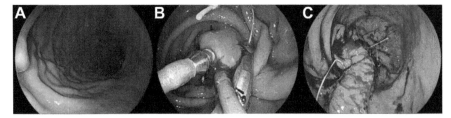

Fig. 9. (A) Dilated SG, (B) distal belt plications at the incisura to reduce the width of the sleeve, and (C) sleeve body immediately after plication SIS.

administer a dose of intravenous haloperidol prior to extubation. Additionally, patients receive opioid-sparing analgesics, such as intravenous acetaminophen and/or ketorolac prior to completion of the procedure. It is recommended that patients refrain from consuming anything by mouth for the reminder of the procedure day with intravenous fluid support and then advance to a protein-rich, liquid diet for 45 days. All patients are started on open-capsule proton pump inhibitors, sucralfate, and all medications are converted to a liquid or crushable form for 45 days. All patients are then followed up in a multidisciplinary bariatric clinic.

SUMMARY

Weight regain after MBS is multifactorial and requires a comprehensive approach to management. Lifestyle and behavioral modifications should be encouraged, and psychological and social support should be offered to all patients. As an adjunct to these interventions, endoscopic revision of MBS is being increasingly performed for the treatment of weight regain given its safety and efficacy. Early data on combination therapy of endoscopic revision with pharmacotherapy is promising with its efficacy approaching that of surgical revision of MBS with a better safety profile. As endoscopic therapies continue to advance, ongoing efforts should be directed toward personalizing interventions for patients experiencing weight regain following MBS.

CLINICS CARE POINTS

- Weight regain following MBS is a complex and multifactorial condition that necessitates a multidisciplinary and personalized approach to management.
- Understanding the anatomic changes and postoperative complications that may contribute to weight regain is essential for tailoring the most effective endoscopic revision approach.
- The fundamental objective of endoscopic revision for RYGB is to decrease the diameter of the GJA to approximately 8 mm, while also addressing pouch elongation in cases of a longer pouch. This can be achieved through either a suturing or plication technique.
- The fundamental objective of endoscopic revision for SG is to reduce the diameter of the sleeve body with or without shortening its length. Similar to endoscopic revision for RYGB, this can be achieved through either a suturing or plication technique.

DISCLOSURE

D. Szvarca has nothing to disclose. P. Jirapinyo serves as a consultant for Apollo Endosurgery, Boston Scientific, ERBE, Spatz Medical, and receives research support from Boston Scientific, United States, Fractyl, GI Dynamics and USGI Medical, United States.

REFERENCES

1. Noria SF, Shelby RD, Atkins KD, et al. Weight Regain After Bariatric Surgery: Scope of the Problem, Causes, Prevention, and Treatment. Curr Diabetes Rep 2023;23(3):31–42.
2. Brunaldi VO, Jirapinyo P, de Moura DTH, et al. Endoscopic Treatment of Weight Regain Following Roux-en-Y Gastric Bypass: a Systematic Review and Meta-analysis. Obes Surg 2018;28(1):266–76.

3. Jirapinyo P, Thompson CC. Obesity Primer for the Practicing Gastroenterologist. Am J Gastroenterol 2021;116(5):918–34.
4. Sjöström L, Narbro K, Sjöström CD, et al, Swedish Obese Subjects Study. Effects of bariatric surgery on mortality in Swedish obese subjects. N Engl J Med 2007; 357(8):741–52.
5. Monaco-Ferreira DV, Leandro-Merhi VA. Weight Regain 10 Years After Roux-en-Y Gastric Bypass. Obes Surg 2017;27(5):1137–44.
6. Lauti M, Kularatna M, Hill AG, et al. Weight Regain Following Sleeve Gastrectomy-a Systematic Review. Obes Surg 2016;26(6):1326–34.
7. Sjöström CD, Lissner L, Wedel H, et al. Reduction in incidence of diabetes, hypertension and lipid disturbances after intentional weight loss induced by bariatric surgery: the SOS Intervention Study. Obes Res 1999;7(5):477–84.
8. Athanasiadis DI, Martin A, Kapsampelis P, et al. Factors associated with weight regain post-bariatric surgery: a systematic review. Surg Endosc 2021;35(8): 4069–84.
9. Abu Dayyeh BK, Lautz DB, Thompson CC. Gastrojejunal stoma diameter predicts weight regain after Roux-en-Y gastric bypass. Clin Gastroenterol Hepatol 2011; 9(3):228–33.
10. Heneghan HM, Yimcharoen P, Brethauer SA, et al. Influence of pouch and stoma size on weight loss after gastric bypass. Surg Obes Relat Dis 2012;8:408–15.
11. Jensen AB, Renström F, Aczél S, et al. Efficacy of the Glucagon-Like Peptide-1 Receptor Agonists Liraglutide and Semaglutide for the Treatment of Weight Regain After Bariatric surgery: a Retrospective Observational Study. Obes Surg 2023;33(4):1017–25.
12. Sodhi M, Rezaeianzadeh R, Kezouh A, et al. Risk of Gastrointestinal Adverse Events Associated With Glucagon-Like Peptide-1 Receptor Agonists for Weight Loss. JAMA 2023;330(18):1795–7.
13. Fulton C, Sheppard C, Birch D, et al. A comparison of revisional and primary bariatric surgery. Can J Surg 2017;60(3):205–11.
14. Abboud DM, Yao R, Rapaka B, et al. Endoscopic Management of Weight Recurrence Following Bariatric Surgery. Front Endocrinol 2022;13:946870.
15. Mitchell BG, Gupta N. Roux-en-Y Gastric Bypass. In: StatPearls. Treasure Island (FL): StatPearls Publishing; 2023. Available at: https://www.ncbi.nlm.nih.gov/ books/NBK553157/.
16. Seeras K, Sankararaman S, Lopez PP. Sleeve Gastrectomy. In: StatPearls. Treasure Island (FL): StatPearls Publishing; 2023. Available at: https://www.ncbi.nlm. nih.gov/books/NBK519035/.
17. Jirapinyo P, Kumar N, AlSamman MA, et al. Five-year outcomes of transoral outlet reduction for the treatment of weight regain after Roux-en-Y gastric bypass. Gastrointest Endosc 2020;91(5):1067–73.
18. Thompson CC, Jacobsen GR, Schroder GL, et al. Stoma size critical to 12-month outcomes in endoscopic suturing for gastric bypass repair. Surg Obes Relat Dis 2012;8(3):282–7.
19. Thompson CC, Chand B, Chen YK, et al. Endoscopic suturing for transoral outlet reduction increases weight loss after Roux-en-Y gastric bypass surgery. Gastroenterology 2013;145(1):129–37.e3.
20. Kumar N, Thompson CC. Comparison of a superficial suturing device with a full-thickness suturing device for transoral outlet reduction (with videos). Gastrointest Endosc 2014;79(6):984–9.
21. Jirapinyo P, de Moura DTH, Thompson CC. Sleeve in sleeve: endoscopic revision for weight regain after sleeve gastrectomy. VideoGIE 2019;4(10):454–7.

22. Schulman AR, Kumar N, Thompson CC. Transoral outlet reduction: a comparison of purse-string with interrupted stitch technique. Gastrointest Endosc 2018;87(5): 1222–8.
23. de Moura DTH, Jirapinyo P, Thompson CC. Modified-ESD Plus APC and Suturing for Treatment of Weight Regain After Gastric Bypass. Obes Surg 2019;29(6): 2001–2.
24. Jirapinyo P, Slattery J, Ryan MB, et al. Evaluation of an endoscopic suturing device for transoral outlet reduction in patients with weight regain following Roux-en-Y gastric bypass. Endoscopy 2013;45(7):532–6.
25. Jirapinyo P, Kröner PT, Thompson CC. Purse-string transoral outlet reduction (TORe) is effective at inducing weight loss and improvement in metabolic comorbidities after Roux-en-Y gastric bypass. Endoscopy 2018;50(4):371–7.
26. Jirapinyo P, de Moura DTH, Thompson CC. Endoscopic submucosal dissection with suturing for the treatment of weight regain after gastric bypass: outcomes and comparison with traditional transoral outlet reduction (with video). Gastrointest Endosc 2020;91(6):1282–8.
27. Dolan RD, Jirapinyo P, Thompson CC. Endoscopic versus surgical gastrojejunal revision for weight regain in Roux-en-Y gastric bypass patients: 5-year safety and efficacy comparison. Gastrointest Endosc 2021;94(5):945–50.
28. Jirapinyo P, Thompson CC. Combining transoral outlet reduction with pharmacotherapy yields similar 1-year efficacy with improved safety compared with surgical revision for weight regain after Roux-en-Y gastric bypass (with videos). Gastrointest Endosc 2023;98(4):552–8.
29. Jirapinyo P, Thompson CC. Endoscopic gastric plication for the treatment of weight regain after Roux-en-Y gastric bypass (with video). Gastrointest Endosc 2022;96(1):51–6.
30. Horgan S, Jacobsen G, Weiss GD, et al. Incisionless revision of post-Roux-en-Y bypass stomal and pouch dilation: multicenter registry results. Surg Obes Relat Dis 2010;6(3):290–5.
31. Moon RC, Teixeira AF, Neto MG, et al. Efficacy of Utilizing Argon Plasma Coagulation for Weight Regain in Roux-en-Y Gastric Bypass Patients: a Multi-center Study. Obes Surg 2018;28(9):2737–44.
32. Jirapinyo P, de Moura DTH, Dong WY, et al. Dose response for argon plasma coagulation in the treatment of weight regain after Roux-en-Y gastric bypass. Gastrointest Endosc 2020;91(5):1078–84.
33. Brunaldi VO, Farias GFA, de Rezende DT, et al. Argon plasma coagulation alone versus argon plasma coagulation plus full-thickness endoscopic suturing to treat weight regain after Roux-en-Y gastric bypass: a prospective randomized trial (with videos). Gastrointest Endosc 2020;92(1):97–107.e5.
34. Fayad L, Trindade AJ, Benias PC, et al. Cryoballoon ablation for gastric pouch and/or outlet reduction in patients with weight regain post Roux-en-Y gastric bypass. Endoscopy 2020;52(3):227–30.
35. Abu Dayyeh BK, Jirapinyo P, Weitzner Z, et al. Endoscopic sclerotherapy for the treatment of weight regain after Roux-en-Y gastric bypass: outcomes, complications, and predictors of response in 575 procedures. Gastrointest Endosc 2012; 76(2):275–82.
36. Heylen AM, Jacobs A, Lybeer M, et al. The OTSC®-clip in revisional endoscopy against weight gain after bariatric gastric bypass surgery. Obes Surg 2011; 21(10):1629–33.
37. Clapp B, Wynn M, Martyn C, et al. Long term (7 or more years) outcomes of the sleeve gastrectomy: a meta-analysis. Surg Obes Relat Dis 2018;14(6):741–7.

38. Landreneau JP, Strong AT, Rodriguez JH, et al. Conversion of Sleeve Gastrectomy to Roux-en-Y Gastric Bypass. Obes Surg 2018;28(12):3843–50.
39. Maselli DB, Alqahtani AR, Abu Dayyeh BK, et al. Revisional endoscopic sleeve gastroplasty of laparoscopic sleeve gastrectomy: an international, multicenter study. Gastrointest Endosc 2021;93(1):122–30.
40. Bazarbashi AN, Jirapinyo P, Thompson CC. Endoscopic sleeve-in-sleeve versus surgical re-sleeve in patients with weight regain after sleeve gastrectomy: a retrospective comparative analysis. GIE 2020;91(6). Supplement, AB226.

Endoscopic Management of Bariatric Surgery Complications: Fistulas, Leaks, and Ulcers

Abhishek Shenoy, MD, MSc[a],
Allison R. Schulman, MD, MPH, FASGE[a,b],*

KEYWORDS

- Fistulas • Leaks • Ulcerations • Marginal ulcerations • Bariatric endoscopy
- Complications

KEY POINTS

- A growing endoscopic armamentarium exists for the management of leaks and fistulas including closure devices, diversion therapy, septotomy techniques, endoscopic vacuum therapy, and sealants.
- The specific endoscopic technique or device used to treat leaks or fistulas depends on a variety of factors including chronicity, size, and location.
- Marginal ulceration is a common complication following Roux-en-Y gastric bypass surgery and can present with nausea, vomiting, pain, bleeding, or perforation, but also commonly is asymptomatic.
- Proton pump inhibitors are first-line therapy for the treatment of marginal ulceration and should be administered in a soluble form.
- In refractory cases of marginal ulcerations, endoscopic suturing may be an alternative treatment to surgical intervention.

INTRODUCTION

Bariatric surgery is the most effective treatment of patients with obesity and obesity-related comorbidities.[1] Although these interventions are generally safe and effective, adverse events are not uncommon. Moreover, fewer than 1% of patients with obesity who are candidates for bariatric surgery undergo these operations, at least in part due

[a] Division of Gastroenterology and Hepatology, University of Michigan, Ann Arbor, MI, USA;
[b] Department of Surgery, University of Michigan, Ann Arbor, MI, USA
* Corresponding author. 1500 East Medical Center Drive, Taubman Center 3912, Ann Arbor, MI 48109.
E-mail address: arschulm@med.umich.edu
Twitter: @abhi2shenoy (A.S.); @allie_schulman (A.R.S.)

Gastrointest Endoscopy Clin N Am 34 (2024) 655–669
https://doi.org/10.1016/j.giec.2024.06.001
1052-5157/24/© 2024 Elsevier Inc. All rights are reserved, including those for text and data mining, AI training, and similar technologies.

to the high-risk profile.[2–4] Roux-en-Y gastric bypass (RYGB) was traditionally the most frequently performed bariatric surgery; however, lower risk and more simple interventions have continued to evolve. Laparoscopic sleeve gastrectomy is increasingly popular and now has surpassed RYGB as the most commonly performed procedure. Despite its safety, adverse events are still encountered. The focus of this study is the endoscopic management of 3 common complications following bariatric surgery including fistulas, leaks, and anastomotic ulcerations.

FISTULAS

Gastrointestinal (GI) fistulas are defined as abnormal communications between epithelialized surfaces. Fistulas may be external, involving communication between the GI tract and the skin (enterocutaneous), or internal, involving communication between 2 portions of the GI tract (enteroenteric) or the GI tract and another organ system (eg, gastropleural and gastrosplenic).[5] Surgical repair of fistulas may ultimately be required but is technically challenging and carries increased morbidity and mortality. As a result, endoscopic approaches that are less invasive are often employed as first-line intervention.[6]

Localization of fistulas is key to successful endoscopic management. Cross-sectional imaging, upper GI series, and other radiographic and fluoroscopic studies are necessary to determine the location, complexity, and intervenability of these lesions. Endoscopic techniques for localization including the use of methylene blue, carbon dioxide insufflation, and radiopaque contrast injection may also be imperative depending on the site and nature of the fistula.[7,8]

Gastrogastric Fistulas

The most common fistula following bariatric surgery is a gastrogastric fistula, which occurs between the gastric pouch and the excluded stomach after RYGB (**Fig. 1**). These typically occur between the gastric pouch and proximal gastric remnant and can range in size from pinpoint to several centimeters.[9,10] The incidence of gastrogastric fistula has declined overtime with the advent of laparoscopic RYGB due to complete division of the pouch and remnant.[11]

The etiology of these fistulas may be multifactorial. As earlier, fistulas may form as a technical complication from incomplete division of the stomach when the pouch is created. This phenomenon occurs in open gastric bypass procedures. Additionally,

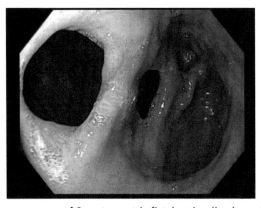

Fig. 1. Endoscopic appearance of 2 gastrogastric fistulas visualized proximal to the GJA.

staple-line failure leading to abscesses or leaks may also promote the creation of gastrogastric fistulas.[9]

Gastrogastric fistulas may be asymptomatic; however, when symptoms occur, they usually include weight regain, borborygmi, reflux, nausea/vomiting, recurrence of diabetes mellitus, and may predispose to ulceration as the acid from the remnant stomach can now freely pass into the gastric pouch without the typical duodenal buffering secretions.[9,12,13]

Historically, symptomatic gastrogastric fistulas were treated surgically; however, endoscopic approaches for closure have become first-line therapy.[6] These transmural defects can be challenging to close given the established epithelial tract and potential proximity to unhealthy tissue. It is critical to de-epithelialize the fistulous tract that can be accomplished using cautery such as argon plasma coagulation (APC) or brush techniques (**Fig. 2**). Following de-epithelialization, closure devices such as cap-mounted clips and endoscopic suturing have become more commonly employed for treatment. Endoscopic submucosal dissection (ESD) prior to defect closure may improve the durability of closure. Other techniques have also been reported including off-label use of cardiac septal occluder devices, tissue sealants, and other biomaterials.[14,15] Early data suggest that ESD of the fistulous tract prior to closure may promote better long-term outcomes.[12,16] Fistulas less than 1 cm in size are associated with increased success rates with endoscopic closure. Despite immediate success, larger fistulas are prone to recurrence.[10] There are increasing data on the success of intervention on the excluded stomach to prevent weight regain and other symptoms for these larger defects. A retrospective matched cohort study of patients with RYGB who underwent endoscopic closure or surgical revision was compared. Endoscopic gastrogastric fistula (GGF) treatment provided greater improvement in abdominal pain, fewer overall, and serious treatment-related adverse events when compared with surgical revision. Success rate of endoscopic closure of gastrogastric fistulas has been reported to be nearly 30% though fistulas less than 10 mm in size have significantly higher sustained closure rates than fistulas greater than 20 mm. In one study involving 95 patients with GGFs, no patients with GGFs over 20 mm in size who underwent endoscopic suturing treatment had sustained closure during the 1 year follow-up period. However, 10 (32%) patients with GGF 10 mm or greater in diameter remained closed at 12 months.[10]

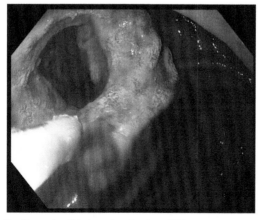

Fig. 2. De-epithelialization of a fistulous tract using APC.

Other Fistulas

Enterocutaneous, digestive–respiratory, entero-visceral, and entero-enteric fistulas have all been reported following bariatric surgery.[17] In patients who have undergone sleeve gastrectomy, these fistulas typically arise in the proximal stomach where the staple line has ruptured that may lead to chronic, untreated leaks from longstanding inflammation.[18] Reported techniques for closure will be reviewed under the "Leak" section. Depending on location, size, and chronicity, these fistulas can lead to high morbidity and may be refractory to endoscopic closure techniques. Depending on symptoms and clinical status, surgical consultation should be considered.

LEAKS AFTER BARIATRIC SURGERY

The most feared complication following bariatric surgery is a postsurgical leak. Leaks are defined as defects leading to communication between intra-luminal and extra-luminal compartments (**Fig. 3**). Symptoms of leaks range from mild nausea and epigastric pain to fever, tachycardia, sepsis, and/or fulminant peritonitis.[19] Symptoms are generally accompanied by objective measures of illness including leukocytosis with left shift, elevated inflammatory markers, including C-reactive protein and erythrocyte sedimentation rate.

Leaks can occur at any time postoperatively. This adverse event arises due to a dehiscence or discontinuity at a surgical anastomosis or the site where tissue is divided. Leaks that occur in the acute postoperative setting have been attributed to technical errors such as stapler misfiring or acute trauma to the tissue.[20] Delayed leaks can result from ischemia to tissue, particularly around anastomotic sites, or due to hematoma or obstruction.[21]

Initial management differs based on patient stability and local expertise. Patients with postsurgical leaks who are clinically unstable should be managed surgically and endoscopic attempts to intervene should be deferred. On the other hand, patients who are clinically stable should undergo an attempt at endoscopic intervention. It is important to note that leaks associated with perigastric or intra-abdominal collections require drainage either via endoscopic, percutaneous, or surgical technique prior to other modalities of treatment. Furthermore, enteral nutrition via nasojejunal tubes should be considered early in patients with postsurgical leaks. Antibiotics also play a major role in management.[22,23]

Endoscopic interventions aimed at leak management are typically performed under general anesthesia and in a fluoroscopy-equipped unit. Timing, chronicity, location,

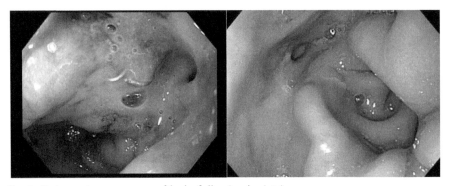

Fig. 3. Endoscopic appearance of leaks following bariatric surgery.

leak size, and available expertise are all important considerations in selecting endoscopic treatment modalities. Acute (<1 week) or early (1–6 weeks) leaks are managed differently than late (6–12 weeks) or chronic (>12 weeks) leaks. Sustained leaks can result in fistulas as previously described.

Endoscopic treatment of postsurgical leaks often requires multiple endoscopic sessions and multimodal therapy is frequently needed. A multicenter, international study evaluating 266 patients with postsurgical leaks noted an endoscopic closure success rate of 80.1%. Leak resolution was achieved by the third and fourth techniques in 70% to 80% of patients, a median of 125 days of endoscopic therapy.[24]

A review of leaks following sleeve gastrectomy and RYGB and common management strategies will be reviewed later.

Leaks Following Sleeve Gastrectomy

Leaks after sleeve gastrectomy are a challenging complication that occurs in a small percentage of patients. One study evaluated 2834 patients who underwent sleeve gastrectomy and the incidence of leak was found to be 1.5% (N = 44).[25] Another review and meta-analysis that included 29 studies and 4888 patients who underwent sleeve gastrectomy reported an overall incidence of 2.4%, with the risk rising to 2.9% in patients with body mass index greater than 50 kg/m^2.[26]

Most leaks following sleeve gastrectomy occur at the proximal aspect of the staple line near the gastroesophageal junction and just below the angle of His.[27] This location tends to be affected due to 2 major factors. First, this is an area of relative ischemia from the takedown of the short gastric arteries during surgery. Second, this is a zone of higher intraluminal pressure. Leaks are known to occur when intragastric pressure exceeds the staple line burst pressure. Distal sleeve stenosis or stricture may precipitate this increased intraluminal pressure, and therefore, realignment of the sleeve axis through dilation of this region should be performed to promote leak closure[28] (**Fig. 4A–D**). Both of these factors, ischemia and increased intraluminal pressure, contribute to the risk of sleeve leak development at the proximal staple line.[29]

Advances in endoscopic approaches have helped create a paradigm shift in the initial management of leaks. Endoscopic treatment has been shown to have lower morbidity and mortality when compared to revisional surgery.[30] Numerous endoscopic interventions have been described, with success rates varying depending on the aforementioned factors.[31] A summary of the most commonly employed technology is reviewed later.

Leaks Following Roux-en-Y Gastric Bypass

Similar to sleeve gastrectomy, leaks following RYGB carry high morbidity and can be life-threatening. This complication occurs less frequently than following sleeve gastrectomy with most studies demonstrating the incidence less than 1%. One study involving the Metabolic and Bariatric Surgery Accreditation and Quality Improvement Data Registry included 77,596 patients and found that the overall leak rate was 0.6% (N = 476). Though low, there was significant morbidity in patients post RYGB due to other complications including reoperation and readmission.[32] Furthermore, factors such as location, chronicity, and size of the leak need to be considered in determining appropriate management strategies.[28] For example, several anatomic locations where leaks can occur following RYGB may not be amenable to endoscopic approaches. Leaks that are amenable to endoscopic intervention are typically proximal in location, and a similar armamentarium of devices and techniques that are employed to manage leaks following sleeve gastrectomy are utilized in this context.

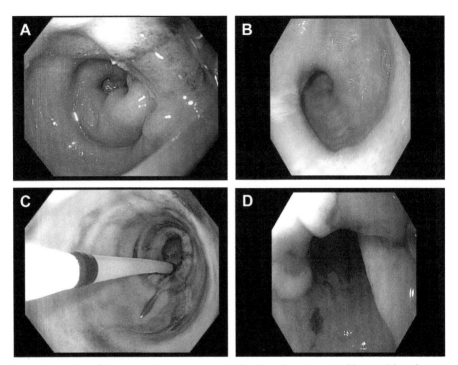

Fig. 4. Examples of sleeve gastrectomy stenosis (*A, B*) and pneumatic dilation (*C*) with post-dilation appearance (*D*).

ENDOSCOPIC ARMAMENTARIUM FOR POST-BARIATRIC SURGICAL LEAKS AND FISTULAS

Despite the advent of many endoscopic options, there remains limited standardized guidance in selection of endoscopic treatment without a formal algorithm. Successful endoscopic management of the patient with a post-bariatric leak or fistulas requires a multidisciplinary team-based approach, local expertise, and availability of closure devices. Common endoscopic options include closure techniques, diversion therapy, internal drainage, septotomy, and endoscopic vacuum-assisted therapy (EVT).

MECHANICAL CLOSURE DEVICES

Closure devices play a role in the management of both fistulas and leaks following bariatric surgery. Ablation of the epithelialized tract is critical prior to the closure of fistulas. For leaks, drainage of a concomitant perigastric collection must be performed before closure is pursued to prevent abscess development. These closure techniques may be more successful in the early/acute phase of leak formation. The more commonly employed closure techniques will be reviewed in the following section.

Endoscopic Suturing Systems

The currently available endoscopic suturing device (OverStitch, Boston Scientific/Apollo Endosurgery, MA, United States) allows for full-thickness apposition of tissue and intraluminal closure of GI fistulas and leak sites.[33,34] This technique can be used for defects of all sizes. Many suture patterns including a variety of running and

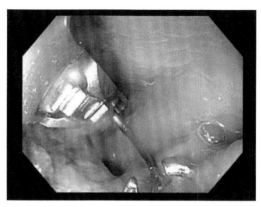

Fig. 5. Endoscopic suturing for management of leak closure.

interrupted patterns have been described for the closure of these defects with smaller lesions leading to more successful sustained results. There are limited data on the consensus approach to technique, though guidelines are in development. The main component of the platform itself includes the needle driver handle and the anchor exchange catheter, with grasping forceps and a tissue retracting helix device being used to aid with full-thickness tissue apposition. Use of this technique requires expertise and advanced training and suturing in these locations may be particularly challenging due to endoluminal space limitations and a tangential orientation of the device (**Fig. 5**). In addition, healthy surrounding tissue is required for best results.

Cap-Mounted Clip

Cap-mounted clips have been described in the closure of various types of GI fistulas and leaks, specifically in the early postoperative period. These devices are biocompatible, made of nitinol, and allow for full-thickness closure of luminal defects up to 2 cm in size. The most widely commercially available system is the over-the-scope clip (Ovesco Endoscopy AG, Tubingen, Germany). Cap-mounted clips have significant advantages over traditional through-the-scope (TTS) clips including their larger size, wider arms, and higher mechanical compression.[35,36] Several studies have suggested that cap-mounted clip closure for fistulas and leaks may be more successful in the early/acute stage. Defects that are more chronic in nature tend to be accompanied by fibrotic edges and scar tissue, which limits the durability and long-term success of cap-mounted clip placement.[37–39]

Through-the-Scope Clips

TTS clips were developed originally for endoscopic hemostasis but have also been used to manage acute perforations and other mucosal defects within the GI tract. While these clips are widely available and easily advanced through the channel of a standard endoscope, they were not designed to close fistulas or leaks.[28] As a result, TTS clips have limited efficacy and are generally not recommended for management of these defects.[10,40]

OTHER TECHNIQUES
Diversion Therapy: Self-Expandable Metal Stents

Endoscopic self-expandable metal stents (SEMS) are commonly used for initial management of acute post-bariatric surgical leaks (**Fig. 6**).[41 42] These stents are deployed

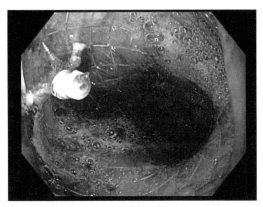

Fig. 6. Leak following placement of self-expanding metal stent with endoscopic suturing fixation.

to seal the defect and divert luminal content to allow for mucosal healing. It is prudent to ensure that any extra-luminal collection has been drained adequately prior to stent placement to avoid abscess development and septic complications. Success rates of SEMS in the upper GI tract have been reported to range from 48% to 75%, with increased success in acute/early leaks.[43,44] One major limitation to the use of SEMS is migration. SEMS migration can occur in up to 40% of patients without fixation techniques like endoscopic suturing or clip placement but still occurs despite fixation in 15.9% of cases.[45] Stent migration may predispose to severe complications including obstruction or perforation.[46] SEMS should generally be avoided in patients with late or chronic leaks due to reduced efficacy and a higher chance of migration.[8]

Newer SEMS designed specifically for patients who have undergone bariatric surgery have predominantly been available outside of the United States. For example, the Mega Stent (Taewoong Medical, Seoul, South Korea) and Nit-S-Beta stent (Taewoong Medical, Seoul, South Korea) are fully covered SEMS with larger phalanges designed to reduce migration and increase flexibility in patients with bariatric surgical anatomy.[47,48]

Septotomy

Endoscopic septotomy is an increasingly popular technique used in the management of chronic leaks where an incision is made to enlarge the fistulous tract between the perigastric collection and the sleeve lumen. This complete division of this tract leads to equalization of the pressure gradient that drives leak formation (**Fig. 7**).

Endoscopic Vacuum Therapy

EVT is a technique that is based on the principles of surgical wound healing. Foam or sponge material is applied to a leak cavity and connected by suction tubing for continuous negative pressure drainage. This technique allows for improvement in microcirculation, promotion of epithelialization, and granulation tissue formation.[14] EVT is popular abroad and has gained increasing excitement within the United States given its efficacy with early studies demonstrating closure success rates approaching 90%.[49] Depending on the size and location of the defect, frequent foam or sponge changes are commonly required leading to the need for multiple procedures and prolonged hospitalizations.

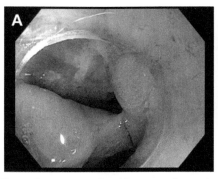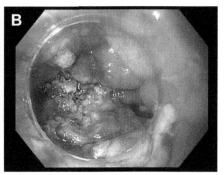

Fig. 7. Septum visualized between the perigastric collection and the gastric lumen (*A*) followed by complete division using septotomy technique (*B*).

Tissue Sealants

Tissue sealants have been described for the management of fistulas and leaks. The 2 most described sealants in the post-bariatric surgical setting are fibrin glue and cyanoacrylate glue.[14] Fibrin glue consists of human fibrinogen and human thrombin reconstituted with calcium chloride. The glue is applied to the defect through a double-lumen catheter and is most efficient in dry areas within the lumen. Cyanoacrylate (n-butyl-2-cyanoacrylate) is a synthetic glue that polymerizes after it has contact with moisture. This reaction causes tissue necrosis and an inflammatory cascade that promotes tissue healing. Sealants have been shown to promote fibroblast and keratinocyte growth but frequently require numerous sessions. This technique has a wide range of reported success in the literature, ranging from 35% to 96.8%. Successful closure appears to increase with lower output fistula and an increasing number of incremental sealant sessions.[50] Another study evaluating the use of fibrin sealants in patients in GI fistula closure, noted success rates closer to 86%, requiring an average of 2.5 endoscopic sessions. Success was seen fare more frequently in fistulas with lower output.[51,52]

ULCERATIONS

Marginal ulceration, or ulceration at the gastrojejunal anastomosis (GJA), is among the most common complication following RYGB. These typically occur on the posterior jejunal aspect of the GJA (**Fig. 8**). The incidence of marginal ulceration ranges from 0.6% up to 16%; however, might approach 50% as many patients are asymptomatic.[53,54] When symptoms do occur, patients commonly present with GI bleeding, abdominal pain, nausea, and/or vomiting. Perforation is encountered less frequently.[55]

Etiology

The etiology of marginal ulceration is multifactorial.[55] The GJA is a low blood flow region prone to tension and tissue ischemia. Surgical technique may also play a role. Furthermore, smoking is an independent risk factor for the development of marginal ulceration, independent of intensity. One study found that light, moderate, and heavy smokers had significant and similar rates of marginal ulcer development (17.4%, 17.1%, 17.9%, respectively).[56]

Another risk for the development of marginal ulceration includes nonsteroidal anti-inflammatory drugs (NSAIDs). One large, retrospective, cross-matched population study across 3 national registries noted that continuous NSAID exposure for 30 days

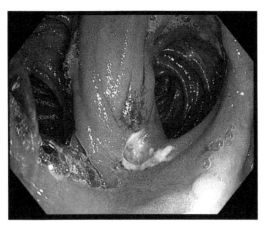

Fig. 8. Endoscopic appearance of a marginal ulceration on the posterior aspect of the GJA in a patient with gastric bypass anatomy.

or more was a significant risk factor for ulcer development following RYGB.[57] Another risk factor is the use of nonabsorbable sutures at the internal layer of the GJA. One study evaluating a total of 3285 patients who underwent RYGB in a 5 year period noted that patients with nonabsorbable suture material at the GJA had an increased incidence of postoperative marginal ulceration.

Finally, *Helicobacter pylori* may play a role in ulcer development. While retrospective studies have had conflicted results, a larger cohort study using the Nationwide Inpatient Sample database found a strong association. In 253,765 patients who underwent bariatric surgery, the prevalence of marginal ulceration across this cohort was 3.9% with 31.2% of patients having *H pylori* infection with an odds ratio of over 11%.[58]

Treatment

Treatment of marginal ulceration consists of high-dose proton pump inhibitors (PPIs). In patients with incomplete response to high-dose open capsule acid suppression therapy, sucralfate may be beneficial to aid in ulcer healing. PPIs should be administered in an opened capsule or soluble formulation, as this has been shown to reduce time to ulcer healing as compared to intact capsules that may be less effective due to decreased absorption in the setting of a small gastric pouch and rapid small-bowel transit.[27] One retrospective study including 164 patients found a median time to ulcer healing of 91 days for the opened capsule PPI group (N = 115) when compared to 342 days in the intact capsule group (N = 49).[58]

Smoking cessation, discontinuation of NSAIDs, and removal of foreign material are imperative in this patient population to promote ulcer healing.[56,57,59] Furthermore, testing for *H pylori* should be performed by either serology in patients who are treatment naïve or stool antigen testing in those with a history of prior infection. Tissue biopsy of the gastric pouch may yield false negative results as *H pylori* may reside in the excluded stomach.[60]

The majority of patients with marginal ulceration respond to aforementioned interventions.[55] In recalcitrant ulcers, endoscopic oversewing has been reported with small case series' demonstrating efficacy and safety. This was first reported in a small case series of 3 patients.[61] A subsequent study including 11 patients with refractory marginal ulceration who underwent endoscopic ulcer oversewing and/or placement of a fully covered SEMS demonstrated technical success in 90% of patients with complete ulcer healing at 8 weeks.[62] Surgical revision is the standard of care for the treatment of refractory marginal ulceration but is associated with high morbidity and recurrence.[63]

SUMMARY

The management of fistulas, leaks, and ulcerations following bariatric surgery continues to evolve. Advances in endoscopic treatment options have created a paradigm shift in the management of these complications, leading to lower morbidity than traditional surgical approaches. Randomized controlled studies comparing the armamentarium of these endoscopic modalities will help individualize patient care and further shape the future of this field.

CLINICS CARE POINTS

- Despite immediate success with fistula closure, there is a high reopening rate in fistula over 1 cm in size.
- Fisutlous tract disruption and de-epithelialization a should be performed prior to other closure techniques to increase long-term success.
- Timing, chronicity, location, leak size and available expertise should all be considered when selecting endoscopic treatment modalities.

DISCLOSURE

Dr A.R. Schulman is a consultant for Apollo Endosurgery, Boston Scientific, Micro-Tech, and Olympus and has received research/grant support from GI Dynamics and Fractyl. A. Shenoy is a consultant Fractyl (including receiving research/grant support from them).

REFERENCES

1. Gasoyan H, Tajeu G, Halpern MT, et al. Reasons for underutilization of bariatric surgery: The role of insurance benefit design. Surg Obes Relat Dis 2019;15(1): 146–51.
2. Spota A, Cereatti F, Granieri S, et al. Endoscopic management of bariatric surgery complications according to a standardized algorithm. Obes Surg 2021; 31(10):4327–37.
3. Chang SH, Stoll CR, Song J, et al. The effectiveness and risks of bariatric surgery: an updated systematic review and meta-analysis, 2003-2012. JAMA Surg 2014; 149(3):275–87.
4. Arterburn DE, Courcoulas AP. Bariatric surgery for obesity and metabolic conditions in adults. BMJ 2014;349:g3961.
5. Kwon SH, Oh JH, Kim HJ, et al. Interventional management of gastrointestinal fistulas. Korean J Radiol 2008;9(6):541–9.
6. Donatelli G, Dumont JL, Cereatti F, et al. Endoscopic internal drainage as first-line treatment for fistula following gastrointestinal surgery: a case series. Endosc Int Open 2016;4(6):E647–51.

7. Kumar N, Larsen MC, Thompson CC. Endoscopic Management of Gastrointestinal Fistulae. Gastroenterol Hepatol 2014;10(8):495–552.

8. de Oliveira VL, Bestetti AM, Trasolini RP, et al. Choosing the best endoscopic approach for post-bariatric surgical leaks and fistulas: Basic principles and recommendations. World J Gastroenterol 2023;29(7):1173–93.

9. Filho AJ, Kondo W, Nassif LS, et al. Gastrogastric fistula: a possible complication of Roux-en-Y gastric bypass. J Soc Laparoendosc Surg 2006;10(3):326–31.

10. Fernandez-Esparrach G, Lautz DB, Thompson CC. Endoscopic repair of gastrogastric fistula after Roux-en-Y gastric bypass: a less-invasive approach. Surg Obes Relat Dis 2010;6(3):282–8.

11. Yao DC, Stellato TA, Schuster MM, et al. Gastrogastric fistula following Roux-en-Y bypass is attributed to both surgical technique and experience. Am J Surg 2010; 199(3):382–5 [discussion 5-6].

12. Dolan RD, Jirapinyo P, Maahs ED, et al. Endoscopic closure versus surgical revision in the management of gastro-gastric fistula following Roux-en-Y gastric bypass. Endosc Int Open 2023;11(6):E629–34.

13. Haddad A, Bashir A, Nimeri A. Gastrogastric Fistula: an Unusual Cause for Severe Bile Reflux Following Conversion of Sleeve Gastrectomy to One Anastomosis Gastric Bypass. Obes Surg 2018;28(7):2151–3.

14. Cereatti F, Grassia R, Drago A, et al. Endoscopic management of gastrointestinal leaks and fistulae: What option do we have? World J Gastroenterol 2020;26(29): 4198–217.

15. de Moura DTH, Sachdev AH, Thompson CC. Endoscopic full-thickness defects and closure techniques. Curr Treat Options Gastroenterol 2018;16(4):386–405.

16. Lafeuille P, Wallenhorst T, Lupu A, et al. Endoscopic submucosal dissection combined with clip for closure of gastrointestinal fistulas including those refractory to previous therapy. Endoscopy 2022;54(7):700–5.

17. Rogalski P, Swidnicka-Siergiejko A, Wasielica-Berger J, et al. Endoscopic management of leaks and fistulas after bariatric surgery: a systematic review and meta-analysis. Surg Endosc 2021;35(3):1067–87.

18. Parmer M, Wang YHW, Hersh EH, et al. Management of staple line leaks after laparoscopic sleeve gastrectomy. J Soc Laparoendosc Surg 2022;26(3).

19. Csendes A, Braghetto I, Leon P, et al. Management of leaks after laparoscopic sleeve gastrectomy in patients with obesity. J Gastrointest Surg 2010;14(9): 1343–8.

20. Clapp B, Schrodt A, Ahmad M, et al. Stapler malfunctions in bariatric surgery: an analysis of the MAUDE database. J Soc Laparoendosc Surg 2022;26(1).

21. Lim R, Beekley A, Johnson DC, et al. Early and late complications of bariatric operation. Trauma Surg Acute Care Open 2018;3(1):e000219.

22. Jacobsen HJ, Nergard BJ, Leifsson BG, et al. Management of suspected anastomotic leak after bariatric laparoscopic Roux-en-y gastric bypass. Br J Surg 2014;101(4):417–23.

23. Praveenraj P, Gomes RM, Kumar S, et al. Management of gastric leaks after laparoscopic sleeve gastrectomy for morbid obesity: A tertiary care experience and design of a management algorithm. J Minim Access Surg 2016;12(4):342–9.

24. Rodrigues-Pinto E, Pereira P, Sousa-Pinto B, et al. Retrospective multicenter study on endoscopic treatment of upper GI postsurgical leaks. Gastrointest Endosc 2021;93(6):1283–12899 e2.

25. Sakran N, Goitein D, Raziel A, et al. Gastric leaks after sleeve gastrectomy: a multicenter experience with 2,834 patients. Surg Endosc 2013;27(1):240–5.

26. Aurora AR, Khaitan L, Saber AA. Sleeve gastrectomy and the risk of leak: a systematic analysis of 4,888 patients. Surg Endosc 2012;26(6):1509–15.

27. Burgos AM, Braghetto I, Csendes A, et al. Gastric leak after laparoscopic-sleeve gastrectomy for obesity. Obes Surg 2009;19(12):1672–7.

28. Schulman AR, Watson RR, Abu Dayyeh BK, et al. Endoscopic devices and techniques for the management of bariatric surgical adverse events (with videos). Gastrointest Endosc 2020;92(3):492–507.

29. Cai JX, Schweitzer MA, Kumbhari V. Endoscopic management of bariatric surgery complications. Surg Laparosc Endosc Percutaneous Tech 2016;26(2): 93–101.

30. Shenoy A, Schulman AR. Advances in endobariatrics: past, present, and future. Gastroenterol Rep (Oxf) 2023;11:goad043.

31. Gjeorgjievski M, Imam Z, Cappell MS, et al. A comprehensive review of endoscopic management of sleeve gastrectomy leaks. J Clin Gastroenterol 2021; 55(7):551–76.

32. Mocanu V, Dang J, Ladak F, et al. Predictors and outcomes of leak after Roux-en-Y gastric bypass: an analysis of the MBSAQIP data registry. Surg Obes Relat Dis 2019;15(3):396–403.

33. Ge PS, Thompson CC. The use of the overstitch to close perforations and fistulas. Gastrointest Endosc Clin N Am 2020;30(1):147–61.

34. Kukreja K, Chennubhotla S, Bhandari B, et al. Closing the gaps: endoscopic suturing for large submucosal and full-thickness defects. Clin Endosc 2018;51(4): 352–6.

35. von Renteln D, Denzer UW, Schachschal G, et al. Endoscopic closure of GI fistulae by using an over-the-scope clip (with s). Gastrointest Endosc 2010; 72(6):1289–96.

36. Piyachaturawat P, Mekaroonkamol P, Rerknimitr R. Use of the over the scope clip to close perforations and fistulas. Gastrointest Endosc Clin N Am 2020;30(1): 25–39.

37. Conio M, Blanchi S, Repici A, et al. Use of an over-the-scope clip for endoscopic sealing of a gastric fistula after sleeve gastrectomy. Endoscopy 2010;42(Suppl 2):E71–2.

38. Niland B, Brock A. Over-the-scope clip for endoscopic closure of gastrogastric fistulae. Surg Obes Relat Dis 2017;13(1):15–20.

39. Lee HL, Cho JY, Cho JH, et al. Efficacy of the over-the-scope clip system for treatment of gastrointestinal fistulas, leaks, and perforations: a korean multi-center study. Clin Endosc 2018;51(1):61–5.

40. Technology Assessment C, Chuttani R, Barkun A, et al. Endoscopic clip application devices. Gastrointest Endosc 2006;63(6):746–50.

41. Freeman RK, Ascioti AJ, Wozniak TC. Postoperative esophageal leak management with the Polyflex esophageal stent. J Thorac Cardiovasc Surg 2007; 133(2):333–8.

42. Freeman RK, Van Woerkom JM, Ascioti AJ. Esophageal stent placement for the treatment of iatrogenic intrathoracic esophageal perforation. Ann Thorac Surg 2007;83(6):2003–7 [discussion 7-8].

43. van Halsema EE, van Hooft JE. Clinical outcomes of self-expandable stent placement for benign esophageal diseases: A pooled analysis of the literature. World J Gastrointest Endosc 2015;7(2):135–53.

44. El H,II, Imperiale TF, Rex DK, et al. Treatment of esophageal leaks, fistulae, and perforations with temporary stents: evaluation of efficacy, adverse events, and

factors associated with successful outcomes. Gastrointest Endosc 2014;79(4):
589–98.

45. Law R, Prabhu A, Fujii-Lau L, et al. Stent migration following endoscopic suture
fixation of esophageal self-expandable metal stents: a systematic review and
meta-analysis. Surg Endosc 2018;32(2):675–81.

46. Ko HK, Song HY, Shin JH, et al. Fate of migrated esophageal and gastroduodenal
stents: experience in 70 patients. J Vasc Intervent Radiol 2007;18(6):725–32.

47. Boerlage TCC, Houben GPM, Groenen MJM, et al. A novel fully covered double-
bump stent for staple line leaks after bariatric surgery: a retrospective analysis.
Surg Endosc 2018;32(7):3174–80.

48. Shehab HM, Hakky SM, Gawdat KA. An endoscopic strategy combining mega
stents and over-the-scope clips for the management of post-bariatric surgery
leaks and fistulas (with videos). Obes Surg 2016;26(5):941–8.

49. Kuehn F, Loske G, Schiffmann L, et al. Endoscopic vacuum therapy for various
defects of the upper gastrointestinal tract. Surg Endosc 2017;31(9):3449–58.

50. Silecchia G, Boru CE, Mouiel J, et al. Clinical evaluation of fibrin glue in the prevention of anastomotic leak and internal hernia after laparoscopic gastric bypass:
preliminary results of a prospective, randomized multicenter trial. Obes Surg
2006;16(2):125–31.

51. Rabago LR, Ventosa N, Castro JL, et al. Endoscopic treatment of postoperative
fistulas resistant to conservative management using biological fibrin glue. Endoscopy 2002;34(8):632–8.

52. Kotzampassi K, Stavrou G, Damoraki G, et al. A four-probiotics regimen reduces
postoperative complications after colorectal surgery: a randomized, double-
blind, placebo-controlled study. World J Surg 2015;39(11):2776–83.

53. Adduci AJ, Phillips CH, Harvin H. Prospective diagnosis of marginal ulceration
following Roux-en-Y gastric bypass with computed tomography. Radiol Case
Rep 2015;10(2):1063.

54. Salame M, Jawhar N, Belluzzi A, et al. Marginal ulcers after roux-en-y gastric
bypass: etiology, diagnosis, and management. J Clin Med 2023;12(13).

55. Azagury DE, Abu Dayyeh BK, Greenwalt IT, et al. Marginal ulceration after Roux-
en-Y gastric bypass surgery: characteristics, risk factors, treatment, and outcomes. Endoscopy 2011;43(11):950–4.

56. Dittrich L, Schwenninger MV, Dittrich K, et al. Marginal ulcers after laparoscopic
Roux-en-Y gastric bypass: analysis of the amount of daily and lifetime smoking on
postoperative risk. Surg Obes Relat Dis 2020;16(3):389–96.

57. Skogar ML, Sundbom M. Nonsteroid anti-inflammatory drugs and the risk of
peptic ulcers after gastric bypass and sleeve gastrectomy. Surg Obes Relat
Dis 2022;18(7):888–93.

58. Schulman AR, Chan WW, Devery A, et al. Opened proton pump inhibitor capsules reduce time to healing compared with intact capsules for marginal ulceration following roux-en-Y gastric bypass. Clin Gastroenterol Hepatol 2017;15(4):
494–500 e1.

59. Sacks BC, Mattar SG, Qureshi FG, et al. Incidence of marginal ulcers and the use
of absorbable anastomotic sutures in laparoscopic Roux-en-Y gastric bypass.
Surg Obes Relat Dis 2006;2(1):11–6.

60. Garcia-Gomez-Heras S, Fernandez-Acenero MJ, Gonzalez G, et al. Involvement
of helicobacter pylori in preoperative gastric findings on a bariatric population. Int
J Environ Res Publ Health 2022;19(15).

61. Jirapinyo P, Watson RR, Thompson CC. Use of a novel endoscopic suturing device to treat recalcitrant marginal ulceration (with videos). Gastrointest Endosc 2012;76(2):435–9.
62. Barola S, Fayad L, Hill C, et al. Endoscopic management of recalcitrant marginal ulcers by covering the ulcer bed. Obes Surg 2018;28(8):2252–60.
63. Nguyen NT, Hinojosa MW, Gray J, et al. Reoperation for marginal ulceration. Surg Endosc 2007;21(11):1919–21.

Endoscopic Sleeve Gastroplasty
Practical Considerations, Current Techniques, and Troubleshooting

Trent Walradt, MD[a], Christopher C. Thompson, MD[b,c],*

KEYWORDS

- Endoscopic sleeve gastroplasty • Stomach tightening • Bariatric endoscopy
- Endoscopic bariatric and metabolic therapies • Obesity

KEY POINTS

- Endoscopic sleeve gastroplasty (ESG) is a minimally invasive treatment for obesity with proven safety and efficacy
- Successful ESG requires placement of an adequate number of full-thickness sutures following a proven pattern
- Effective troubleshooting is a key skill for endoscopic suturing practitioners

INTRODUCTION

Endoscopic bariatric and metabolic therapies have emerged as a solution for the treatment gap that exists between the medical and surgical therapies that are attempting to address the obesity pandemic. Endoscopic sleeve gastroplasty (ESG) is a minimally invasive, endoluminal, and organ-sparing procedure that is performed using an endoscopic suturing device to place full-thickness sutures in the stomach, reducing its size, and altering its motility.[1]

Endoscopic suturing was first used to treat obesity using The Bard EndoCinch Suturing System (C.R. Bard Inc, Marray Hill, NJ, USA) in patients without a durable response to bariatric surgery by Thompson and colleagues, in 2004.[2,3] Fogel and

[a] Division of Gastroenterology, Hepatology and Endoscopy, Brigham and Women's Hospital, Harvard Medical School, 75 Francis Street, Boston, MA 02115, USA; [b] Division of Gastroenterology, Hepatology and Endoscopy, Brigham and Women's Hospital, 75 Francis Street, Boston, MA 02115, USA; [c] Department of Medicine, Harvard Medical School, 25 Shattuck Street, Boston, MA 02115, USA
* Corresponding author. Division of Gastroenterology, Hepatology and Endoscopy, Brigham and Women's Hospital, 75 Francis Street, Boston, MA 02115.
E-mail address: cthompson@hms.harvard.edu
Twitter: @TrentWalradt (T.W.); @MetabolicEndo (C.C.T.)

Gastrointest Endoscopy Clin N Am 34 (2024) 671–685
https://doi.org/10.1016/j.giec.2024.04.005
1052-5157/24/© 2024 Elsevier Inc. All rights reserved.

colleagues then evaluated the concept of transoral suturing for gastric volume reduction in normal anatomy in a single-center study in 2008.[4] This procedure was performed along the lesser curvature of the stomach emulating the surgical vertical banded gastroplasty. Effective working length (EWL) at 1 year in this study was 58.1% plus minus 19.9%, though these results were not reproducible. An alternative endoscopic procedure mimicking surgical gastric imbrication, focusing on the greater curvature, was being developed simultaneously. This procedure utilized the RESTORe Suturing System (Bard/Davol, Warwick, RI, USA) to place multiple running sutures along the greater curvature of the stomach. A pilot study (TRIM trial) including 18 patients demonstrated a 12-month EWL of 27.7% plus minus 21.9%.[5] Twelve-month endoscopy, however, revealed partial or complete release of plications in 13 of 18 patients, likely because of the partial-thickness nature of the suture placement. Nonetheless, the major principle developed from this procedure was the reduction of gastric volume by placement of running sutures along the greater curvature, which inspired the modern ESG.

The technical features of ESG have progressed over time. Thompson and Hawes used the Apollo OverStitch (Boston Scientific, Marlborough, MA, USA) to perform the first ESG in 2012.[6] Running sutures were placed in a triangular pattern at the anterior wall, greater curvature, and posterior wall of the stomach during these initial procedures. An alternative technique in which 2 parallel rows of interrupted sutures were placed from the prepyloric antrum to the gastroesophageal junction was reported by Abu Dayyeh and colleagues, which were incorporated into modern techniques as reinforcing sutures.[7] Additional modifications to the procedure have been reported including the number of sutures, orientation of sutures, and type of reinforcing sutures.[8] Recently, a running suture consisting of several stitches in a "U" pattern has been used in an effort to distribute suture tension, and minimize the total number of sutures needed and many of the more recent publications are using a version of this pattern.[9] Nevertheless, the defining feature of ESG is the placement of running sutures along the greater curvature in the body of the stomach to reduce its volume and alter motility, regardless of pattern or number of sutures.

OverStitch is a suturing device capable of placing full-thickness sutures. It is currently the only endoscopic suturing device that is Food and Drug Administration (FDA)-approved for an obesity indication. Two versions of the device are available. The Over-Stitch SX device can be mounted on a single-channel endoscope, while the original OverStitch device requires a double-channel therapeutic endoscope. The device consists of a curved needle driver and an anchor exchange catheter. The needle driver is connected to a handle that is attached near the instrument channel port. Closing the handle advances the needle driver allowing the needle to be transferred back and forth between the needle driver and the anchor exchange catheter. A tissue helix can be passed through the working channel to grab tissue, facilitating suture placement. When suturing is complete, the suture is secured and cut using a cinching device.

Successful ESG requires a nuanced understanding of the suturing device, sound technique, and the ability to troubleshoot. This article focuses on the details of how to perform an ESG, the common pitfalls of the procedure, and how to address/avoid them.

PRE-PROCEDURE PLANNING

ESG is approved by the United States FDA for adult patients with obesity with a body mass index (BMI) of 30 kg/m to 50 kg/m.[10] Nevertheless, recent studies have shown that higher BMI predicts greater weight loss after ESG.[9] Before ESG, patients should undergo education regarding lifestyle modifications including diet and exercise. Care should be taken to discuss the transitional diet immediately after the procedure to prevent early suture disruption. It is crucial that patients understand ESG is not a panacea, but rather one component of a holistic treatment plan for obesity. Patients should also undergo laboratory testing including vitamin and micronutrient levels, as well as *Heliobacter pylori* (with treatment and test of cure if positive). An upper gastrointestinal series can be obtained to screen for contraindications to the procedure including hiatal hernia, surgically altered anatomy, and ulcerations or stenosis.

PREP AND PATIENT POSITIONING

- ESG is performed with general anesthesia and endotracheal intubation.
- The patient is placed in the supine or lazy left lateral position.
- Patients are given one dose of IV antibiotics during the procedure. The authors do not discharge patients on oral antibiotics after ESG.
- Equipment and Materials
  - Double channel endoscope for OverStitch or single channel endoscope for OverStitch SX
  - 120 cc of saline with simethicone
  - Water jet with saline for lavage
  - Overtube
  - OverStitch device
  - Tissue helix
  - 2-0 sutures (ensure adequate number available)
  - Cinching devices
  - Lubricant
  - Alcohol swabs
  - Long Q-tips
  - Toothbrush
  - Rat tooth forceps
  - Kelly clamp
  - Wire cutters
  - Veress needle, sterile saline syringe, sterile drape, and ChloraPrep

PROCEDURAL APPROACH

- General principles
  - ESG should be performed in the proper environment with an experienced team. All equipments should be identified and confirmed to be available before patient sedation, including troubleshooting equipment. Carbon dioxide should always be used for insufflation throughout the procedure. Saline should be used for lavage instead of sterile water to minimize mucus production and enhance visualization. End-tidal carbon dioxide ($ETCO_2$) and peak airway pressure (P_{peak}) should be monitored throughout the procedure to allow early complication management.
- Diagnostic endoscopy
  - This is performed to evaluate for any contraindications including ulcerations, varices, active bleeding, malignancy, large esophageal hernia, or surgically altered anatomy. In addition, the size and shape of the stomach are assessed. Optionally, instill 120 cc of simethicone into the stomach and distal duodenum at the end of the diagnostic endoscopy to facilitate visualization during suturing and minimize bloating during post-procedure recovery.

- Marking
  - This is an optional step that the authors do not perform. This can be helpful, however, early in the learning curve. The anterior and posterior walls of the stomach can be marked using thermal coagulation to help guide placement of sutures. This may be less helpful in the latter stages of the ESG as the gastric anatomy becomes progressively distorted.
- Overtube placement
  - This is another optional step but is prudent for endoscopists without significant experience performing ESG. The overtube protects the oropharynx and esophagus from trauma because of repeated intubations with the OverStitch in place and can aid in device removal if the suturing arm becomes bent or damaged. Remember to keep the OverStitch closed whenever inserting or removing the device. It is critical to never move the endoscope against resistance within the overtube as this could lead to esophageal perforation.
- Suturing
  - Attach the OverStitch and pass the endoscope into the stomach
    - Before inserting the endoscope, the authors perform a complete loading and unloading cycle with the suture to confirm the device is functioning properly and minimize complications during the procedure.
    - Ensure the actuation cable is straight along the shaft of the endoscope
  - Pattern: Variable suture patterns are utilized during ESG. The authors currently perform the following pattern: running, interrupted, 'U', interrupted, 'U', interrupted, 'U', 'J' moving from the distal to proximal stomach with an optional medial running suture (**Figs. 1** and **2**). There is variability in this pattern based on an individual patient's anatomy.
    - Running: 5 to 10 stitches
      - Identify the greater curvature portion of the incisura and place the first stitch anterior and proximal to this location. There should be enough space so that 2 to 3 stitches can be placed before reaching the incisura. Stitches are generally placed 5 mm to 10 mm apart. Descend along the greater curvature, staying opposite the incisura, toward the lesser

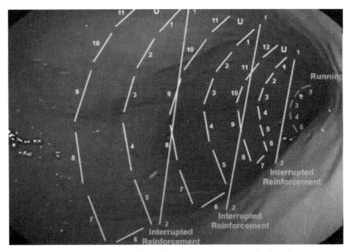

Fig. 1. Endoscopic sleeve gastroplasty (ESG) suture pattern with distal running suture and 3 sets interrupted and 'U' sutures.

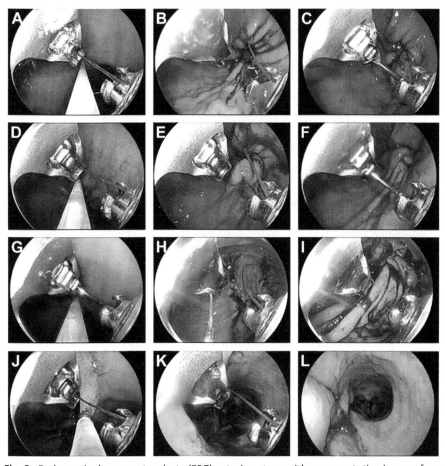

Fig. 2. Endoscopic sleeve gastroplasty (ESG) suturing steps with representative images from the start of each suture pattern, after completion of suturing, and after cinching. *(A–C)* Running suture pattern; *(D–F)* Interrupted suture pattern; *(G–I)* 'U' suture pattern; *(J–L)* 'J' suture pattern.

curvature. This suture creates a "neo-pylorus" and may contribute to delayed gastric emptying.
- Interrupted: 2 stitches
  - Two gastric folds are created by the initial running suture: an anterior fold and a posterior fold. The first stitch is placed in the anterior fold and the second stitch is placed in the posterior fold.
- 'U' or 'V': 8 to 14 stitches
  - This suture is started lateral to the anterior fold, as anteriorly as possible. The first leg of the 'U' descends from the anterior surface of the greater curvature onto the posterior surface, staying as close as possible to the prior suture row. At the bottom of the 'U', the OverStitch device is rotated 180° by torquing the endoscope. The device will now be pointing up along the greater curvature toward the anterior surface. This maneuver prevents the formation of alpha loops, or looping of the suture, which may lead to increased suture tension, ischemia and earlier stitch loss (**Fig. 3**). This

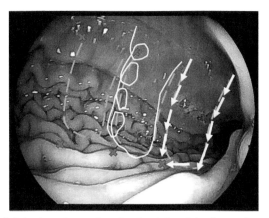

Fig. 3. Depiction of alpha loop formation. On the right of the figure the yellow arrows show the orientation of the OverStitch device as suturing is performed during a 'U'. The yellow line in the middle of the figure depicts the shape of the suture – the suture is straight during the first half of the 'U', but forms a loop with every stitch during the second half of the 'U'.

technique tends to produce more of a 'V' appearance to these sutures. 'U' or 'V' sutures reduce both the width and length of the stomach.

- ■ 'J': 6 to 8 stitches
  - • The purpose of this suture is to close off the opening to the fundus and promote early satiety. The endoscope is rotated counterclockwise, and a stitch is placed in the superior, proximal aspect of the fundus. Stiches are placed distally until the prior reinforcing suture is reached at which point sutures are continued proximally along the posterior surface.
- ■ Medial suture: 6 to 10 stitches
  - • This suture is placed to further reduce sleeve diameter if the sleeve is too wide or if there are gaps in the prior suture lines. The suture is placed from distal to proximal, joining the anterior and posterior surface of the sleeve.
  - ○ Full-thickness stitch placement
    - ■ It is important to use the tissue helix which allows one to pull the gastric mucosa into the Overstitch device and obtain full-thickness bites. It is also important to avoid over-insufflating the stomach that makes it more difficult to pull the tissue into the device. Tactile feedback is important to confirm full-thickness stitch placement. As the needle passes through the serosal surface, there is a characteristic "pop" that should be felt in the hand contacting the handle.
- • Second-look endoscopy
  - ○ The purpose of this step is to assess the final sleeve configuration and take measurements, evaluate for gaps necessitating addition sutures, and to assess for bleeding.
- • Procedure duration: 40 minutes to 90 minutes

TROUBLESHOOTING

- • Suture wrapped around the OverStitch tower
  - ○ This is an issue than can arise when there is too much suture slack and is best prevented by keeping the suture trim (**Fig. 4**). This issue can be resolved by passing the suture to the anchor exchange catheter, rotating the endoscope

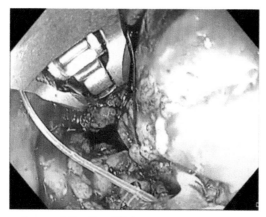

Fig. 4. Suture wrapped around the OverStitch tower.

clockwise, partially closing the handle, and pulling the suture out of the working channel. It is a key to recognize this problem before cinching.

- Suture break or cut before cinching
  - Several factors can lead to suture breakage. First, the suture can become frayed if it rubs against the OverStitch. This can also occur if the cinch is pulled into the working channel. Finally, if cinching is performed too quickly the suture can be cut before it is locked in place. Pre-tightening the suture before cinching is a key preventative measure. Once the cinch is in place, it is important to provide counter pressure and be gentle with the suture. In addition to facilitating successful cinch release, maintaining a straight cinch catheter and closing the cinch handle slowly also prevent suture breakage. If suture breakage does occur, the broken suture should be removed and a new suture placed in the same location.
- Crossed or knotted suture
  - It is important to use an open and running suture. If the suture becomes crossed or knotted the suture tension will become too great and prevent adequate tissue coaptation. This can be prevented by careful control of suture slack. If knotting or crossing does occur, it should be addressed immediately. If identified too late, and tissue apposition is compromised, the suture should be cut and replaced.
- Broken suture loading tab
  - The suture loading tab is fragile and can break if handled too forcefully or if it is not pulled in the same axis as the cinch catheter when loading a suture. If breakage does occur the suture can be manually threaded through the peak collar in the distal end of the catheter. It is also prudent to save loading tablets for reuse in case one breaks.
- Anchor exchange catheter not aligned with needle driver
  - Misalignment of the anchor exchange catheter and needle driver prevents needle exchange and can result in damage to the needle or OverStitch device. When this occur the anchor exchange catheter should be pulled back a few centimeters into the working channel, rotated, then carefully pushed back out.
- Inability to release the cinch
  - This can be caused by closing the cinch handle when the cinch catheter is not straight or closing the cinch handle too quickly. These actions can cause the

inner wire of the cinch to fail to release from the plug. The solution is to manually break, or use wire cutters, to cut through the cinch handle and catheter, then use pliers or a Kelly clamp to pull the inner wire until the cinch releases. This can require a significant amount of force.

- Needle damaging the endoscope
  - The anchor exchange catheter should be pushed out of the working channel, away from the distal tip of the endoscope when the needle/suture is dropped because the needle or T tag can damage the working channel. Additionally, if the suture is dropped, the T tag should never be pulled through the working channel of the endoscope.
- Inability to release the tissue helix
  - It is important to ensure the helix is completely released from the tissue before it is retracted. Failing to do so can result in tissue damage. The individual operating the helix should keep count of the number of clockwise turns during tissue capture and perform the same number of counterclockwise turns during tissue release. The minimum number of turns necessary should be used. In addition, excess pressure on the helix and over insufflation of the stomach should be avoided as both actions may lead to capture of adjacent extragastric structures. Finally, keeping the helix free of debris and cleaning periodically is important. The authors clean the helix with a tooth brush every time cinching is performed.
- Bent needle
  - A bent needle is potentially the most serious complication because it can prevent removal of the OverStitch device without risking serious damage to the esophagus (**Fig. 5**). When the needle is on the needle driver and the handle is being closed, it is important to ensure the anchor exchange catheter is fully within the working channel. If the anchor exchange catheter is protruding out of the working channel this can result bending of the needle or suture arm.[11] If bending occurs, a rat-toothed forceps can be inserted through the working channel and used to bend the suturing arm back into position or remove the needle.
- Bleeding
  - Minor bleeding is a relatively common occurrence during ESG. Intraluminal bleeding is usually addressed by holding tension on the suture for tamponade. In most cases, suturing can then resume. In selected cases, it is necessary to cinch to achieve hemostasis. When a stitch breaks, it results in multiple

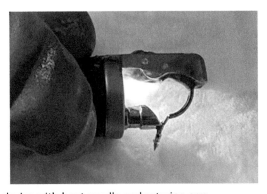

Fig. 5. OverStitch device with bent needle and suturing arm.

perforations from the needle at risk for uncontrolled bleeding. Therefore, it is important to place a new stitch as close as possible to the prior suture site to tamponade the area. Hemodynamic instability and dropping hemoglobin levels post-procedurally should raise suspicion for extra-gastric bleeding. This should prompt computed tomography (CT) for evaluation.

- Perforation
  - Perforation is an extremely rare, but serious potential complication of ESG. Early detection is critically important. Therefore, frequent abdominal examinations should be performed evaluating for distension and crepitus. In addition, $ETCO_2$ andP_{peak} should be monitored. The normal range for $ETCO_2$ is 35 mm Hg to 45 mm Hg and P_{peak} is 25 cmH_2O to 30 cmH_2O. A rise in either of these levels should raise suspicion for perforation. If a perforation is identified, a Veress needle can be used for decompression after which the defect can be closed endoscopically. The procedure can usually still be completed after perforation is addressed.
- Leaks
  - Leak is another rare complication of ESG.[9,12] The clinical presentation of a leak is nonspecific, but the most common findings include tachycardia, leukocytosis, and an elevated C-reactive protein.[13] Imaging options include abdominal CT with oral contrast and an upper gastrointestinal series, though the later study has poor sensitivity.[14] Several technical practices can help prevent leak. Suturing in the fundus, which has the thinnest wall in the stomach and is adjacent to the spleen, should be avoided.[15] Using the OverStitch to take tissue bites efficiently is also important. The needle driver should be aligned with the anchor exchange catheter to prevent repeated passes through tissue without effective pickup. The needle driver should not be passed through tissue without the needle attached. Additionally, the appropriate amount of insufflation should be used as under-insufflation can lead to excessively thick folds or acquisition of multiple tissue folds that prevents needle passage. The needle driver should be kept in the tissue as little time as possible. Finally, pulling the helix out of tissue without releasing it and failing to remove any lost or broken sutures also predispose to leaks. If a leak does occur the management will depend on the timing and location of the leak, but often requires drain placement.
- Stenosis
  - Stenosis usually results from being too "greedy", that is, placing sutures too close to the lesser curvature of the stomach. Although less common, an intramural hematoma, can also cause stenosis (**Fig. 6**). In the short term, a nasojejunal tube can be placed for feeding. If symptoms persist past 6 weeks, these patients can be treated endoscopically with balloon dilation or by cutting and removing sutures.

RECOVERY & REHABILITATION

- Periprocedural
  - The Enhanced Recovery After Surgical Endoscopy (ERASE) protocol has been shown to decrease post-anesthesia care unit length of stay and 30-day readmissions.[16] Key tenets of this protocol include:
    - Carbohydrate rich beverages the day before the procedure
    - Initiation of a scopolamine patch upon admission
    - Fluid management: aim for greater than or equal to 3 L of lactated ringers IV perioperatively

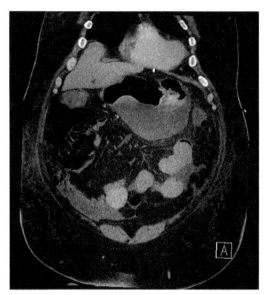

Fig. 6. Gastric hematoma (*red arrow*) in a patient with a mechanical aortic valve on anticoagulation after ESG.

- ■ Multimodal post-operative nausea and vomiting prophylaxis: administer aprepitant, dexamethasone, and ondansetron before extubation
- ■ Opioid-sparing analgesia: administer IV acetaminophen and IV ketorolac before extubation
- Post discharge
  - ○ Diet:
    - ■ Day of procedure: Nil per os
    - ■ Post-procedure day 1: Clear liquid diet
    - ■ Post-procedure day 2 to 45: Protein shakes
    - ■ Post-procedure day 46 to 55: Soft proteins
    - ■ Post-procedure day 56 onwards: Regular diet
  - ○ Medications:
    - ■ Omeprazole 40 mg twice a day open capsule for 8 weeks
    - ■ Liquid acetaminophen 650 mg every 6 hours as needed for pain
      - • The authors do not discharge patients on opioids. If their pain is not controlled with non-opioid analgesics after the procedure they are admitted to the hospital.
    - ■ Ondansetron 8 mg disintegrating tablet every 6 hours as needed for nausea
    - ■ Optionally, liquid carafate 1 g three times a day for up to 6 weeks
      - • If liquid formulation is not covered by insurance patients can use tablets and crush and mix with 3 oz to 5 oz of water
    - ■ All home medications should be converted to liquid or crushable form for 6 weeks after ESG
  - ○ Follow-up:
    - ■ The patients see a registered Dietitian 2 weeks after ESG with access to monthly group visits and quarterly individual visits. Follow-up in bariatric endoscopy clinic is scheduled at 1 month, 3 months, 9 months, and 12 months, respectively.

OUTCOMES

Numerous studies have demonstrated the safety and efficacy of ESG. The MERIT trial, a randomized, multi-center, and open-label study including 209 participants demonstrated 13.6% plus minus 8.0% total weight loss (TWL) in the ESG group and 0.8% plus minus 5.0% in the control group at 52 weeks.[17] The serious adverse event (SAE) rate was 2% and comprised 1 case of upper gastrointestinal bleeding managed conservatively, 1 case of abdominal abscess managed endoscopically, and 1 case of malnutrition requiring ESG reversal. In a meta-analysis of 8 observational studies totaling 1772 patients TWL 6 months after ESG was 15.1% (95% CI, 14.3–16.0), 16.5% (95% CI, 15.2–17.8) at 12 months, and 17.2% (95% CI, 14.6–19.7) at 18 months to 24 months.[18] The SAE rate was 2.2%, and included upper gastrointestinal bleeding, pain or nausea requiring hospitalization, and peri-gastric leak or fluid collection. The durability of weight loss after ESG has also been evaluated. A single center prospective cohort study demonstrated a 5-year TWL of 15.9% (95% CI, 11.7–20.5), and the 10-year data were recently presented confirming persistent durability.[19,20]

In addition to weight loss, ESG also leads to improvement in the metabolic sequelae of obesity. Patients who underwent ESG in the MERIT trial were more likely than controls to have improvement in multiple metabolic outcomes including glycated hemoglobin ($HgbA_{1c}$), blood pressure, triglycerides, waist-to-hip ratio, and transaminases.[17] A retrospective study of 139 patients who underwent ESG outside of a controlled trial showed a significant decrease in fasting glucose, $HgbA_{1c}$, total cholesterol, triglycerides, and transaminases.[21] Finally, a registry study of 118 patients with metabolic dysfunction associated steatotic liver disease those who underwent ESG, demonstrated significant improvements in hepatic steatosis as estimated by the hepatic steatosis index, as well as hepatic fibrosis as estimated by the NAFLD fibrosis score.[22]

TRAINING

Achieving proficiency in ESG requires a stepwise approach. Trainees should begin by developing cognitive skills through readings, live cases, and conferences. Technical skills can be honed through the use of ex-vivo simulators and assisting during procedures.[23] The authors recommend trainees learn transoral outlet reduction (TORe) prior to ESG, as TORe is a shorter and safer procedure. Once trainees progress to ESG, the authors start with interrupted sutures, followed by running, and finally the 'U'. In addition, suturing should begin in the distal body as this location is generally less challenging than the proximal body. Although the precise number of cases needed to achieve competence is variable, a single-operating learning curve analysis revealed efficiency for ESG was attained after 38 procedures and mastery was attained after 55 procedures.[24] Finally, it is the key to have access to an experienced mentor throughout the training process.

FUTURE DIRECTIONS

ESG has also been combined with other techniques to augment weight loss. Gastroplasty with endoscopic myotomy involves submucosal tunneling to perform a pylorus-sparing antral myotomy before traditional ESG. A pilot study including 6 patients demonstrated decreased gastric emptying with $T_{1/2}$ increasing from 90 plus minus 58 minutes at baseline to 204 plus minus 18 minutes at 2 weeks.[25] In addition, TWL at 3 months was 14.8% plus minus 2.5%, with all patients achieving at least 10%

TWL. Additionally, argon plasma coagulation has also been used in combination with ESG to induce tissue fibrosis and improve durability. Itani and colleagues demonstrated the feasibility of this technique.[26]

In addition to OverStitch, other platforms have also been developed for gastric plication. The Endomina system (Endo Tools Therapeutics SA, Gosselies, Belgium) is an endoscopic plication platform that can be used with any endoscope. The system includes 2 channels, 1 of which can be bent perpendicularly to facilitate suture passage through tissue. Grasping forceps are used to pull tissue into the Endomina after which a dedicated needle (TAPES, Endo Tools Therapeutics SA, Gosselies, Belgium) loaded with 2 anchors connected by suture is passed. The anchors are then tightened leading to serosa-to-serosa apposition. A multi-center and single-arm prospective trial of 51 patients revealed a 12 month TWL of 7.4% plus minus 7.0 with no SAE.[27] A subsequent randomized study including 71 subjects revealed a 6-month TWL of 11.0% (95% CI 8.9–13.2) in the Endomina group compared with 2.7% (95% CI 0.1–5.4) in the control group.[28] There were no SAEs. The intraocular pressure (IOP) (USGI Medical, San Clemente, CA) is another plication platform consisting of 4 devices: the Transport Endoscopic Guide, a maneuverable 54 French tube that contains working channels for the other tools, as well as an ultra slim endoscope, the g-Lix, a tissue grasper, the g-Prox EZ, for approximating tissue, and the g-Cath, for deploying tissue anchors. A US pivotal, randomized, and sham-controlled trial (ESSENTIAL trial) including 332 patients demonstrated 5.0% plus minus 7.0% TWL in the POSE arm compared with 1.4% plus minus 5.6% TWL in the sham arm at 12 months.[29] A modified procedure, known as Distal POSE or POSE 2.0, was subsequently developed that involves placement of plications only within the gastric body, sparing the fundus. This technique resulted in greater weight loss with initial studies reporting 15.0% TWL at 6 months and 15.7%–17.8% at 12 months.[30–32] Both the Endomina system and IOP are FDA-approved for tissue approximation but have not yet been approved for an obesity indication. Finally, robotic endoscopy is an emerging tool that promises improved visualization, control, and ergonomics compared with traditional endoscopy. Initial studies have shown that endoscopic suturing is feasible using an endoscopic robotic platform.[33]

SUMMARY

The performance of ESG has evolved substantially over the past decade from the time it was first described. In this article, the authors reviewed its history and the evidence supporting its use for the treatment of obesity and its related metabolic complications. The authors detailed the key steps of this procedure, as well as the management of patients before and after undergoing ESG. Finally, the authors described the common pitfalls endoscopists face when performing ESG, how to avoid them, and how to address them when they occur.

CLINICS CARE POINTS

- The combination of a proven suture pattern, an adequate number of sutures, and full-thickness stitch placement are required for a successful and durable ESG.
- Knowledge of the common pitfalls associated with endoscopic suturing and their management is the key to improving efficiency and decreasing adverse outcomes.
- Incorporating the ERASE protocol may decrease length of stay and readmissions.

DISCLOSURE

T. Walradt has nothing to disclose. C.C. Thompson has served as a consultant for Apollo Endosurgery, Boston Scientific, EnVision Endoscopy, Fujifilm, USGI Medical, Medtronic/Covidien, and Olympus/Spiration; has served as an advisory board member for USGI Medical; has received research grants and support from USGI Medical, United States, Apollo Endosurgery, Boston Scientific, United States, ERBE, FujiFilm, Olympus, Japan/Spiration; and has served as a founder for EnVision Endoscopy.

REFERENCES

1. Vargas EJ, Rizk M, Gomez-Villa J, et al. Effect of endoscopic sleeve gastroplasty on gastric emptying, motility and hormones: a comparative prospective study. Gut 2023;72(6):1073–80.
2. Thompson CC, Carr-Locke D. Novel Endoscopic Approaches to Common Bariatric Postoperative Complications. ASGE Video Forum. New Orleans, LA: Digestive Diseases Week; 2004.
3. Thompson CC, Slattery J, Bundga ME, et al. Peroral endoscopic reduction of dilated gastrojejunal anastomosis after Roux-en-Y gastric bypass: a possible new option for patients with weight regain. Surg Endosc 2006;20(11):1744–8.
4. Fogel R, De Fogel J, Bonilla Y, et al. Clinical experience of transoral suturing for an endoluminal vertical gastroplasty: 1-year follow-up in 64 patients. Gastrointest Endosc 2008;68(1):51–8.
5. Brethauer SA, Chand B, Schauer PR, et al. Transoral gastric volume reduction for weight management: technique and feasibility in 18 patients. Surg Obes Relat Dis 2010;6(6):689–94.
6. Mo1155 Endoscopic Sleeve Gastroplasty for Primary Therapy of Obesity: Initial Human Cases - ClinicalKey. Available at: https://www-clinicalkey-com.ezp-prod1.hul.harvard.edu/#!/content/playContent/1-s2.0-S0016508514620710?returnurl=null&referrer=null. [Accessed 26 August 2023].
7. Abu Dayyeh BK, Rajan E, Gostout CJ. Endoscopic sleeve gastroplasty: a potential endoscopic alternative to surgical sleeve gastrectomy for treatment of obesity. Gastrointest Endosc 2013;78(3):530–5.
8. Kumar N, Abu Dayyeh BK, Lopez-Nava Breviere G, et al. Endoscopic sutured gastroplasty: procedure evolution from first-in-man cases through current technique. Surg Endosc 2018;32(4):2159–64.
9. Barrichello S, Hourneaux de Moura DT, Hourneaux de Moura EG, et al. Endoscopic sleeve gastroplasty in the management of overweight and obesity: an international multicenter study. Gastrointest Endosc 2019;90(5):770–80.
10. Health C for D and R. Weight-loss and weight-management devices. FDA; 2023. Available at: https://www.fda.gov/medical-devices/products-and-medical-procedures/weight-loss-and-weight-management-devices. [Accessed 10 December 2023].
11. Yu JX, Schulman AR. Complications of the Use of the OverStitch Endoscopic Suturing System. Gastrointest Endosc Clin N Am 2020;30(1):187–95.
12. Alqahtani A, Al-Darwish A, Mahmoud AE, et al. Short-term outcomes of endoscopic sleeve gastroplasty in 1000 consecutive patients. Gastrointest Endosc 2019;89(6):1132–8.
13. Schulman AR, Thompson CC. Complications of Bariatric Surgery: What You Can Expect to See in Your GI Practice. Am J Gastroenterol 2017;112(11):1640–55.

14. Musella M, Cantoni V, Green R, et al. Efficacy of Postoperative Upper Gastrointestinal Series (UGI) and Computed Tomography (CT) Scan in Bariatric Surgery: a Meta-analysis on 7516 Patients. Obes Surg 2018;28(8):2396–405.

15. Rawlins L, Rawlins MP, Teel D. Human tissue thickness measurements from excised sleeve gastrectomy specimens. Surg Endosc 2014;28(3):811–4.

16. D'Ascanio C, Schuler E, Jirapinyo P, et al. Implementation of an Enhanced Recovery After Surgical Endoscopy protocol to improve outcomes following endoscopic sleeve gastroplasty. iGIE 2023. https://doi.org/10.1016/j.igie.2023.08.001.

17. Abu Dayyeh BK, Bazerbachi F, Vargas EJ, et al. Endoscopic sleeve gastroplasty for treatment of class 1 and 2 obesity (MERIT): a prospective, multicentre, randomised trial. Lancet 2022;400(10350):441–51.

18. Hedjoudje A, Abu Dayyeh BK, Cheskin LJ, et al. Efficacy and Safety of Endoscopic Sleeve Gastroplasty: A Systematic Review and Meta-Analysis. Clin Gastroenterol Hepatol 2020;18(5):1043–53.e4.

19. Sharaiha RZ, Hajifathalian K, Kumar R, et al. Five-Year Outcomes of Endoscopic Sleeve Gastroplasty for the Treatment of Obesity. Clin Gastroenterol Hepatol 2021;19(5):1051–7.e2.

20. Jirapinyo P, Kumar N, Shaikh S, et al. Ten-Year Efficacy of Endoscopic Sleeve Gastroplasty (ESG). Gastrointest Endosc 2023;97(6):AB34–5.

21. Annan KA, Sayegh L, Gala K, et al. Weight-loss and metabolic outcomes of endoscopic sleeve gastroplasty (ESG) in the clinical setting. Gastrointest Endosc 2023;97(6):AB35.

22. Hajifathalian K, Mehta A, Ang B, et al. Improvement in insulin resistance and estimated hepatic steatosis and fibrosis after endoscopic sleeve gastroplasty. Gastrointest Endosc 2021;93(5):1110–8.

23. Jirapinyo P, Thompson CC. Development of a novel endoscopic suturing simulator: validation and impact on clinical learning curve (with video). Gastrointest Endosc 2024;99(1):41–9.

24. Saumoy M, Schneider Y, Zhou XK, et al. A single-operator learning curve analysis for the endoscopic sleeve gastroplasty. Gastrointest Endosc 2018;87(2):442–7.

25. Thompson CC, Jirapinyo P, Shah R, et al. Gastroplasty With Endoscopic Myotomy (GEM) for the Treatment of Obesity: Preliminary Efficacy and Physiologic Results. Gastroenterology 2022;163(5):1173–5.

26. Itani MI, Farha J, Sartoretto A, et al. Endoscopic sleeve gastroplasty with argon plasma coagulation: A novel technique. J Dig Dis 2020;21(11):664–7.

27. Huberty V, Machytka E, Boškoski I, et al. Endoscopic gastric reduction with an endoluminal suturing device: a multicenter prospective trial with 1-year follow-up. Endoscopy 2018;50(12):1156–62.

28. Huberty V, Boskoski I, Bove V, et al. Endoscopic sutured gastroplasty in addition to lifestyle modification: short-term efficacy in a controlled randomised trial. Gut 2020. https://doi.org/10.1136/gutjnl-2020-322026. gutjnl-2020-322026.

29. Sullivan S, Swain JM, Woodman G, et al. Randomized sham-controlled trial evaluating efficacy and safety of endoscopic gastric plication for primary obesity: The ESSENTIAL trial. Obesity (Silver Spring) 2017;25(2):294–301.

30. Jirapinyo P, Thompson CC. Endoscopic gastric body plication for the treatment of obesity: technical success and safety of a novel technique (with video). Gastrointest Endosc 2020;91(6):1388–94.

31. Lopez Nava G, Asokkumar R, Laster J, et al. Primary obesity surgery endoluminal (POSE-2) procedure for treatment of obesity in clinical practice. Endoscopy 2021;53(11):1169–73.

32. Lopez Nava G, Arau RT, Asokkumar R, et al. Prospective Multicenter Study of the Primary Obesity Surgery Endoluminal (POSE 2.0) Procedure for Treatment of Obesity. Clin Gastroenterol Hepatol 2023;21(1):81–9.e4.

33. Moura DTH de, Aihara H, Thompson CC. Robotic-assisted surgical endoscopy: a new era for endoluminal therapies. VideoGIE 2019;4(9):399–402.

Intragastric Balloons
Practical Considerations

D.T.H. de Moura, MD, MSc, PhD, Post-PhD[a,b,*],
Sergio A. Sánchez-Luna, MD[c], Adriana Fernandes Silva, MD[b],
Alexandre Moraes Bestetti, MD[a,b]

KEYWORDS

- Obesity • Endoscopy • Balloon • Intragastric balloon

KEY POINTS

- Obesity is a pandemic with increasing incidence.
- The treatment of obesity requires personalized attention.
- Intragastric balloons are an effective and minimally invasive measure in treating obesity.

 Video content accompanies this article at http://www.giendo.theclinics.com.

INTRODUCTION

The World Health Organization advocates for therapeutic measures targeting a 5% to 10% reduction in body weight, offering benefits in improving metabolic parameters and reducing morbidity and mortality.[1] Intragastric balloons (IGB) emerge as a minimally invasive therapy, widely used and approved by regulatory bodies around the world, including the Food and Drug Administration and European Commission (EC).[2,3] IGBs, regardless of type, often meet the requirements set by professional societies, ensuring at least 25% excess weight loss (%EWL) and less than 5% severe adverse events (SAEs).[4–7] In the context of obesity management, IGBs play a pivotal role, achieving total body weight loss (%TWL) up to 18% in short-term follow-up with a favorable safety profile.[8]

This review highlights the significance of IGBs in managing obesity and associated comorbidities. The low uptake of bariatric surgery underscores the need for alternative

[a] Gastrointestinal Endoscopy Division, Instituto DOr de Pesquisa e Ensino (IDOR), Hospital Vila Nova Star, R. Dr. Alceu de Campos Rodrigues, 126 - Vila Nova Conceição, São Paulo, São Paulo 04544-000, Brazil; [b] Gastrointestinal Endoscopy Unit, Department of Gastroenterology, Hospital das Clínicas da Faculdade de Medicina da Universidade de São Paulo, Av. Dr. Enéas de Carvalho Aguiar, 255 Cerqueira César, 05403-000, Brazil; [c] Division of Gastroenterology & Hepatology, Department of Internal Medicine, Basil I. Hirschowitz Endoscopic Center of Excellence, The University of Alabama at Birmingham Heersink School of Medicine, 510 20th Street S, LHFOT 1203, Birmingham, AL 35294, USA
* Corresponding author. R. Dr. Alceu de Campos Rodrigues, 126 - Vila Nova Conceição, São Paulo, São Paulo 04544-000, Brazil.
E-mail addresses: dthmoura@hotmail.com; diogo.moura@hc.fm.usp.br

Gastrointest Endoscopy Clin N Am 34 (2024) 687–714
https://doi.org/10.1016/j.giec.2024.04.013
1052-5157/24/© 2024 Elsevier Inc. All rights reserved.

giendo.theclinics.com

approaches, and IGBs offer a promising option. The subsequent sections briefly outline the historical development and technological evolution of IGBs, emphasizing their crucial role in addressing the challenges posed by obesity.

HISTORY

The development of IGBs began in the 1980s as a non-surgical approach to the management of obesity. The first United States-approved IGB, the Garren-Edwards Gastric Bubble, had several SAEs, leading to its withdrawal from the market in 1992. The SAEs were associated with its cylindrical balloon model, which had a rough surface, causing damage to the gastric mucosa, as well as the low filling volume, consisting of only 220 mL of air. This often led to spontaneous deflation, followed by migration and intestinal obstruction.[9,10] In response, experts outlined the ideal characteristics of IGBs in 1987, including a smooth surface, ease of endoscopic placement and removal, radiopaque markers, elasticity, and a circumferential shape. In 1991, the BioEnterics Corporation (BIB, Inamed, Santa Barbara, CA, USA) introduced an IGB, now called Orbera (Apollo Endosurgery, Austin, TX, USA), that met these criteria. Over 2 decades of global experience, the efficacy and safety of this model have been well-established in the literature.[11] The technology of IGBs has expanded globally, from air-filled to adjustable IGBs, and recently to swallowable IGBs that do not require endoscopic procedures for placement and removal.

MECHANISM OF ACTION

The mechanism of action of IGBs still needs to be entirely understood. Several mechanisms have been proposed for this space-occupying device, including mechanical, physiologic, and neurohormonal pathways. The IGB creates intermittent mechanical pseudo-obstruction and volume restriction in the stomach, causing delayed gastric emptying and early satiety.[12,13] A recent meta-analysis showed a 2-hour delay in gastric emptying after placing a fluid-filled IGB.[14]

The balloon's contact with the gastric fundus wall may stimulate parasympathetic mechanoreceptors, further contributing to early satiety. Additionally, appetites and gastric emptying are also influenced by hormones such as ghrelin and cholecystokinin (CCK). There is a decrease in ghrelin level, while CCK level increases due to the device placed in the gastric fundus. While some studies[15,16] show a reduction in plasma ghrelin levels, others suggest that mechanical effects from IGBs do not significantly impact its levels.[17,18] Regarding the neurogenic mechanism, it is suggested that IGB stimulates the central portion of the paraventricular nucleus of the solitary tract through vagal afferent stimulation.[19]

INDICATIONS AND CONTRAINDICATIONS

The indications and contraindications of IGB placement (**Table 1**) are slightly different between countries and centers.[12,17,20,21]

In the authors' clinical practice, the authors do treat *Helicobacter pylori* infection and confirm eradication before IGB placement to reduce the risk of ulcers developing during the IGB dwell time.

INTRAGASTRIC BALLOON TYPES

The most used IGB devices are described below.[22–50] Additionally, **Tables 2** and **3** summarize their individual characteristics. **Table 2** details the most used devices and **Table 3** some novel and obsolete devices.

Table 1
Intragastric balloons indications and contraindications

Indications	Body Mass Index (BMI) >27 kg/m² after conservative measures fail and/or with comorbidities BMI >35 kg/m² for patients who declined bariatric surgery BMI >50 kg/m² as a bridge therapy for bariatric surgery
Absolute Contraindications	Previous esophageal and/or gastric surgery Active peptic ulcer disease Gastroesophageal varices Hiatal hernia >4 cm Eating disorders (eg, anorexia nervosa, bulimia nervosa) Uncontrolled psychiatric disorders Drug addiction Use of non-discontinuable anticoagulants and non-steroidal anti-inflammatory drugs Coagulopathies Structural abnormalities in the esophagus or pharynx Pregnancy
Relative Contraindications	Gastroesophageal varices Hiatal hernia <4 cm Erosive esophagitis (Los Angeles Classification B, C, and D) Uncontrolled eosinophilic esophagitis Human immunodeficiency virus infection Breastfeeding (<6 mo) BMI <27 kg/m² Refusal to follow up with a multidisciplinary team Active *Helicobacter pylori* infection Patients <18-year-old (only with parents' consent and after a multidisciplinary evaluation)

Orbera (Apollo Endosurgery, Austin, TX, USA)

This is the most traditional IGB, which has been used for more than 20 years, with several names but the same characteristics, with recognized safety and effectiveness as proved by a meta-analysis including only randomized controlled trials (RCTs) (evidence level 1A).[17] This study demonstrated that fluid-filled IGB greater than 400 mL is more effective than sham/diet in achieving BMI loss, absolute weight loss, and % EWL. In a large retrospective study including more than 30,000 patients using this device, the adverse event (AE) rate was only 2%, with less than 0.05% of ulcers, proving its satisfactory safety profile[22] (**Fig. 1**). On the other hand, in 2017, following the FDA approval, the FDA has issue two letters to healthcare providers alerting them to AEs associated with ORBERA and ReShape IGBs, including several deaths (Tate CM, Geliebter A. Intragastric Balloon Treatment for Obesity: FDA Safety Updates. Adv Ther. 2018 Jan;35(1):1-4. doi: 10.1007/s12325-017-0647-z. Epub 2017 Dec 28. PMID: 29285708.). The different outcomes between U.S. and non-U.S. countries are not completely understood. Factors that may be related includes close follow-up (messages and phone calls direct between endoscopist and patient), local and personal experience, and patient's behavior.

Heliosphere (Hélioscópie Medical Implants, Vienne, France)

Air-filled IGBs are recognized to present fewer adaptative side effects such as emesis, nausea, and dehydration.[23] Although it provides a better tolerance profile, the device is more rigid than other IGB types and thus makes placement and removal more technical challenging. Additionally, it is associated with high rates of early deflation.[23–25] In

Table 2
Summary of the characteristics and outcomes of the most used intragastric balloons

Intragastric Balloons Types	Company	FDA Approved/CE Approved	Material Shape/Capacity	Number of Intragastric Balloons	Duration (mo)	Insertion/Retrieval	Best Available Evidence	Efficacy/Safety	Advantages	Disadvantages
Orbera[4]	Apollo Endosurgery, Austin, TX, USA	Yes/Yes	Silicone Spherical Saline: 400–700 mL	1	6–12	Endoscopic/Endoscopic	Meta-Analysis of RCTs	TWL: 13.16% EWL: 25.44% SAE: 2%	Recognized effectiveness and safety	Non-negligible early removal rate during adaptation
Heliosphere[45]	Helioscopie Medical Implants, Vienne, France	No/Yes	Polyurethane and silicone Spherical (Air 550 mL)	1	6	Endoscopic/Endoscopic	Prospective cohort	TWL: 13.4% EWL: 33% SAE: 5.5%	Weighs <30 g	Difficult placement
Spatz 3[27]	Spatz FGIA, Great Neck, NY, USA	Yes/Yes	Silicone/Spherical with an adjustable catheter Filled fluid 400–900 mL	1	12	Endoscopic/Endoscopic	RCT	TWL: 15% EWL: 25% SAE: 4%	Adjustable for improved tolerance. Reduced early removals due to intolerance. Increased volume for enhanced satiety and weight loss	Catheter use raises ulcer incidence
ReShape Duo Integrated Dual Balloon System[29]	ReShape Lifesciences, San Clemente, CA	Yes/Yes	Silicone Bi-lobal Saline: 375–450 mL each intragastric balloon (IGB) (total: 750–900 mL)	2	6	Endoscopic/Endoscopic	RCT	TWL: 7.6% EWL: 25.1% SAE: 7.5%	Potential for enhanced weight loss as, in the event of one of the devices rupturing, the second remains inflated, allowing continued treatment and reducing the risk of migration	High rates of ulcer-related to the device Withdrawn from market

Device	Company	CE/FDA		Composition		Delivery/Removal	Study	Outcomes	Advantages	Disadvantages
Obalon[44]	Obalon Therapeutics, Carlsbad, CA, USA	Yes/Yes	1–3	Gelatin capsule Spherical Gas nitrogen-sulfur hexafluoride: 250 mL	3–6	Deglutable/ Endoscopic	RCT	TWL: 7.1% EWL: 26% SAE: 0.3%	No need for sedation during placement Only mild adaptation symptoms	possible lower weight loss than fluid filled balloons Multiple[3] sessions for placement
Allurion[38]	Allurion Technologies, Wellesley, MA, USA	No/Yes	1	Polymer film Spherical Proprietary solution Filled fluid 550 mL	4	Deglutable/ Natural excretion	Meta-analysis of cohort studies	TWL: 12% EWL: 49.1% SAE: 2.3%	Insertion and removal without sedation and 1-year follow-up through the multidisciplinary program of Allurion, via the app associated with the bioimpedance scale	No endoscopic evaluation prior to IGB placement

Abbreviations: SAE, adverse events; ATIIP, adjustable totally implantable intragastric prosthesis; CE, Conformité Européenne; CO_2, carbon dioxide; EWL, excess weight loss; FDA, food and drug administration; RCT, randomized controlled trial; TWL, total weight loss.

Table 3
Summary of the characteristics and outcomes of the several types of intragastric balloons

Intragastric Balloons Types	Company	FDA Approved/ CE Approved	Material Shape/ Capacity	Number of Intragastric Balloons	Duration (mo)	Insertion/ Retrieval	Best Available Evidence	Efficacy/ Safety	Advantages	Disadvantages
Medicone[22]	Medicone, Cachoeirinha, Brazil	No/No	Silicone Spherical Saline 300–700 mL + methylene blue	1	6	Endoscopic/ Endoscopic	Retrospective analysis	TWL: 18.4% AE: 3%	Variability in filling during endoscopy	Higher rate of early withdrawal during the adaptation phase
MedSil[46]	CSC MEDSIL, Moskovskaya Oblast, Russia	No/Yes	Silicone Saline 400–700 mL	1	6	Endoscopic/ Endoscopic	Prospective cohort	EWL: 19.3%	The biocompatibility of the silicone compound enhances tolerance	Reports of complications, such as cardiac arrhythmias
LexBal[47]	Lexel Medical, Buenos Aires, Argentina	No/Yes	Silicone Saline 500–800 mL	1	6	Endoscopic/ Endoscopic	Prospective cohort	AWL: 25.2 ± 13.5 kg AE: 6.35%	Encased in a silicone sheath	Clinical intolerance
End-ball[49]	Endalis, Brignais, France	No/Yes	Polyurethane Spherical (Air/Saline 600 mL)	1	6	Endoscopic/ Endoscopic	Retrospective analysis	TWL: 17.1% EWL: 36.5% AE: 7%	Balloon inflation with air or saline solution	Lower weight loss, difficult removal

ATIIP (EndogAst[48])	Districlass Medical, Chaponnay, France	No/No	Polyurethane Oval (Air 300 cm³)	1	Endoscopic-surgical/ Not removed	Prospective cohort	6–12	EWL: 39.2% AE: 5.2%	Device connected to a subcutaneously implanted prosthesis, enabling volume adjustment and reducing balloon migration	Combined procedure with surgical complications, including subcutaneous infection
Silimed[50]	Silimed, Rio de Janeiro, Brazil	No/No	Silicone Saline 650 mL + methylene blue	1	Endoscopic/ Endoscopic	Prospective cohort	6	EWL: 46.5% AE: 6%	Thin silicone sheath and improved traction-based insertion and removal technique	Recalled by the ANVISA due to particle contamination

Abbreviations: ATIIP, adjustable totally implantable intragastric prosthesis; AWL, absolute weight loss; CE, Conformité Européenne; CO_2, carbon dioxide; EWL, excess weight loss; FDA, food and drug administration; TWL, total weight loss.

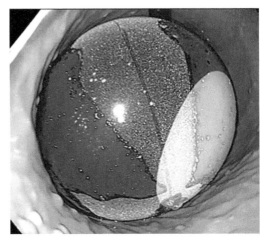

Fig. 1. Fluid-filled balloon after placement in the stomach (Orbera).

the authors' experience, this type of IGB is less effective than the fluid-filled IGBs. However, it is still superior to diet alone as reported by a meta-analysis showing a reduction of the body mass index (BMI) with an average difference of 2.40 kg/m^2 compared to the control group, with a statistically significant difference[26] (**Fig. 2**).

Spatz3 Adjustable Balloon System (Spatz Medical, Great Neck, NY, USA)

This is the only IGB in the market that allows volume adjustment. This feature is possible due to a catheter connected to the IGB, also known as the "tail." The catheter, despite providing several benefits, can potentially trigger the development of gastric ulcers. The ability to reduce the volume decreases early removal rates as the patient can choose a lower filling volume in the event of intractable adaptive side effects.[27,28] Additionally, increasing the volume allows for a higher weight loss as more volume may improve satiety. Furthermore, the adjustment is beneficial in keeping the patient close to the multidisciplinary team and, thus, improving outcomes. The Food and Drug Administration (FDA) recently approved this adjustable IGB after an RCT proved its benefits. Spatz3 reached a 15% TWL compared to 3.3% in the control group. In addition, upward volume adjustment facilitated an additional TWL of 5.2%. Furthermore, downward

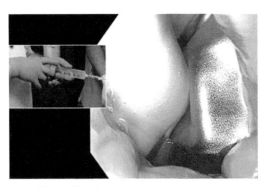

Fig. 2. Air-filled balloon (Heliosphere).

volume adjustment allowed 75% of patients to improve compliance and complete the treatment[27] (**Fig. 3**).

ReShape Duo (ReShape Medical Inc, San Clemente, CA, USA)

This device comprises two fluid-filled silicone spheres connected by a short, central flexible silicone shaft, with the primary purpose of reducing the risk of migration.[26,34–36] A RCT[34] showed satisfactory weight loss, represented by 28% of EWL and 7.6% of TWL. One of the most frequent AE associated with this IGB is the occurrence of gastric ulceration, especially in the incisura, due to the distal tip of the device, with an incidence that can reach up to 35% of cases.[34] Despite design modifications, with eliminating the distal tip floret in exchange for a smooth recessed tip end, the incidence of this complication remained high (10%). In December of 2018 the ReShape Duo was purchased by Apllo Endosurgery from ReShape Medical, and due to already having a balloon, they did not manufacture the balloon or continue compliance with FDA regulatory requirements, leading to withdrawal from the market (**Fig. 4**).

Obalon (Obalon Therapeutics Inc, Carlsbad, CA, USA)

This device consists of a swallowable gelatin capsule gas-filled with nitrogen-sulfur hexafluoride gas with a capacity of 250 mL. Three IGBs can be used with a total volume of up to 750 mL. It is important to note that the IGBs are inserted sequentially. The second IGB can be swallowed after 2 weeks, and the third after 4 to 8 weeks of the first one. Thus, the 3 IGBs can be placed within the first 3 months of treatment. The IGB is packaged in a capsule with a long catheter. After swallowing, fluoroscopy or a dedicated device is used to confirm its position. After confirming the intragastric position, the IGB is inflated using a gas-contained canister, and the catheter is then removed.[32–34] One European series demonstrated a high rate of deflation with an early generation of the device that was placed for 3 months, however deflation was rare in both the US randomized controlled trial and large registry series with the 6 month balloon. The main advantage of this IGB is placement without the need for an esophagogastroduodenoscopy (EGD). However, an EGD is required to remove the IGBs 6 months after the first IGB insertion.[33,35] A meta-analysis demonstrated advantages in its results compared to conservative measures, as this device achieved a %TWL of 3.20% and a %EWL of 11.50%, however

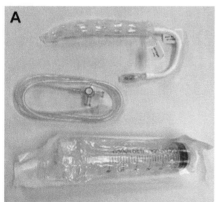 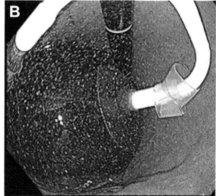

Fig. 3. Adjustable fluid-filled balloon (Spatz). (*A*) Pre-procedure; (*B*) After placement in the stomach.

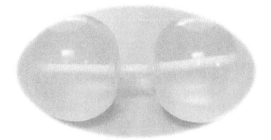

Fig. 4. Double (Bi-lobal) balloon (ReShape).

this only included data from the sham-controlled US RCT. Data from a prospective US registry of 1343 patients demonstrated $10.0 \pm 6.1\%$ TWL and an SAE rate of 0.19%. The SAE rate was comparable to the US pivotal trial and is the lowest across US trials.[26] Although approved by the FDA, the device is not commercially available due to company financial issues (**Fig. 5**).

Allurion (Allurion Technologies, Wellesley, MA, USA)

This is the only device that does not require EGD for either placement or removal. This swallowable IGB comprises a capsule with a polymer film connected to a slender catheter. After swallowing the capsule, fluoroscopy is used to verify the placement of the radiopaque valve within the gastric chamber. Once a suitable position is confirmed, the IGB is filled with a proper solution. Subsequently, a second radiological assessment is performed before removing the catheter.[36,37]

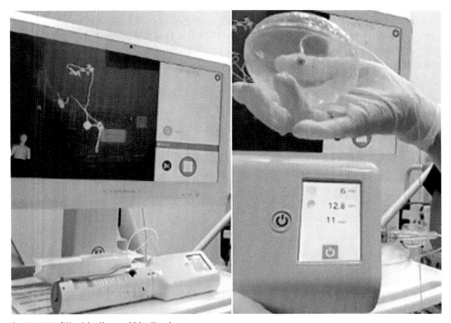

Fig. 5. Air-filled balloon (Oballon).

This IGB achieved significant weight loss, similar to other balloons, as demonstrated by a meta-analysis including 1770 patients receiving this swallowable IGB, resulting in an average %TWL of 14.2% and %EWL of 67% at 4 months follow-up.[36] The most recent meta-analysis demonstrated a significantly higher acceptance rate during the adaptation phase of this device compared to other IGB types, such as the Orbera and ReShape Duo, represented by a lower prevalence of nausea, vomiting, and abdominal pain, consequently reducing the early withdrawal rate due to clinical intolerance.[38] The most recent study by Ienca actually shows 0.2%. This is important to note because the balloon and manufacturing process have been updated multiple times resulting in a very low rate of incomplete balloon deflation, which is what causes the SBOs.[4,38] The Allurion balloon has a special follow-up program for patients using the IGB, including multidisciplinary team consultations, a mobile app, and a scale. The program allows better follow-up, facilitating patients and multidisciplinary team contact and hence overall adherence to treatment (**Fig. 6**).

EFFICACY

Data regarding IGB effectiveness is heterogeneous due to the different profiles of patients included in the studies from patients with overweight to patients with class III obesity. Thus, a significant difference between outcomes is expected. For example, a patient with a BMI of 28 kg/m^2 will have a %EWL greater than a patient with a BMI greater than 50 kg/m^2. Additionally, the time of follow-up varies. As post-IGB removal patients have high rates of weight regain, studies with long-term potentially present worse outcomes than studies with a short follow-up period. Therefore, careful interpretation of the results is necessary.

Weight Loss

Alterable weight loss
IGBs are more effective than lifestyle interventions for short-term and medium-term weight loss. An illustrative example of its effectiveness is provided by a meta-analysis of RCTs including only patients receiving fluid-filled IGB with a volume higher than 400 mL, showing a pooled mean difference between the IGB group and the sham/diet group of 3.55 kg [(95% CI -6.20 to −.90), $P = .009$, $I^2 = 0\%$] greater with IGB group.[17]

Body mass index loss
Another meta-analysis of RCTs published by the authors' group showed the effectiveness of different IGB types (Orbera, Heliosphere, ReShape, Obalon, and Spatz3)

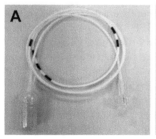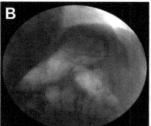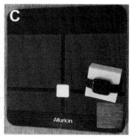

Fig. 6. Fluid-filled swallowable balloon (Allurion). (*A*) Swallowable balloon capsule; (*B*) Fluoroscopic image showing adequate placement (intragastric); (*C*) Follow-up program includes an application connected to a bioimpedance scale.

comparing IGBs and lifestyle modification versus lifestyle modification alone. The mean difference was 2.13 kg/m^2 favoring the IGB group.[26]

% total weight loss
A meta-analysis evaluated the effectiveness of several types of IGBs in RCTs and revealed a mean difference in TWL of 4.4% between the IGB group and the control group, which solely received lifestyle interventions.[26] Despite all IGBs having favorable outcomes, the %TWL was predominantly determined by the adjustable IGB results.

% estimated weight loss
An evidence 1A meta-analysis[26] reported a mean difference in %EWL of 17.98% [(95% CI, 8.37–27.58), $P<.00001$, $I^2 = 98\%$] across the various IGB models. However, in this analysis, there was no significant difference between the IGB types.

Metabolic Parameters and Obesity-Associated Comorbidities

Type 2 diabetes mellitus
Endoscopic therapy with IGBs has demonstrated favorable changes in metabolic parameters and reduction of obesity-associated comorbidities. In a recent meta-analysis involving 5668 patients from 10 RCTs, significant results were reported, including a reduction in fasting blood glucose (12.7 mg/dL) and triglyceride levels (19 mg/dL) as well as dyslipidemia (OR: 1.4), and diabetes remission at 6 months (OR: 1.4).[39] In addition, a 0.17% decrease in hemoglobin A1c levels and a significant reduction of 2.23 points in homeostasis model assessment of insulin resistance values were reported by other meta-analyses.[40]

Hypertension
A recent meta-analysis reported significant improvement in systolic blood pressure levels following treatment with the IGB, resulting in an average systolic blood pressure reduction of 7.27 mm Hg.[40] Another meta-analysis also provided evidence of the quality of improvement in diastolic blood pressure, resulting in a reduction of 2.9 mm Hg in diastolic blood pressure.[39]

Abdominal circumference
Abdominal circumference is an important parameter of the metabolic syndrome. A meta-analysis revealed an average reduction of 12.12 cm in abdominal circumference after 6 months of IGB use.[40] Additionally, a prospective study also demonstrated relevance by achieving a 6.5 cm decrease in waist circumference, along with a 19.5% reduction in body fat percentage.[41]

Metabolic dysfunction-associated fatty liver disease
Improvement in metabolic and anthropometric parameters has a positive impact on the management of metabolic dysfunction-associated fatty liver disease (MAFLD). A meta-analysis assessed the impact of weight loss following IGB therapy on liver volume reduction presenting an average reduction of 303 cm^3 after 6 months of IGB use without statistical significance.[40] Another study demonstrated that hepatic improvement was relevant in the short term, with a significant decrease in liver volume during the first and second months. However, the results worsened again during the last 3 months.[42] A recent study demonstrated improvements in steatohepatitis and fibrosis following treatment with the IGB, achieving outcomes approved by the FDA for nonalcoholic steatohepatitis resolution and fibrosis improvement. Additionally, histologic improvement through the Non-Alcoholic Fatty Liver Disease Activity Score (reduction from a score of 4 to1 with a $P<.001$) and recovery in hepatic fibrosis measured by nuclear magnetic resonance after 6 months of IGB use was reported.[43]

MANAGEMENT

The key factor that will significantly impact the success of weight loss is not closely associated with IGB placement or removal. These are straightforward endoscopic procedures without significant technical challenges. In addition to intrinsic factors related to the patient, the management and maintenance of the treatment are of utmost importance to achieve clinical success.

Patients suffering from obesity pose a challenge to manage due to this being a complex and multifaceted disease and thus a multidisciplinary team approach is mandatory. Close follow-ups are needed to improve outcomes and prevent complications. Patient complaints need to be considered seriously. The endoscopist must be prepared to perform EGD when necessary and promote early removal when cases of extreme intolerance occur (eg, emergency room visits, and hospital admission for dehydration).[39]

It is essential that treatment planning involves the complete understanding and consent of the patient regarding the procedure, along with its possible adverse events and complications. The consent needs to include the benefits, risks, advantages, and disadvantages of the procedure. The endoscopic procedure for the insertion of the IGB is typically performed on an outpatient basis with discharge between 2 and 4 hours after the procedure.[22]

Patient selection is the key as it has a significant impact on weight loss, complications, and overall outcomes. Additionally, IGB type selection should be individualized.

BMI is not the most appropriate measure to evaluate obesity as it is used to grade obesity. A BMI above 40 kg/m^2 usually suggests that a surgical approach may be more suitable, mainly when associated with T2DM. IGB may be useful as a bridge to a surgical approach, as the higher the BMI, the greater the risk of surgical and anesthesia-related complications.

Additionally, during the anamnesis, it is essential to investigate issues related to cardiac, endocrine, and infectious diseases. It is also relevant to identify any history of psychological or psychiatric disorders, as well as significant eating disorders that could affect the effectiveness of weight loss or pose a risk for complications from the procedure. Gathering information about previous endoscopic procedures, behavior during sedation, and potential allergic reactions to medications is crucial. It is imperative to rule out any contraindications, whether absolute or relative. Furthermore, females of childbearing age need to exclude the possibility of pregnancy at the beginning of the treatment.[4,51]

During the initial consultation, the use of anti-obesity medications, lifestyle changes performed, previous IGB use, and most importantly, previous gastrointestinal surgery should be interrogated. It is essential to assess the patient's level of knowledge about the treatment, ascertain whether they prefer a specific type of IGB, and understand their expectations regarding weight loss. We must align patient's expectations with the reality. During the consultation, it is imperative to investigate the causes of weight gain and the timeframe in which it occurred and evaluate the patient's commitment to serious and regular follow-up visits with a multidisciplinary team, including nutritionists and psychologists. It is also relevant to inquire if the patient is already participating in a physical activity program and to assess the level of social support in the decision-making process, as this will play a crucial role in cases of potential treatment failure and complications.

Once the patient is selected and the procedure is scheduled, the following steps are recommended:

1. Initiate the use of proton pump inhibitors (PPIs) 1 week prior to IGB placement;
2. Use prokinetics and adopt a liquid diet 48 hours before the procedure;

3. Provide the informed consent a few days in advance, so that the patient can read it carefully and sign it;
4. Prepare the patient for the adaptation period, prescribing an adequate diet and medications;
5. Standard preprocedural fasting for 12 hours is recommended except for prescription medications and sips of water.

Regardless of the type of IGB, in the first days, adaptative symptoms such as nausea, vomiting, and abdominal pain are expected to occur. These symptoms represent a physiologic response to the foreign body placed in the gastric chamber. Air-filled IGBs are typically associated with less pronounced symptoms, suggesting that they are more related to the weight of the IGB rather than its size (to increase the IGB diameter by 1 cm, an additional 300 mL of fluid is required).

Patients should not wait for symptoms to develop to start medications (antispasmodics, antiemetics, etc.), as this can delay or reduce their overall tolerance. Antiemetics, analgesics, and antispasmodics are recommended and should be taken scheduled and not as needed during the early stages of treatment after IGB placement. Additionally, medications to reduce stomach acidity, such as PPIs, are required to reduce the risk of ulcers and gastroesophageal reflux. The use of PPIs is extremely important and essential for the treatment because the presence of the device stimulates continuous and excessive production of hydrochloric acid. The use of PPI reduces dyspeptic symptoms, reduces damage to the IGB wall from a foreign object, and delays food digestion time.[52,53]

Patients must stay well-hydrated and follow an appropriate diet before and after IGB implantation (**Table 4**). The progression of the diet should not consider only the amount but also the levels of micro and macronutrients. A nutritionist is essential during follow-up to indicate the best diet plan for each patient. The diet must be hypocaloric, preferably with less than 1200 kcal/day, without compromising adequate nutrition. The American Gastroenterology Association (AGA) suggests daily supplementation with 1 to 2 adult dose multivitamins after IGB placement.[54] Nutritionist goals should include gradual weight loss, dietary re-education, and healthy nutrition promotion.[55,56] These should be long-term goals aimed to linger beyond IGB removal.

After IGB removal, patients should continue with a monthly dietary follow-up visit to ensure weight loss maintenance.

Following IGB implantation, close contact with the patient is recommended. In authors' practice, the authors provide all multidisciplinary team contacts (personal mobile phone). They believe that this measure reduces the risk of complications and early removal. Given the likelihood of these patients visiting the emergency department in the initial phase, it is a good practice to provide a letter for the patient to present to the emergency department personnel, with predictability symptoms and recommendations. Strenuous physical activities are typically allowed after the first month of post-IGB placement.

Table 4		
Diet plan during intragastric balloon treatment		
Time Period	**Diet**	**Calorie Limit**
Days 1 and 3	Clear liquids only	600 kcal/day
Days 4–14	Complete liquid diet	700 kcal/day
Days 15–28	Mechanical soft diet	750–1200 kcal/day
After 28 d	Normal textured foods	1200 kcal/day

When an adjustable IGB is preferred, a readjustment is considered between the third and fourth months to increase volume for enhanced satiety and weight loss, mainly for patients with poor weight loss. Typically, an increased volume of 200 to 300 mL is preferred.

Box 1 summarizes recommendations for the management of patients during the IGB treatment phase.

IGB is safe and effective for obesity. Nevertheless, complications can occur even in experienced hands, however, when early intervention is done, satisfactory outcomes are usually expected. On the other hand, patients without close follow-up can have undesired outcomes.

PLACEMENT AND REMOVAL

Each type of IGB has its own placement and removal technique details. In the following sections, the authors describe, step-by-step the placement (**Table 5**) and removal (**Table 6**) of non-swallowable fluid-filled IGBs.

SAFETY PROFILE

The IGB is a widely used endoscopic bariatric and metabolic technique in the primary treatment of obesity and is considered a device with a low-risk of SAEs.[24,57]

Box 1
Recommendations for the management of patients during intragastric balloon treatment phase and related conditions

A. Regular consultation with a dietician is mandatory. The main symptoms during intragastric balloon (IGB) treatment after adaptation are related to diet.

B. Sleeping on the left lateral position. This position usually reduces reflux and discomfort during sleeping due to the stomach's conformation and IGB position.

C. Pregnancy risk:
  • Due to gastric stasis, medication absorption is altered, thus, oral contraceptive pills malabsorption can occur. Changes in the menstrual cycle, such as menorrhagia, are common.
  • Significant weight loss can increase fertility, which may result in pregnancy during treatment. If this occurs, the authors recommend waiting until the first trimester for removal.

D. Changes in bowel habits: Stagnant food and delayed digestion can affect the intestinal microbiome, leading to sporadic episodes of diarrhea during treatment. Constipation is more common at the beginning of treatment due to a low-fiber diet and the use of antispasmodics.

E. Alcohol abuse: Although not recommended, alcohol consumption is not prohibited. Due to its composition and carbonation, beer should be avoided. Alcohol can irritate the gastric mucosa, which, combined with the presence of the IGB, may increase the risk of peptic ulcer disease. The authors strongly recommend moderation in alcohol consumption.

F. IGB rupture: Although extremely rare, it can occur. Methylene blue mixed in the injectate is recommended during the placement as in cases of leakage, the patient will repeatedly urinate greenish urine. The authors advise the patient not to panic but to immediately inform the authors' team. They recommend IGB removal as soon as possible whenever this occurs. Antispasmodics are prescribed when immediate removal is not possible.

G. Physical activities: It is recommended. However, some strenuous exercises that increase intra-abdominal pressure may cause discomfort.

H. Late adjustment: Not recommended after the eighth month of placement due to the risk of rupture related to the weakening of the IGB elasticity and compliance.

Table 5
Step-by-step fluid-filled balloon placement

Step-by-step *fluid-filled balloon (traditional igb) placement*	
1	Insert the empty silicon IGB through the mouth like a nasogastric tube until it reaches the gastric chamber. The entire procedure lasts approximately 15 min.
2	Before proceeding with balloon inflation, ensure the correct positioning to avoid complications like esophageal and duodenal rupture or antral impaction. The IGB should be inflated 2 cm below the esophagogastric junction under direct endoscopic visualization.
3	To inflate the IGB, the guidewire of the catheter is removed and then the catheter is connected to a tube connected to the fluid solution for inflation. The authors strongly recommend the use of methylene blue (1 cc per 100 cc of saline) (Video 1) as it can "warn" about IGB leak or rupture as urines becomes blue or green (**Fig. 7**).
4	Fill the IGB with the adequate amount of solution based on the physician's discretion. Volume should be individualized, but always respecting the manufacturer's recommendation. The catheter is then removed along with the endoscope with a continuous traction maneuver.
5	Repeat EGD to rule out complications (ie, esophageal tear), confirm correct placement, and to evaluate for any IGB valve leak.
6	An additional IGB should be readily available in case of any manufacturer defects. Furthermore, a removal kit must be available for cases of leak after insertion.
Step-By-Step Adjustable IGB Placement	
1	The IGB insertion kit consists of the adjustable IGB itself, a 60 mL syringe, an IGB sealing cap, a device for IGB inflation, and a silicone sheath. The IGB is attached to the tip of the gastroscope, and the silicone sheath fixes both ends.
2	Connect the inflation valve to the catheter attached to the solution that will fill the IGB. Then, under direct endoscopic visualization introduce the system into the gastric chamber. Once in the distal body/antrum, a U turn maneuver is performed to ensure the IGB [inflation catheter (tail)] is completely inside the stomach.
3	Using a 60-mL syringe, a solution (methylene blue with saline is preferred) is inserted until the desired volume is achieved (450–900 mL). Usually, the authors start with 500–600 mL. Then, the IGB valve connected to the catheter is removed through the mouth. The system is disconnected, the valve is closed (sealed), and the catheter is positioned into the stomach or duodenum using a grasper forceps hooked to the nylon suture attached to the tip of the catheter.
4	The authors recommend orotracheal intubation for adjustable IGBs during placement or adjustments to avoid adverse events such as aspiration.

Although most patients tolerate the duration of the IGB treatment without complications, some experience intense adaptive symptoms or complications that require its early removal. Among the adaptive symptoms, persistent nausea, vomiting, abdominal pain or discomfort, and reflux symptoms are noteworthy. These symptoms are common but tend to be self-limiting. AGA[54] suggests the use of perioperative antiemetics and also a scheduled antiemetic regimen for 2 weeks after IGB placement. Aggressive treatment of these symptoms is mandatory as patients can experience severe dehydration episodes and electrolyte imbalances needing emergency room (ER) visits or even admission for treatment during these episodes.

A systematic review,[58] including 6101 patients from 26 studies undergoing treatment with the fluid-filled or air-filled IGB, demonstrated the following rates of AEs related to the use of IGB: nausea and vomiting (23.9%), abdominal pain (19.9%), gastroesophageal reflux disease (14.3%), diarrhea or constipation (10.4%), among others. The rate of early removal was 3.5% with abdominal pain (17.3%), and

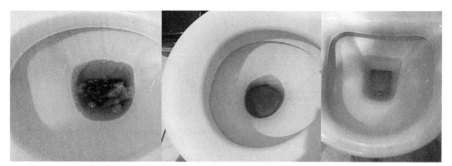

Fig. 7. Diagnosing a leakage of the fluid-filled intragastric balloon (IGB) due to the bluish coloration of the urine because of the excretion of methylene blue.

nausea and vomiting (18.3%) being the leading causes. In the authors' practice, the rates of nausea and vomiting as well as abdominal pain during the adaptative symptoms are considerably higher than the reported rates, except for the early removal rate.

Although rare, IGB-related complications can occur (**Fig. 11**), including gastrointestinal obstruction, bacterial contamination, fungal colonization, lacerations, bleeding, esophageal or gastric ulcers, perforation, pancreatitis, and others (**Box 3, Table 7**).[58–78]

Although extremely rare, fatal complications during the use of the IGB have been reported in the literature. Deaths related to IGB use are likely to occur only when there is no follow-up or poor adherence to a treatment plan. Without adequate follow-up, adverse events such as ulcers, perforation, hyperinflation, antral impaction, obstruction, and bleeding can become catastrophic events.[65–67,74–78] In cases of complications, early intervention is key to improving outcomes. For example, a patient with a gastric perforation treated 12 hours after symptom onset will likely have a more favorable outcome than a patient presenting with a 3-day history of a perforation complicated with peritonitis and sepsis. It is imperative to have a high index of suspicion for any IGB-related complication. Keep in mind that complications will occur, but that timely recognition and adequate treatment are likely to have a positive outcome.

WEIGHT REGAIN

Weight regain is common after IGB removal.[75] Obesity is a chronic and recidivant disease, therefore, weight regain is expected and patients should be aware of this.[76,79] Thus, subsequent weight loss or maintenance interventions such as dietary

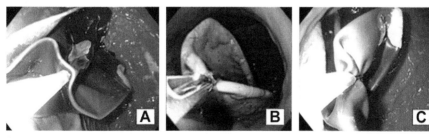

Fig. 8. IGB removal using the conventional technique. (*A*) IGB puncture and emptying using the aspiration needle catheter; (*B*) Foreign body forceps grasping the IGB; (*C*) IGB captured by the polypectomy snare.

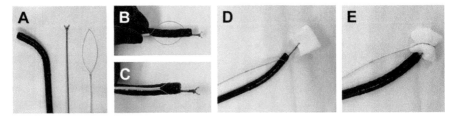

Fig. 9. The step-by-step IGB removal using a single channel gastroscope. (*A*) Devices: foreign body forceps and polypectomy snare; (*B*) close the polypectomy snare in the distal tip of the gastroscope ("over-the-scope snare"); (*C*) insert and use the foreign body forceps through the working channel; (*D*) grasp the IGB with the foreign body forceps passed through the working channel; (*E*) open the snare and grasp the IGB for subsequent removal.

interventions, pharmacotherapy, repeat IGB placement, endoscopic bariatric and metabolic therapies, or bariatric surgery are recommended and should be considered in these cases.[54] The choice of interventions is determined based on the patient's context and comorbidities following a shared decision-making approach.

FUTURE PERSPECTIVES

The increasing incidence of obesity has prompted the medical field to develop various less-invasive therapeutic interventions aimed at ameliorating the morbidity and mortality associated with this chronic disease. Despite technological advancements in various treatment modalities, there is no standardized treatment protocol. The IGB remains the most widely used endoscopic bariatric and metabolic therapy, with level 1A evidence confirming its satisfactory efficacy compared to sham or lifestyle interventions for weight loss in patients with overweight and obesity, along with an adequate safety profile.

The role of the IGB as a "bridge therapy" is being recognized more for patients suffering from obesity who need to lose weight before undergoing complex surgeries. This has been shown to reduce cardiorespiratory severe adverse events during anesthesia. A recent study showed that IGB use allowed more than 75% of patients to undergo joint replacement or hernia repair at an ideal weight, making it a viable

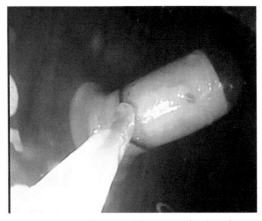

Fig. 10. Inner valve grasping for challenging IGB removal using the eversion technique.

Box 2
Intragastric balloon toolbox

Aspiration needle catheter

Foreign body forceps (Grasper)/Rat-toothed forceps

Polypectomy snare

Endoscopic scissors

Canola oil

Magill forceps

Double channel gastroscope

Esophageal overtube

Table 6
Step-by-step fluid-filled intragastric balloon removal

Step-by-step *fluid-filled balloon (traditional IGB) removal*

1	Fasting for 12 h is recommended after a 72-h period of exclusive clear fluid intake. Carbonated beverages (eg, Coca-Cola, Sprite) are generally recommended for IGB cleaning. Prokinetics may be prescribed for 5–7 d prior to the procedure.
2	Orotracheal intubation is strongly encouraged. However, experienced endoscopists prefer sedation to reduce costs. In these cases, one must ensure a clear stomach before removal. If not, intubation or rescheduling is necessary. In the authors' practice, as patient safety is the authors' top priority, they routinely intubate all patients for IGB removal.
2	Under direct endoscopic visualization and using a needle catheter, the IGB is punctured after adequate position is encountered. The gastroscope must be stable and close to the IGB (no more than 1 cm away). The needle and the catheter should be inserted 5 cm into the IGB.
3	Then, remove the needle and aspirate the fluids through the catheter. Using powerful surgical aspirators with effective and rapid suction is recommended, reducing procedural time and, consequently, its potential risks. The aspirated volume should be measured to ensure complete emptying.
4	After complete aspiration of fluid is performed, use a foreign body forceps, rat-toothed forceps, or a polypectomy snare to capture the IGB on the opposite side of the valve (**Fig. 8**). Then, with continuous traction, remove the IGB, keeping the IGB close to the tip of the gastroscope. In the authors' practice, the authors use an over-the-scope polypectomy snare and a grasper forceps for IGB removal as detailed in **Fig. 9**.
5	Sometimes IGB removal can be challenging, and other techniques are necessary such as the eversion technique (**Fig. 10**). The authors strongly recommend an IGB toolbox for IGB placement and removal (**Box 2**).
5	After IGB removal, a revisional EGD is recommended to rule out complications such as mucosal tears and perforations.

Step-by-Step Adjustable IGB Removal

1	Two approaches: one is similar to the non-adjustable fluid-filled IGB and the other one, besides puncturing the IGB with the aspiration needle catheter, involves capturing the catheter valve and removing it through the mouth for aspiration until the IGB becomes empty.
2	After the adjustable IGB is empty, it can be easily removed using the conventional technique or using its own catheter for removal. In the authors' practice, the authors use an aspiration needle catheter for emptying the IGB and then they use a polypectomy snare to grasp the catheter and remove it. The adjustable IGB is usually easier to remove than the traditional fluid-filled balloon.

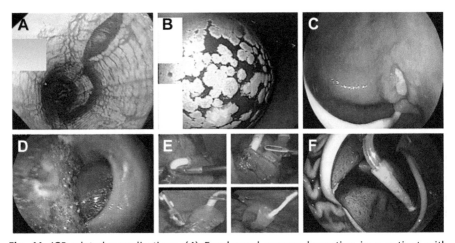

Fig. 11. IGB-related complications. (*A*) Esophageal mucosa laceration in a patient with eosinophilic esophagitis; (*B*) Fungal contamination; (*C*) Gastric ulcer; (*D*) Antral impaction/obstruction; (*E*) Migration requiring laparoscopic-assisted surgical removal; (*F*) Spontaneous rupture.

endoscopic therapy for those needing weight loss before elective surgery.[80] The use of IGB before laparoscopic vertical gastrectomy in patients suffering from severe obesity has proven to be more advantageous when compared to medication use, as this endoscopic therapy achieved higher percentages of %EWL and %TWL compared to the liraglutide group.[7]

Endoscopic device combinations applied simultaneously or sequentially, that employ different mechanisms of action and combination with pharmacotherapies are now actively being studied to enhance weight loss. A study evaluating the combination of IGBs and the duodenal jejunal bypass liner (DJBL) showed that combination therapies are feasible and may improve outcomes. In this study, outcomes were superior compared to the insertion of the IGB or the DJBL alone. Additionally, there was a trend of higher postprandial glucagon-like peptide 1 for the combination group.[81] A recent study evaluated a novel device, named Sleeveballoon, which is a combination of a large IGB with a duodenal jejunal bypass liner, and showed a reduction in peripheral and hepatic insulin resistance, weight loss, and visceral adipose tissue, with similar results to Roux-en-Y gastric bypass.[82]

Box 3
Rare intragastric balloon-related complications

Complications related to anesthesia or deep sedation

Pharynx trauma and/or inflammation

Wernicke's syndrome, related to poor nutritional status—is reversible when diagnosed early

Esophageal mucosa laceration, mainly related to esophageal disorders

Allergies to intragastric balloon (IGB) components or methylene blue (extremely rare)

Acute pancreatitis

Ischemia or diffuse necrosis of the gastric wall

Table 7
Summary of the most reported adverse events related to intragastric balloon

Gastrointestinal Symptoms	Approximately 90% of patients will experience gastrointestinal symptoms in the first 3–7 d, including nausea, abdominal pain, vomiting, dyspepsia, constipation, and reflux. Most of them respond to aggressive medical treatment. A meta-analysis[70] reported rates of 63.33% of nausea and 55.29% of vomiting after IGB placement.
Early removal	Early balloon removal due to clinical intolerance is expected in <5% of patients. A review[61] reported a 3.5% early removal rate.
Ulcers	Occurs in <1% of patients using IGB. Diagnosed during EGD after patients complain of abdominal pain or bleeding. Higher rates in non-spherical IGBs (Reshape Duo and Spatz). In the authors' practice, when non-spherical IGBs are used, the authors immediately perform EGD if patients complain of abdominal pain.[71] Spherical shape, flat surface, and volume <700 mL reduce the incidence of ulcers. Bleeding is extremely rare with a rate <0.1%.
Gastric Perforation	This is a rare adverse event, and early diagnosis is crucial when it occurs. The therapeutic approach depends not only on the patient's clinical condition but also on cross-sectional imaging findings. In the absence of free fluid in the cavity, endoscopic treatment may be an option as reported by the authors' group.[72] Perforation can also occur during both IGB placement and removal. In these cases, endoscopic treatment is usually performed with high rates of successful closure.
Hyperinflation and Fungal contamination	Rare (1%) and still not well understood. One possible etiology is the overgrowth of microorganisms such as Candida sp. or Klebsiella pneumoniae inside the IGB related to the use of medications that reduce gastric acidity such as proton-pump inhibitors (PPIs). Permeability of the IGB may be the cause of hyperinflation, which results in the entry of fluids and gases by osmosis, or due to the presence of gas-producing anaerobic bacteria. There is no evidence to support the routine use of antibiotics or antifungals. IGB removal is recommended if this is encountered. However, for non-adjustable IGBs, deflation followed by refilling can be considered. Nevertheless, in the authors' experience, hyperinflation is likely to reoccur. Therefore, the authors recommend IGB removal even for adjustable IGBs.
Deflation, Migration, and Obstruction	Deflation and subsequent migration of the IGB and even gastrointestinal obstruction can occur during IGB use. Deflation is more common for air-filled IGBs. Prolonged IGB use is a significant risk factor as well as its volume (>600 mL). Common sites of impaction are the duodenum and terminal ileum. Thus, early intervention is the key to avoiding undesired outcomes.

(continued on next page)

Table 7 *(continued)*	
	There is a fear regarding the use of the Allurion IGB which may increase the rates of obstruction. However, a systematic review reported similar rates of bowel obstruction compared to other IGB types[73]
Aspiration	Aspiration can occur during placement and mainly during IGB removal. Therefore, the authors strongly recommend orotracheal intubation, especially for IGB removal. For patients with obstructive symptoms, orotracheal intubation is imperative.

As new IGB types are being developed and others are under development, several areas can be addressed to improve outcomes. We are already seeing device improvements to simplify its placement and removal, such as the Allurion IGB, and to improve its effectiveness and durability, such as the adjustable IGB and the 12-month IGBs. Recently, a study disclosed a new device, named the vibrating ingestible bioelectronic stimulator pill, which aims to activate gastric mechanoreceptors, resulting in stomach distension and influencing satiety, potentially leading to reduced appetite and minimizing weight gain in animals.[83] This new technology could contribute to the development of new vagal stimulation modalities in the treatment of obesity.

As new IGB types are being developed, standardized training and credentialing processes will be required to ensure patient safety and maintain good clinical outcomes.[84] Furthermore, patient selection is always an important consideration for optimizing patient outcomes. Based on the authors' experience, the optimal candidates for the IGB are patients with a BMI lower than 32, without a history of childhood obesity, and without genetic risk factors.

Finally, clinical success is correlated with dietary and behavioral changes and should be carried out by a multidisciplinary team. It is important to emphasize that the procedure does not mark the end of obesity treatment, but rather the beginning of a period of long-term behavioral and dietary changes that can have a positive effect on the well-being of our patients.

SUMMARY

In summary, considering the worsening obesity epidemic and the increasing demand for less invasive endoscopic bariatric and metabolic therapies, IGBs offer a minimally invasive outpatient approach with favorable clinical short-term outcomes supported by systematic reviews and meta-analyses of randomized controlled trials. Placement of an IGB is not a procedure to substitute any bariatric surgery, but it is another device in the armamentarium that we can offer to patients in the early stages of obesity. Furthermore, it is crucial to recognize the complexity of obesity treatment, emphasizing the necessity of a multidisciplinary approach.

CLINICS CARE POINTS

- Multidisciplinary management and close follow-up are essential for achieving satisfactory outcomes.

- The intragastric balloon, when combined with a proper lifestyle modification, is an effective and safe method for treating overweight and obesity (evidence 1A).
- Each type of balloon has specific considerations regarding placement and removal. Physicians should have a comprehensive understanding of these aspects before performing the procedure.

DISCLOSURES

All the authors have nothing to disclose.

SUPPLEMENTARY DATA

Supplementary data related to this article can be found online at https://doi.org/10.1016/j.giec.2024.04.013.

REFERENCES

1. World obesity atlas. 2023. Available at: https://www.worldobesity.org/resources/resource-library/world-obesity-atlas-2023.
2. Food and Drug Administration. FDA activities: weight-loss and weight-management devices. Available at: https://www.fda.gov/intragastric+balloon. Accessed November 15, 2023.
3. Gollisch KSC, Raddatz D. Endoscopic intragastric balloon: a gimmick or a viable option for obesity? Ann Transl Med 2020;8(Suppl 1):S8. PMID: 32309412; PMCID: PMC7154325.
4. ASGE Bariatric Endoscopy Task Force and ASGE Technology Committee, Abu Dayyeh BK, Kumar N, Edmundowicz SA, et al. ASGE bariatric endoscopy task force systematic review and meta-analysis assessing the ASGE PIVI thresholds for adopting endoscopic bariatric therapies. Gastrointest Endosc 2015; 82(3):425–38.e5. Epub 2015 Jul 29. PMID: 26232362.
5. Bawahab MA, Abbas KS, Maksoud WMAE, et al. Factors affecting weight reduction after intragastric balloon insertion: a retrospective study. Healthcare (Basel) 2023;11(4):600. PMID: 36833134; PMCID: PMC9957044.
6. Lee KG, Nam SJ, Choi HS, et al. Korean research group for endoscopic management of metabolic disorder and obesity. efficacy and safety of intragastric balloon for obesity in Korea. Clin Endosc 2023;56(3):333–9. Epub 2022 Dec 13. PMID: 36510655; PMCID: PMC10244150.
7. Martines G, Dezi A, Giove C, et al. Efficacy of intragastric balloon versus Liraglutide as bridge to surgery in super-obese patients. Obes Facts 2023;16(5):457–64. Epub 2023 Aug 14. PMID: 37579738; PMCID: PMC10601677.
8. Goyal D, Watson RR. Endoscopic bariatric therapies. Curr Gastroenterol Rep 2016;18(6):26. PMID: 27098813.
9. Nieben OG, Harboe H. Intragastric balloon as an artificial bezoar for treatment of obesity. Lancet 1982;1(8265):198–9. PMID: 6119560.
10. Hogan RB, Johnston JH, Long BW, et al. A double-blind, randomized, sham-controlled trial of the gastric bubble for obesity. Gastrointest Endosc 1989;35(5): 381–5. PMID: 2792672.
11. Gleysteen JJ. A history of intragastric balloons. Surg Obes Relat Dis 2016;12(2): 430–5. Epub 2015 Oct 16. PMID: 26775045.

12. Ribeiro IB, APST Kotinda, Sánchez-Luna SA, et al. Adverse events and complications with intragastric balloons: a narrative review (with Video). Obes Surg 2021; 31(6):2743–52. Epub 2021 Mar 30. PMID: 33788158.

13. Lopez-Nava G, Jaruvongvanich V, Storm AC, et al. Personalization of endoscopic bariatric and metabolic therapies based on physiology: a prospective feasibility study with a single fluid-filled intragastric balloon. Obes Surg 2020;30(9):3347–53. PMID: 32285333.

14. Vargas EJ, Bazerbachi F, Calderon G, et al. Changes in time of gastric emptying after surgical and endoscopic bariatrics and weight loss: a systematic review and meta-analysis. Clin Gastroenterol Hepatol 2020;18(1):57–68.e5. Epub 2019 Apr 4. PMID: 30954712; PMCID: PMC6776718.

15. Mion F, Napoléon B, Roman S, et al. Effects of intragastric balloon on gastric emptying and plasma ghrelin levels in non-morbid obese patients. Obes Surg 2005;15(4):510–6. PMID: 15946431.

16. Konopko-Zubrzycka M, Baniukiewicz A, Wróblewski E, et al. The effect of intragastric balloon on plasma ghrelin, leptin, and adiponectin levels in patients with morbid obesity. J Clin Endocrinol Metab 2009;94(5):1644–9. Epub 2009 Mar 3. PMID: 19258408.

17. Moura D, Oliveira J, De Moura EG, et al. Effectiveness of intragastric balloon for obesity: A systematic review and meta-analysis based on randomized control trials. Surg Obes Relat Dis 2016;12(2):420–9. Epub 2015 Oct 20. PMID: 26968503.

18. Mathus-Vliegen EM, Eichenberger RI. Fasting and meal-suppressed ghrelin levels before and after intragastric balloons and balloon-induced weight loss. Obes Surg 2014;24(1):85–94. PMID: 23918282.

19. Kotzampassi K, Shrewsbury AD. Intragastric balloon: ethics, medical need and cosmetics. Dig Dis 2008;26(1):45–8. Epub 2008 Feb 15. PMID: 18600015.

20. Genco A, Lorenzo M, Baglio G, et al. Italian Group for Lapband and BIB (GILB). Does the intragastric balloon have a predictive role in subsequent LAP-BAND(®) surgery? Italian multicenter study results at 5-year follow-up. Surg Obes Relat Dis 2014;10(3):474–8. Epub 2013 Dec 6. PMID: 24680759.

21. Laing P, Pham T, Taylor LJ, et al. Filling the void: a review of intragastric balloons for obesity. Dig Dis Sci 2017;62(6):1399–408. Epub 2017 Apr 18. PMID: 28421456.

22. Neto MG, Silva LB, Grecco E, et al. Brazilian Intragastric Balloon Consensus Statement (BIBC): practical guidelines based on experience of over 40,000 cases. Surg Obes Relat Dis 2018;14(2):151–9. Epub 2017 Sep 28. PMID: 29108896.

23. De Castro ML, Morales MJ, Del Campo V, et al. Efficacy, safety, and tolerance of two types of intragastric balloons placed in obese subjects: a double-blind comparative study. Obes Surg 2010;20(12):1642–6. PMID: 20390374.

24. Mion F, Gincul R, Roman S, et al. Tolerance and efficacy of an air-filled balloon in non-morbidly obese patients: results of a prospective multicenter study. Obes Surg 2007;17(6):764–9. Erratum in: Obes Surg. 2007;17(7):996. PMID: 17879576.

25. Genco A, Dellepiane D, Baglio G, et al. Adjustable intragastric balloon vs nonadjustable intragastric balloon: case-control study on complications, tolerance, and efficacy. Obes Surg 2013;23(7):953–8. PMID: 23526067.

26. Kotinda APST, de Moura DTH, Ribeiro IB, et al. Efficacy of intragastric balloons for weight loss in overweight and obese adults: a systematic review and meta-analysis of randomized controlled trials. Obes Surg 2020;30(7):2743–53. PMID: 32300945.

27. Abu Dayyeh BK, Maselli DB, Rapaka B, et al. Adjustable intragastric balloon for treatment of obesity: a multicentre, open-label, randomised clinical trial. Lancet

2021;398(10315):1965–73. Epub 2021 Nov 15. Erratum in: Lancet. 2021 Nov 27;398(10315):1964. PMID: 34793746.

28. Machytka E, Klvana P, Kornbluth A, et al. Adjustable intragastric balloons: a 12-month pilot trial in endoscopic weight loss management. Obes Surg 2011;21(10):1499–507. PMID: 21553304; PMCID: PMC3179587.

29. Ponce J, Woodman G, Swain J, et al. REDUCE Pivotal Trial Investigators. The reduce pivotal trial: a prospective, randomized controlled pivotal trial of a dual intragastric balloon for the treatment of obesity. Surg Obes Relat Dis 2015;11(4):874–81. Epub 2014 Dec 16. PMID: 25868829.

30. Suchartlikitwong S, Laoveeravat P, Mingbunjerdsuk T, et al. Usefulness of the ReShape intragastric balloon for obesity. SAVE Proc 2019;32(2):192–5. PMID: 31191125; PMCID: PMC6541059.

31. Kim SH, Chun HJ, Choi HS, et al. Current status of intragastric balloon for obesity treatment. World J Gastroenterol 2016;22(24):5495–504. PMID: 27350727; PMCID: PMC4917609.

32. Bazerbachi F, Sawas T, Vargas EJ, et al. Bariatric surgery is acceptably safe in obese inflammatory bowel disease patients: analysis of the nationwide inpatient sample. Obes Surg 2018;28(4):1007–14. PMID: 29019151.

33. Mion F, Ibrahim M, Marjoux S, et al. Swallowable Obalon® gastric balloons as an aid for weight loss: a pilot feasibility study. Obes Surg 2013;23(5):730–3. PMID: 23512445.

34. Turkeltaub JA, Edmundowicz SA. Endoscopic bariatric therapies: intragastric balloons, tissue apposition, and aspiration therapy. Curr Treat Options Gastroenterol 2019;17(2):187–201. PMID: 30963378.

35. De Peppo F, Caccamo R, Adorisio O, et al. The Obalon swallowable intragastric balloon in pediatric and adolescent morbid obesity. Endosc Int Open 2017;5(1):E59–63. PMID: 28180149; PMCID: PMC5283171.

36. Ienca R, Al Jarallah M, Caballero A, et al. The procedureless elipse gastric balloon program: multicenter experience in 1770 consecutive patients. Obes Surg 2020;30(9):3354–62. Erratum in: Obes Surg. 2020 May 5;: Erratum in: Obes Surg. 2020 Nov;30(11):4691-4692. PMID: 32279182; PMCID: PMC7458897.

37. Genco A, Ernesti I, Ienca R, et al. Safety and efficacy of a new swallowable intragastric balloon not needing endoscopy: early italian experience. Obes Surg 2018;28(2):405–9. PMID: 28871497.

38. Ramai D, Singh J, Mohan BP, et al. Influence of the elipse intragastric balloon on obesity and metabolic profile: a systematic review and meta-analysis. J Clin Gastroenterol 2021;55(10):836–41. PMID: 33394629.

39. Popov VB, Ou A, Schulman AR, et al. The impact of intragastric balloons on obesity-related co-morbidities: a systematic review and meta-analysis. Am J Gastroenterol 2017;112(3):429–39. Epub 2017 Jan 24. PMID: 28117361.

40. de Freitas Júnior JR, Ribeiro IB, de Moura DTH, et al. Effects of intragastric balloon placement in metabolic dysfunction-associated fatty liver disease: A systematic review and meta-analysis. World J Hepatol 2021;13(7):815–29. PMID: 34367502; PMCID: PMC8326158.

41. Donadio F, Sburlati LF, Masserini B, et al. Metabolic parameters after bioenterics intragastric balloon placement in obese patients. J Endocrinol Invest 2009;32(2):165–8. PMID: 19411817.

42. Sekino Y, Imajo K, Sakai E, et al. Time-course of changes of visceral fat area, liver volume and liver fat area during intragastric balloon therapy in Japanese super-obese patients. Intern Med 2011;50(21):2449–55. Epub 2011 Nov 1. PMID: 22041341.

43. Bazerbachi F, Vargas EJ, Rizk M, et al. Intragastric balloon placement induces significant metabolic and histologic improvement in patients with nonalcoholic steatohepatitis. Clin Gastroenterol Hepatol 2021;19(1):146–54.e4. Epub 2020 Apr 30. PMID: 32360804; PMCID: PMC8106130.

44. Sullivan S, Swain J, Woodman G, et al. Randomized sham-controlled trial of the 6-month swallowable gas-filled intragastric balloon system for weight loss. Surg Obes Relat Dis 2018;14(12):1876–89. Epub 2018 Sep 29. PMID: 30545596.

45. Lecumberri E, Krekshi W, Matía P, et al. Effectiveness and safety of air-filled balloon Heliosphere BAG® in 82 consecutive obese patients. Obes Surg 2011; 21(10):1508–12. PMID: 21221835.

46. Bužga M, Evžen M, Pavel K, et al. Effects of the intragastric balloon MedSil on weight loss, fat tissue, lipid metabolism, and hormones involved in energy balance. Obes Surg 2014;24(6):909–15. PMID: 24488758; PMCID: PMC4022986.

47. Żurawiński W, Sokołowski D, Krupa-Kotara K, et al. Evaluation of the results of treatment of morbid obesity by the endoscopic intragastric balloon implantation method. Wideochir Inne Tech Maloinwazyjne 2017;12(1):37–48. Epub 2017 Mar 30. PMID: 28446931; PMCID: PMC5397553.

48. Gaggiotti G, Tack J, Garrido AB Jr, et al. Adjustable totally implantable intragastric prosthesis (ATIIP)-Endogast for treatment of morbid obesity: one-year follow-up of a multicenter prospective clinical survey. Obes Surg 2007;17(7):949–56. PMID: 17894156.

49. Keren D, Rainis T. Intragastric balloons for overweight populations-1 year post removal. Obes Surg 2018;28(8):2368–73. PMID: 29497962.

50. Carvalho GL, Barros CB, Okazaki M, et al. An improved intragastric balloon procedure using a new balloon: preliminary analysis of safety and efficiency. Obes Surg 2009;19(2):237–42. Epub 2008 Jun 26. PMID: 18581191; PMCID: PMC7419478.

51. Ashrafian H, Monnich M, Braby TS, et al. Intragastric balloon outcomes in super-obesity: a 16-year city center hospital series. Surg Obes Relat Dis 2018;14(11): 1691–9. Epub 2018 Aug 2. PMID: 30193905.

52. Papademetriou M, Popov V. Intragastric balloons in clinical practice. Gastrointest Endosc Clin N Am 2017;27(2):245–56. PMID: 28292403.

53. Abu Dayyeh BK, Edmundowicz S, Thompson CC. Clinical practice update: expert review on endoscopic bariatric therapies. Gastroenterology 2017;152(4): 716–29. Epub 2017 Jan 29. PMID: 28147221.

54. Muniraj T, Day LW, Teigen LM, et al. AGA clinical practice guidelines on intragastric balloons in the management of obesity. Gastroenterology 2021;160(5): 1799–808. PMID: 33832655.

55. Melissas J. IFSO guidelines for safety, quality, and excellence in bariatric surgery. Obes Surg 2008;18(5):497–500. PMID: 18340500.

56. Nunes GC, Pajecki D, de Melo ME, et al. Assessment of weight loss with the intragastric balloon in patients with different degrees of obesity. Surg Laparosc Endosc Percutaneous Tech 2017;27(4):e83–6. PMID: 28731953.

57. Alsabah S, Al Haddad E, Ekrouf S, et al. The safety and efficacy of the procedureless intragastric balloon. Surg Obes Relat Dis 2018;14(3):311–7. Epub 2017 Dec 9. PMID: 29305305.

58. de Almeida LS, Bazarbashi AN, de Souza TF, et al. Modifying an Intragastric Balloon for the Treatment of Obesity: a Unique Approach. Obes Surg 2019; 29(4):1445–6. PMID: 30737762.

59. Bennett MC, Badillo R, Sullivan S. Endoscopic management. Gastroenterol Clin N Am 2016;45(4):673–88. Erratum in: Gastroenterol Clin North Am. 2017 Jun;46(2): xvii. PMID: 27837781.

60. Deshpande K, Pandya Y. Advances in endoscopic balloon therapy for weight loss and its limitations. World J Gastroenterol 2017 28;23(44):7813–7. PMID: 29209122; PMCID: PMC5703910.

61. Yorke E, Switzer NJ, Reso A, et al. Intragastric balloon for management of severe obesity: a systematic review. Obes Surg 2016;26(9):2248–54. PMID: 27444806.

62. Smigielski JA, Szewczyk T, Modzelewski B, et al. Gastric perforation as a complication after BioEnterics intragastric balloon bariatric treatment in obese patients–synergy of endoscopy and videosurgery. Obes Surg 2010;20(11):1597–9. Epub 2009 Oct 28. PMID: 19862583.

63. Oztürk A, Akinci OF, Kurt M. Small intestinal obstruction due to self-deflated free intragastric balloon. Surg Obes Relat Dis 2010;6(5):569–71. Epub 2009 Dec 11. PMID: 20226743.

64. Moszkowicz D, Lefevre JH. Deflated intragastric balloon-induced small bowel obstruction. Clin Res Hepatol Gastroenterol 2012;36(1):e17–9. Epub 2011 Jul 23. PMID: 21783455.

65. Drozdowski R, Wyleżoł M, Frączek M, et al. Small bowel necrosis as a consequence of spontaneous deflation and migration of an air-filled intragastric balloon - a potentially life-threatening complication. Wideochir Inne Tech Maloinwazyjne 2014;9(2):292–6. Epub 2013 Oct 11. PMID: 25097704; PMCID: PMC4105657.

66. Mohammed AE, Benmousa A. Acute pancreatitis complicating intragastric balloon insertion. Case Rep Gastroenterol 2008 20;2(3):291–5. PMID: 21490858; PMCID: PMC3075186.

67. Issa I, Taha A, Azar C. Acute pancreatitis caused by intragastric balloon: A case report. Obes Res Clin Pract 2016;10(3):340–3. Epub 2015 Sep 26. PMID: 26410462.

68. Spyropoulos C, Katsakoulis E, Mead N, et al. Intragastric balloon for high-risk super-obese patients: a prospective analysis of efficacy. Surg Obes Relat Dis 2007; 3(1):78–83. PMID: 17241940.

69. Koutelidakis I, Dragoumis D, Papaziogas B, et al. Gastric perforation and death after the insertion of an intragastric balloon. Obes Surg 2009;19(3):393–6. Epub 2008 Oct 2. PMID: 18836786.

70. Trang J, Lee SS, Miller A, et al. Incidence of nausea and vomiting after intragastric balloon placement in bariatric patients - A systematic review and meta-analysis. Int J Surg 2018;57:22–9. Epub 2018 Jul 20. PMID: 30031839.

71. Bazerbachi F, Haffar S, Sawas T, et al. Fluid-filled versus gas-filled intragastric balloons as obesity interventions: a network meta-analysis of randomized trials. Obes Surg 2018;28(9):2617–25. PMID: 29663250.

72. Barrichello Junior SA, Ribeiro IB, Fittipaldi-Fernandez RJ, et al. Exclusively endoscopic approach to treating gastric perforation caused by an intragastric balloon: case series and literature review. Endosc Int Open 2018;6(11):E1322–9. Epub 2018 Nov 7. PMID: 30410952; PMCID: PMC6221813.

73. Vantanasiri K, Matar R, Beran A, et al. The efficacy and safety of a procedureless gastric balloon for weight loss: a systematic review and meta-analysis. Obes Surg 2020;30(9):3341–6. PMID: 32266698.

74. Barrichello S, de Moura DTH, Hoff AC, et al. Acute pancreatitis due to intragastric balloon hyperinflation (with video). Gastrointest Endosc 2020;91(5):1207–9. Epub 2019 Dec 19. PMID: 31866316; PMCID: PMC8752042.

75. Sander BQ, Alberti LR, MOURA DTH, et al. Analysis of long-term weight regain in obese patients treated with intragastric balloon. Acta Sci Gastroint Disord 2019; 10(2):08–10.

76. de Moura DTH, Dantas ACB, Ribeiro IB, et al. Status of bariatric endoscopy-what does the surgeon need to know? A review. World J Gastrointest Surg 2022;14(2): 185–99. PMID: 35317547; PMCID: PMC8908340.
77. Lari E, Burhamah W, Lari A, et al. Intra-gastric balloons - The past, present and future. Ann Med Surg (Lond) 2021;63:102138. PMID: 33664941; PMCID: PMC7903294.
78. Madeira M, Madeira E, Guedes EP, et al. Symptomatic bacterial contamination of an intragastric balloon. Gastrointest Endosc 2013;78(2):360–1 [discussion 361].
79. Singh S, de Moura DTH, Khan A, et al. Intragastric balloon versus endoscopic sleeve gastroplasty for the treatment of obesity: a systematic review and meta-analysis. Obes Surg 2020;30(8):3010–29. PMID: 32399847; PMCID: PMC7720242.
80. Abbitt D, Netsanet A, Kovar A, et al. Losing weight to achieve joint or hernia surgery: is the intragastric balloon the answer? Surg Endosc 2023;37(9):7212–7. Epub 2023 Jun 26. PMID: 37365392.
81. Ghoz H, Jaruvongvanich V, Matar R, et al. A preclinical Animal study of combined intragastric balloon and duodenal-jejunal bypass liner for obesity and metabolic disease. Clin Transl Gastroenterol 2020;11(9):e00234. PMID: 33094961; PMCID: PMC7508443.
82. Casella-Mariolo J, Castagneto-Gissey L, Angelini G, et al. Simulation of gastric bypass effects on glucose metabolism and non-alcoholic fatty liver disease with the Sleeveballoon device. EBioMedicine 2019;46:452–62. Epub 2019 Aug 7. PMID: 31401193; PMCID: PMC6712366.
83. Srinivasan SS, Alshareef A, Hwang A, et al. A vibrating ingestible bioelectronic stimulator modulates gastric stretch receptors for illusory satiety. bioRxiv [Preprint] 2023. https://doi.org/10.1101/2023.07.17.549257. 07.17.549257.
84. de Moura DTH, de Moura EGH, Neto MG, et al. To the editor. Surg Obes Relat Dis 2019;15(1):155–7. Epub 2018 Oct 18. PMID: 30477752.

Small Bowel Therapies for Metabolic Disease and Obesity

Ivo Boškoski, MD, PhD, FESGE[a,b], Loredana Gualtieri, MD[a,b],
Maria Valeria Matteo, MD[a,b],*

KEYWORDS

- Small bowel • Endoscopy • Obesity • Type 2 diabetes mellitus • Metabolic diseases

KEY POINTS

- Data from bariatric surgery suggest that the small intestine plays a pivotal role in the pathogenesis of metabolic diseases.
- Endoscopic bariatric metabolic treatments (EBMTs) targeting the small bowel have been recently developed as minimally invasive procedures to treat obesity and its related metabolic comorbidities.
- Small bowel EBMTs have been developed and investigated in several clinical trials, showing promising short-term results for the treatment of metabolic disease, especially type 2 diabetes mellitus.
- Further evidence from randomized controlled trials with long-term follow-up is necessary to validate current results and, eventually, for the introduction in routine clinical practice on a large scale.

INTRODUCTION

Bariatric/metabolic surgery is the most effective treatment for obesity, providing satisfactory and prolonged weight loss as well as sustained improvements in patients with metabolic comorbidities, including type 2 diabetes mellitus (T2DM) and metabolic dysfunction-associated steatotic liver disease (MASLD)/ non-alcoholic fatty liver disease (NAFLD).[1–6] Recent animal and human studies have reported that the small intestine plays a key role in metabolic homeostasis and in the pathophysiology of metabolic diseases.[7,8] It has been shown that a diet high in fat and carbohydrates leads to a hypertrophy of the mucosa and an endocrine hyperplasia that seems to trigger an alteration of the cellular and hormonal signal resulting in a "dismetabolic" state characterized by peripheral insulin resistance.[9–11]

[a] Digestive Endoscopy Unit, Fondazione Policlinico Universitario Agostino Gemelli IRCCS, Largo A. Gemelli 8, 00168, Roma, Italy; [b] Università Cattolica del Sacro Cuore, Roma 00168, Italy
* Corresponding author. Digestive Endoscopy Unit, Fondazione Policlinico Universitario Agostino Gemelli IRCCS, Largo A. Gemelli, 8, Rome 00168, Italy.
E-mail addresses: mariavaleria.matteo@unicatt.it; m.valeria.matteo@gmail.com

Gastrointest Endoscopy Clin N Am 34 (2024) 715–732
https://doi.org/10.1016/j.giec.2024.06.002   giendo.theclinics.com

Data from bariatric surgery point out the pivotal role of the small intestine, in particular of the duodenum, in glucose and metabolic homeostasis.[9,12,13] Bariatric surgeries that bypass the duodenum and the upper part of the small intestine exert favorable metabolic effects preventing the contact of nutrients with their mucosal surface, with reduction of abnormal hormone secretion, improvement of insulin sensitivity, and of β-cell function.[9,12,13] Although bariatric/metabolic surgery is the best option in terms of efficacy and durability of results, its use is restricted by its invasiveness, non-negligible morbidity and mortality as well as elevated costs.[14]

Endoscopic metabolic bariatric treatments (EMBTs) have emerged and spread as minimally invasive tools to bridge the huge therapeutic gap for obesity and related metabolic diseases.[15] Indeed, the duodenum and the small intestine can be readily reachable by endoscopy, thus being an appealing therapeutic target for metabolic disorders preventing the anatomic disruption related to bariatric/metabolic surgery. As such, small bowel-targeted EBMTs have the potential to treat metabolic disorders related to obesity including T2DM and MASLD.

Several devices have been developed and investigated in multiple clinical trials, though none of them is currently marked and approved by the Food and Drug Administration (FDA). This article provides an updated and detailed overview of the indications and outcomes of currently available small intestine-targeted EBMTs for metabolic diseases and obesity.

ABLATIVE TECHNIQUES
Duodenal Mucosal Resurfacing

Duodenal Mucosal Resurfacing (DMR) consists of hydrothermal ablation and subsequent regeneration of the duodenal mucosa aimed at reducing the aberrant signals from the duodenum thus restoring peripheral insulin sensitivity.[16]

The procedure

The DMR procedure employs the Revita device (Fractyl Laboratories, Lexington, MA), which consists of a disposable hydrothermal balloon catheter designed to inject saline solution into the submucosa and to burn the duodenal mucosal surface by heated water recirculating within the balloon. Currently, the device has CE marking for use in Europe.

The whole DMR procedure is performed under endoscopic and fluoroscopic guidance.[17] First, a standard esophagogastroduodenoscopy using a pediatric colonoscope is performed to exclude contraindications (ie, ulcers, strictures, telangiectasia) and to mark the position of the Vater papilla by applying a hemostatic clip on the contralateral wall, as a reference to avoid the thermal damage of the papilla itself (**Fig. 1**A). Next, a 0.035' guide wire is introduced under fluoroscopic control beyond the Treitz ligament to aid the DMR balloon catheter placement distal to the papilla (**Fig. 1**B, C). Next, circumferential submucosal injection of saline solution and methylene blue is performed using 3 balloon-integrated needle injectors oriented 120° from each other around the circumference of the balloon. This generates a thermal barrier to avoid transmural damage and a homogeneous ablation surface. After submucosal lifting, mucosal ablation is performed by inflating the balloon with hot water (80–90°C) for about 10 seconds. The balloon is then deflated and advanced to treat the downstream duodenal segment. Starting 1 cm distal from the Vater papilla, 9 cm to 10 cm of duodenal mucosal are treated with at least 5 consecutive ablations (**Fig. 1**D). All stages, from submucosal injection to hot water circulation and subsequent cooling of the balloon, are automatically controlled by an electronic device. Initially, the injection and the ablation were performed with 2 different catheters, positioned sequentially with the help of a guidewire.[18]

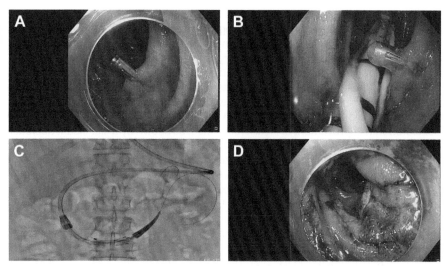

Fig. 1. (A) Marking the position of the Vater papilla with a clip on the contralateral wall; (B) insertion of the device into the duodenum (endoscopic view); (C) Placement of the device over a guide wire (fluoroscopic view); (D) Final result of Duodenal Mucosal Resurfacing.

The device was subsequently improved by creating a single integrated catheter capable of performing both injection and ablation, thus reducing procedure time and ensuring that ablation occurs precisely in the injection segment, to avoid damage to the adjacent non-injected mucosa.[17] The mean duration of the DMR procedure is about 60 minutes to 70 minutes.

DMR can be performed under general anesthesia or deep sedation, according to local guidelines and the endoscopists' preference. We suggest that the patient should be in a supine position to ensure proper positioning of the catheter under fluoroscopic guidance. Patients are usually discharged within 24 hours, according to local guidelines. If necessary, intravenous paracetamol or similar drugs can be administered post-procedure to manage any gastrointestinal symptoms or abdominal pain. In the postoperative phase, patients are prescribed a liquid diet with a progressive transition to a semi-solid diet over 2 weeks.

Outcomes

Efficacy

The main evidence available on DMR concerns the treatment of non-insulin dependent T2DM.

The first-in-human study published in 2016 included 39 patients with T2DM on at least 1 oral antidiabetic medication who underwent DMR with the initial dual-catheter system.[18] The authors reported a 1.2% reduction in glycated hemoglobin (Hb1Ac) at 6 months after DMR ($P<.001$) in the entire cohort. Out of 39 patients, 11 received a short-segment ablation (SS-DMR, length < 6 cm) and 28 a long-segment ablation (LS-DMR, length > 9 cm), as a result of further development of the technique during the study. Better results were observed in the LS-DMR group, with a 2.5% reduction in Hb1Ac at 3 months (vs 1.2% SS-DMR group, $P<.05$) and 1.4% at 6 months (vs 0.7% in the SS-DMR group, $P = .3$) despite a reduction in oral antidiabetic medications in half of LS-DMR patients.

A subsequent multicenter, prospective, open-label study (REVITA-1) investigated the feasibility and the safety of the DMR as well as the impact on glycemic control in non-insulin-dependent T2DM subjects.[19] Out of the 46 included patients, 37 received a complete DMR (ie, ablation length 9–10 cm) and 36 were included in the efficacy analysis. DMR was incomplete in 9 patients because of technical issues, such as catheter failure (n = 4/9), difficulty with positioning the catheter (n = 3/9), duodenal tortuosity (n = 1/9), or inadequate lifting (n = 1/9), while 1 patient was excluded from the efficacy analysis due to the need for insulin use post-DMR. The authors reported a reduction of Hb1Ac and fasting blood glucose (FPG) by 10±2 mmol/mol (P<.001) and 1.2±0.9 mmol/L (P<.001) at 24 weeks, respectively. DMR was also associated with improvement of insulin resistance, as shown by a significant decrease in the Homeostatic Model Assessment for Insulin Resistance (HOMA-IR) by 3.3±0.9 at 12 months as well as reduction of alanine transaminase (ALT) levels from 40±4U/L to 30±3U/L at 12 months follow-up (P<.001). Further, DMR resulted in a mild but significant weight loss of −2.5±0.6 kg at 24 weeks and −2.4±0.7 kg at 12 months (P<.001), although not related to Hb1Ac decrease. Eventually, patients reported an improvement in diabetes treatment satisfaction.

A subsequent multicenter, double-blind, sham-controlled randomized trial (REVITA-2) including 108 subjects from Europe and Brazil reported a median reduction in Hb1Ac of −10.4 (IQR 18.6) mmol/mol in the DMR group (n = 56) compared with −7.1 (IQR 16.4) mmol/mol in the sham group (n = 52) at 24 weeks follow-up (P = .147).[20] However, a post-hoc analysis showed that in patients with high baseline fasting plasma glucose (FPG ≥10 mmol/L) the median decrease in HbA1c was significantly higher in the DMR group compared with the sham group (−14.2 (IQR 17.5) mmol/mol versus −4.4 mmol/mol (IQR 15.3) mmol/mol, P = .002). On the other hand, no statistically significant differences between the 2 cohorts were detected in patients with lower basal FPG. A post-hoc analysis stratifying by region showed a significant reduction in the DMR group compared with the sham group in the European cohort (−6.6 mmol/mol vs −3.3 mmol/mol, P=.033), while no differences were found in the Brazilian one (−20.1 mmol/mol vs −12.5 mmol/mol, P=.104). In patients with NAFLD, defined by a liver MRI proton density fat fraction (MRI-PDFF) greater than 5, the procedure resulted in a drop in MRI-PDFF by −5.4 (IQR 5.6) % in the DMR group versus −2.9 (IQR 6.2) % in the sham group (P = .096) at 12 weeks follow-up. Similar to Hb1Ac, patients with baseline FPG greater than or equal to 10 mmol/L showed a significant liver-fat change after DMR compared to the sham cohort (−7.6 vs 3.1, P =.01), while in those with low FPG, the difference was not statistically significant (DMR -3.2 vs sham 2.8, P = .273). In the European cohort, weight loss at 24 weeks was significantly higher in the DMR group compared with the sham group (−2.4 kg vs −1.4 kg, P= .005). Despite weight loss in the Brazilian cohort being almost twice as much as in the European cohort, no differences were found between the DMR and sham group (−4.1 vs 2.1 kg, P = .388). According to the authors, this may be a consequence of a more intensive approach to diabetes with a larger sham effect in the Brazilian subjects.

Focusing on glycemic control, a recent meta-analysis of 4 studies, including 127 non-insulin dependent T2DM patients undergoing DMR, confirmed significant improvements in glycemic control, with a decrease of HbA1c, respectively by 1.72% (P = .02) and 0.94% (P<.001) at 3 and 6 months post-DMR.[21]

Furthermore, a small feasibility study investigated the role of DMR combined with a glucagon-like peptide-1 receptor agonist (GLP-1RA) introduction in 16 insulin-dependent patients with T2DM (Hb1Ac ≤ 8% and peptide-C ≥ 5 nmol/L). The rate of insulin withdrawal was 69% of cases with Hb1Ac values less than 7.5% at 6 months, confirmed in 56% and in 53% at 12 and 18 months from DMR.[22]

Despite the limited number of available studies and the short follow-up, these data suggest that a single DMR session can result in a substantial drop in glycemic values maintained for up to 6 months to 12 months in patients with poorly controlled T2DM (HbA1c > 7.5%) despite at least 3 months of 1 or more oral anti-diabetic medications. A one-shot procedure seems to be comparable to many oral anti-diabetic medications taken for 6 months with no need to ensure therapy adherence. As such, DMR could offer a synergistic action in the management of T2DM, with the potential of reducing oral and possibly insulin therapy, thus improving patient compliance and quality of life.

Data from the abovementioned studies suggest that DMR may also play a role in the treatment of MASLD, which is strongly related to obesity and T2DM. Van Baar and colleagues reported in 85 patients with T2DM a significant reduction in transaminase at 6 months after DMR (ALT from 41± 3 IU/L to 29±2 IU/L at 6 months; AST from 30±2 IU/L to 23±1 IU/L, P<.001), associated with a reduction in the (FIB- 4).[23]

In a prospective pilot study, 11 patients with biopsy-proven nonalcoholic steatohepatitis (NASH) showed no resolution of NASH on biopsy at 12 months after DMR, and 3 patients (27%) had marginal improvement in fibrosis with no worsening of NASH.[24] Similarly, no significant improvement in secondary endpoints (ie, serum aminotransferase levels, fibrosis 4 index [Fib-4 score], NAFLD fibrosis score, vibration-controlled transient elastography, MRI-PDFF, HB1Ac, HOMA-IR) or significant weight changes were observed at 12 months follow-up. Based on this limited evidence, no conclusions can be drawn on the therapeutic role of DMR in the treatment of steatotic liver disease.

Safety

According to the studies published so far, DMR has an excellent safety profile. Adverse events reported (ie, gastrointestinal symptoms, abdominal pain, general malaise, and fever) are mostly mild, transient, and can be managed conservatively.[19,20] In the first-in-human study, 3 cases of duodenal stenosis occurred 2 weeks to 6 weeks post-DMR, all successfully treated with endoscopic pneumatic dilatation.[18] These adverse events were attributed to overlapping ablation or to ablation of non-injected mucosa. The introduction of the single catheter, a greater submucosal injection, and the improvement of the technique (ablation proximal-distal, instead of distal-proximal) allowed for the improvement of the intraprocedural mucosal visualization, thus avoiding improper ablation.[17,25] In the REVITA-2 study, 2 procedure-related serious adverse events in the Brazilian population were reported, namely an episode of mild haematochezia probably related to a visible external hemorrhoid and an intra-procedural perforation requiring surgery, both resolved without sequelae. No clinical or laboratory signs of malabsorption, anemia, biliary complications, pancreatitis, or infections were found in any case treated.[20] Further, follow-up endoscopies with biopsies showed complete mucosal healing after 1 month from DMR.[18,20]

Most relevant data on the technique are summarized in **Table 1**.

DUODENAL RE-CELLULARIZATION VIA ELECTROPORATION THERAPY

Electroporation therapy (ReCET) is a novel endoscopic technique aimed at inducing duodenal mucosal regeneration by using pulsed electric fields. The ReCET Technology (Endogenex Inc.) employs a specialized catheter that is positioned under endoscopic control into the duodenum. Once placed, a small coil is deployed from the device and intermittent electric fields are delivered to the duodenal mucosa. This controlled electric current induces cell apoptosis and regeneration with subsequent improvement of cellular signaling involved in glucose homeostasis.[26] The procedure duration is about 60 minutes.[26]

The ReCET Procedure is currently under investigation in clinical trials to evaluate its safety and efficacy when used in subjects with T2DM to improve glycemic control and is not currently approved for use in the United States or outside of the United States.

Table 1
Safety and efficacy of the current available duodenal regenerative techniques

Procedure	Study	Study Design	N. Patients	Indication	Patients Characteristics	Main Efficacy Outcomes	Procedure-Related SAEs
Duodenal Mucosal Resurfacing (Revita device)	REVITA-1[19]	Prospective, open-label, single arm	46	T2DM on oral glucose-lowering mediations	BMI: 31.6 (4.3) kg/m² Hb1Ac 70 (9) mmol/mol	Hb1Ac: -10±2 mmol/mol at 24 wk WL: −2.5±0.6 kg at 24 wk	0%
Duodenal Mucosal Resurfacing (Revita device)	REVITA-2[20]	Double-blind, sham-controlled randomized trial	108 (56 DMR; 52 sham)	T2DM on oral glucose-lowering mediations	BMI: • DMR: 31.5 (4.7) BMI kg/m² • Sham: 30.7 (5.7) kg/m² Hb1Ac • DMR: 65.6 (8.7) mmol/mol • Sham: 66.1 (10.4) mmol/mol	DMR: Hb1Ac −10.4 (18.6) mmol/mol WL: −2.5 kg (4.5) Sham: Hb1Ac −7.1 (16.4) mmol/mol WL −1.5 kg (3.3	3.5%
Duodenal Mucosal Resurfacing (Revita device) + GLP1RA (liraglutide)	Van Baar et al,[22] 2021	Pilot, prospective, single-arm	16	T2DM on insulin therapy	BMI: 28.8 (26.5–31.7) kg/m² Hb1Ac: 7.5% (7.1–7.9)	Insulin withdrawal rate (Hb1Ac < 7.5): 69% at 6 mo 56% at 12 mo 53% at 18 mo Hb1Ac: 6.7 (6.6–7.0) at 6 mo vs 7.5 (7.1–7.9) at baseline (P = .009) WL: 80.6 (77.7–92.7) at 6 mo vs 87.8 (80.2–99.7) at baseline (P = .004)	0%

Duodenal Mucosal Resurfacing (Revita device)	Hadefi et al,[24] 2024	Pilot, prospective, single arm (interim results)	11	NASH	BMI 32.1 (28.6–34.8) kg/m² Hb1Ac: 6.5% (6.4–6.8)	No resolution of NASH at 12 mo No significant weight loss, no changes in marker of liver fibrosis	2/14
Electroporation Therapy (ReCET™)	Sartoretto el al,[26] 2023	First in human, prospective, single arm (interim results)	18	T2DM on oral glucose-lowering mediations	BMI: 32.2 ± 3.9 kg/m² Hb1Ac: 8.6%±0.9	HbA1c 7.5% ± 1.1% vs 8.4% ± 1.0% at baseline (P<.01)	0
Electroporation Therapy (ReCET™) + GLP1RA (semaglutide)	EMINENT[27]	First in human, prospective, single arm	14	T2DM on insulin therapy	BMI: 28.8 (25.1–31.2) kg/m² Hb1Ac: 7.2% (7.0–7.4)	Insulin withdrawal rate: 86% at 6 mo	0

Abbreviations: BMI, body mass index; DMR, duodenal mucosal resurfacing; GLP1RA, glucagon-like peptide 1 receptor agonist; T2DM, type 2 diabetes mellitus; WL, weight loss.

Preliminary results from a first-in-human multicenter, open-label study including patients with poorly controlled T2DM on non-insulin glucose-lowering medications have been recently published.[26] Of 30 treated subjects, the first 12 received a single energy application, and the remaining received a double energy application. Technical success was met at 100%, with a mean length of treated mucosa of 11.0 ± 1.9 cm. The procedure resulted in only mild or moderate adverse events (ie, transient sore throat and diarrhea), with no device or procedure-related serious adverse events. Follow-up endoscopy at 4 weeks showed total mucosal healing. Further, the authors reported a clinically significant reduction in Hb1Ac at 24 weeks (7.5 ± 1.1% vs 8.4 ± 1.0% at baseline, $P<.05$) in 14 patients treated with double energy application.

The ReCET procedure combined with a glucagon-like peptide 1 receptor agonist (GLP1RA) has also been evaluated in 14 insulin-dependent T2DM patients in a single-center study with the goal of withdrawing insulin therapy.[27] Technical success was 100% (mean treatment length of 12 cm), with no severe adverse events (SAEs) reported. At 6 months, the procedure resulted in a significant improvement in glycemic control and metabolic parameters, with 12 (86%) patients being able to stop insulin therapy.

These preliminary results, summarized in **Table 1**, suggest that the ReCET procedure has the potential to improve the management of T2DM.

BYPASS TECHNIQUES
EndoBarrier Duodenal-Jejunal Bypass Liner

The procedure
The Duodeno-Jejunal Bypass Liner (DJBL, GI Dynamics, Lexington, MA), also called EndoBarrier, is a bariatric and metabolic endoscopic device designed to treat patients with obesity and T2DM.[28] It consists of a 60-cm fluoropolymer liner with a proximal 5.5 cm nitinol self-expandable stent with spikes (**Fig. 2**). The device is placed under endoscopic and fluoroscopic control to guarantee a correct placement. A catheter-based delivery system is inserted into the duodenal bulb over a guidewire and then the liner is deployed. The proximal end is anchored within the duodenal bulb, while the distal end reaches the proximal jejunum. Once the liner is deployed, the contact between the nutrients and the proximal part of the small intestine is prevented, simulating surgical bypass. According to the foregut and the hindgut hypotheses, bypass of the proximal small bowel results in the reduction of presumed diabetogenic signaling (foregut hypothesis), while the early contact of the nutrients with the distal small intestine results in increased secretion of incretins like GLP1 (hindgut hypothesis).[13] The device implantation can last up to 12 months; then, the device is removed endoscopically. Both placement and removal procedures require general anesthesia.

Outcomes

Efficacy
Over the years, numerous multicenter randomized controlled trials have been conducted and demonstrated the effectiveness of the DJBL in the management of obesity and T2DM.[29–32]

A meta-analysis including 14 studies and 412 patients with T2DM and obesity showed a reduction in Hb1Ac by 1.3% [95% confidence interval (CI) (1.0–1.6)] and in HOMA-IR by 4.6 [95% CI (2.9, 6.3)] after a mean implantation time of 8.4 ± 4.0 months.[33] Notably, HbA1c was still 0.9% [95% CI (0.6, 1.2)] below the baseline value at 6 months after DJBL removal. At the time of removal, patients experienced mean total body weight loss (TBWL) and excess weight loss (EWL) of 18.9% and 36.9%, respectively. At 1 year after removal, weight loss remained significant, with mean %TBWL of 7% and %EWL of 27.7%.[33]

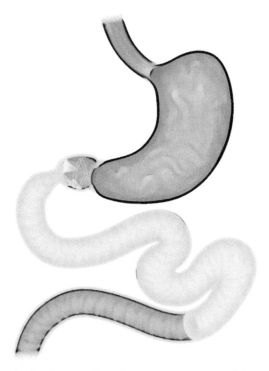

Fig. 2. The Duodenal-Jejunal Bypass liner. (Image Courtesy F.B. Calabretta.)

Beneficial effects of DJBL on NAFLD and cardiovascular risk were also observed. A prospective study including 71 patients with obesity and T2DM undergoing DJBL implantation evaluated the impact on NAFLD.[34] The mean duration of DJBL in situ was 8.8 ± 3.5 months. The authors reported a significant decrease in Fatty Liver Index (FLI) at the time of explantation (FLI 93.4 vs 98.2 at baseline, P<.001), and after 6 months of follow-up (90.37 at 6 months vs 93.4 at explantation, P<.001). An improvement in NAFLD score was also observed, with the score dropping from 0.186 ± 1.31 at baseline to −0.831 ± 1.35 at removal (P<.001), as well as a reduction of alanine aminotransferase levels (29.03 vs 42.29 U/L, P<.0001), maintained at 6 months follow-up. Another recent study showed a significant improvement in cardiovascular serologic biomarkers and a reduction of the estimated cardiovascular risk in patients with T2DM and metabolic syndrome undergoing DBJL.[35]

Safety
Despite the observed beneficial effects, the safety of the Endobarrier device is currently debated, to the extent that its use has been restricted worldwide. A systematic review reported a total of 891 adverse events in 1056 subjects; of these, 3.7% were classified as SAEs. The most frequent SAEs were hepatic abscess which occurs in 33.3% of SAE cases (n = 11), gastrointestinal bleeding in 24.2% (n = 8), and esophageal perforation in 12.1% (n = 4).[36] Further, the randomized sham-controlled pivotal trial (the ENDO trial) was prematurely stopped because of the high incidence (3.5%) of liver abscess.[30] As a result, the device did not obtain FDA approval, and the CE mark was retired.

Recently pyogenic liver abscess risk has been related to the use of Proton Pump Inhibitors (PPIs), probably due to gut microbiome alteration and morphologic changes in the bile duct.[37] As such, avoiding PPI use during Endobarrier treatment may reduce the incidence of liver abscesses. Currently, a new System Pivotal Trial (STEP-1) of the EndoBarrier is ongoing (NCT04101669) to further evaluate the safety and efficacy of the device.[38]

TONGEE DUODENAL-JEJUNAL BYPASS SLEEVE
The Procedure

The TONGEE Duodenal Jejunal Bypass Sleeve (Tangji Medical, Hangzhou, China) is a new endoscopic system, which is similar to the Endobarrier developed with the aim to improve materials, anchoring, and delivery system.[39] It consists of a 60-cm polyethylene sleeve with an anchoring system at the proximal end. The implantation and explantation of the TONGEE DJBS are performed endoscopically without the need for fluoroscopic guidance, due to the improvements in the delivery and retrieval systems.[39] Further, the barbs of the proximal anchoring system were modified to reduce duodenal injuries and the biomaterials were improved to provide better barrier properties, thus reducing the proliferation of harmful bacteria responsible for liver abscesses.[39]

Outcomes

Efficacy
Currently, 1 study evaluating the efficacy and safety of TONGEE DJBS in 26 patients with obesity and NAFLD has been published.[39] Patients were evaluated during device treatment (3 months) and at 6 months after removal. The TONGEE DJBS system resulted in TBWL and EWL of 8.9 ± 4.0% and 47.9 ± 32.1% ($P<.001$) at 3 months follow-up, respectively. At 6 months post-explantation, weight loss remained significant ($P<.01$). Further, the procedure was associated with improvement in liver steatosis and glycemic profile. At 3 months, the steatosis degree improved in 63.6% of patients, as measured by the controlled attention parameter. Further, liver enzymes and Hb1Ac were significantly reduced at 3 months follow-up. Improvements in hepatic and metabolic parameters remained statistically significant at 6 months post-explantation.

Safety
The authors reported only 1 severe adverse event, namely a gastrointestinal bleeding treated with device removal and endoscopic hemostasis.[39] Some mild-to-moderate adverse events were described, including abdominal pain (42.3%), nausea (30.8%), and vomiting (26.9%). Despite the promising results in terms of safety and efficacy, further clinical studies are needed.[39]

GASTRO-DUODENO-JEJUNAL BYPASS SLEEVE
The Procedure

The Gastro-Duodeno-Jejunal Bypass Sleeve (ValenTx, Inc. Carpinteria, CA, USA) is a 120-cm-long fluoropolymer with the proximal end anchored at the esophago-gastric junction and the distal end delivered in the proximal jejunum (**Fig. 3**).[40] The placement of the device requires general anesthesia and is performed under endoscopic and fluoroscopic control to ensure proper deployment of the device along the small intestine and correct cuff attachment at the gastro-esophageal junction by full-thickness suture-anchors.[40,41] The device is left in place for 12 weeks and then removed endoscopically.[40]

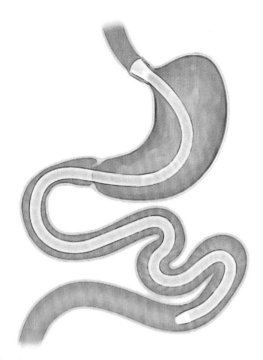

Fig. 3. The gastro-duodeno-jejunal bypass sleeve. (Image Courtesy F.B. Calabretta.)

Outcomes

Efficacy
A pilot study including 13 patients showed a mean EWL of 54% at 1 year, as well as a reduction in HbA1c levels of more than 1% point and in fasting blood glucose values of 38% in patients with T2DM.[42] Improvement in blood pressure values and lipid levels were also observed.[42] A prospective, multicenter clinical trial including 32 patients with obesity (mean BMI 42.3 kg/m^2) showed an EWL of 44.8% and a TBWL of 17.6% at 12 months follow-up.[41] In addition, serum levels of HbA1c and fasting glucose dropped by 1.1% points and 29 mg/dL in patients with T2DM, respectively.

Safety
The most frequent adverse events reported were mild-to-moderate and included epigastric pain, heartburn, regurgitation, vomiting, dysphagia, and nausea (70% of total adverse events).[41] No SAEs occurred, but the procedure resulted in 6 (19%) serious adverse device effects, including inability to retain liquids, food impaction and knotting of the sleeve in the stomach.[41]

Despite the favorable obtained results, no further clinical studies are ongoing, probably because of the procedural complexity.

THE INCISIONLESS MAGNETIC ANASTOMOSIS SYSTEM
The Procedure

The Incisionless Magnetic Anastomosis System (IMAS) (GI Windows, Westwood, MA, USA) consists of self-assembling octagonal magnets endoscopically delivered into the proximal jejunum and the terminal ileum, via enteroscopy and colonoscopy, to create a jejunal-ileal anastomosis (**Fig. 4**).[43] The result is a partial jejunal diversion (PJD) allowing a part of nutrients to bypass most of the small bowel, maintaining the native path still open.[43] The procedure is performed under general anesthesia. The device is made up of a nitinol exoskeleton that allows the insertion in a linear configuration through the working channel of the scope; once fully deployed in the small bowel lumen, it takes the shape of an octagonal ring.[43] Laparoscopy assistance is required to assess to correct site of the connection and to help with the magnets' assembling process. Once the anastomosis is formed because of tissue necrosis, the magnets naturally pass by stools.

Outcomes

Efficacy

Machytka E. and colleagues reported the results of the first-in-human pilot study evaluating PJD with IMAS in 10 patients with obesity.[43] According to the study protocol, the procedure was performed as described above, an abdominal X-ray was performed within 48 hours to assess the magnets' position and patients were instructed to eat a liquid/soft diet for the first 2 weeks. The procedure resulted in a TBWL of 14.6% at 1-year follow-up, as well as a significant reduction in Hb1Ac in all patients with diabetes (−1.9%) and pre-diabetes (−1.0%).

Safety

No SAEs were reported after IMAS. No leaks or strictures were observed at the upper GI series performed at 2 weeks. Similarly, endoscopic follow-up at 2, 6, and 12 months

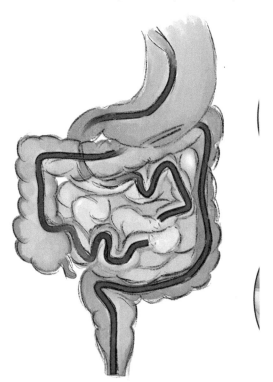

Fig. 4. The incisionless magnetic anastomosis system. (Image Courtesy F.B. Calabretta.)

confirmed patent anastomoses with healthy-appearing mucosa in all cases. It is worth mentioning that the anastomosis cannot be reversed, and currently, there are no data about potential long-term malabsorption. However, as noted in the procedure description, there is only partial diversion of nutrients into the bypass and the native path still receives a portion of ingested food.

SATISPHERE

The SatiSphere device (Endosphere, Columbus, OH) consists of a nitinol wire with pigtail ends and several polyethylenterephthalat spheres along the wire (**Fig. 5**).[44] The device is implanted endoscopically under general anesthesia and placed into the stomach and duodenum for 3 months with the aim of delaying gastric emptying in the duodenum. Only 1 pilot study has been conducted so far on 31 patients (21 patients for Satisphere group; 10 patients for control group).[44] Device migration occurred in 10 of 21 total patients. Mean weight loss was 6.7 kg at 3-month follow-up in patients who completed the treatment. The SatiSphere implantation was also associated with delayed glucose uptake and changes in insulin secretion and GLP-1 levels.[44] In view of the high migration rate, device modifications and further clinical studies proving more data on the efficacy and safety of this device are needed.

Future Perspectives

Minimally invasive endoscopic techniques for the treatment of obesity and metabolic comorbidities are of extreme interest and rapidly evolving.

For instance, the possibility to perform a fully endoscopic bypass has been investigated in animal models (Landrace pigs) with the Natural Orifice Translumenal Endoscopic Surgery (NOTES) technique.[45–47] In more detail, the NOTES technique is an endoscopic technique which provides access to the peritoneal cavity by natural orifices, avoiding the percutaneous approach through the abdominal wall. The technique

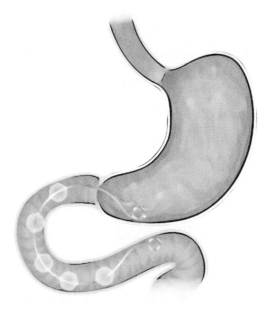

Fig. 5. The StatiSphere device illustrated. (Image Courtesy F.B. Calabretta.)

has been described in pilot feasibility study including 6 growing pigs.[48] A dedicated light beacon inserted into the jejunal is used to measure the length of the bypassed limb (150 cm). By using a double channel gastroscope, an endoscopic gastrostomy is performed by a needle knife, then the jejunal loop detected by the light is caught by a dedicated grasper, pulled back toward the gastrostomy and a 20 mm dedicated lumen-apposing metal stent (LAMS) is inserted between the stomach and the targeted jejunum thus obtaining a gastro-jejunal anastomosis.[48] Eventually, the pylorus is occluded by a dedicated device (duodenal exclusion device, DED) after 2 weeks. Procedural technical success was met at 100%. However, the migration of the gastro-jejunal LAMS and DED was observed in a half of the treated animals. Further, transient diarrhea (3/7), asymptomatic partial duodenal stenosis 28.6% (2/7), small wall abscesses in the muscularis externa (2/5), early death (1/5) were reported. However, the authors described a weight gain significantly lower in the pigs treated endoscopic bypass procedures than expect for age.[48] Despite the long way to go due to the high rate of adverse events and the technical challenges, this is a minimally invasive technique with great potential to further develop in the next future.

Given the high level of interest in bariatric and metabolic endoscopy, the development of devices is rapidly growing as well as the number of clinical trials. In parallel, novel and potentially more effective anti-obesity medications, such as multireceptor agonists, are under investigation.[49,50] Further, as alterations in the gut microbiota have been related to the obesity and metabolic comorbidities pathogenesis,[51,52] microbiota manipulation may offer a promising approach to treat obesity, and this will be evaluated in future studies.[53] Considering this dynamic scenario, there will be soon the opportunity of combined treatments to fight an extremely complex multifactorial disease.

SUMMARY

In conclusion, the small bowel plays a pivotal role in the pathogenesis of obesity and metabolic diseases. In recent years, several small intestine-targeted EBMTs have been developed and investigated in several trials. Current evidence suggests that these techniques may have a concrete therapeutic role. However, it is unquestionable the need for more safety and efficacy data from larger randomized trials with long-term follow-up before marketing and application in routine clinical practice. However, clinical research is progressing very quickly, and we expect that this will happen in the next future. Further, the combination with restrictive gastric procedures, and other novel non-invasive approaches (ie, anti-obesity medications and microbiota modulation) may represent the new frontier in the minimally invasive treatment of obesity and metabolic diseases.

CLINICS CARE POINTS

- Small bowel-targeted EBMTs are generally under general anesthesia or deep sedation, according to local guidelines and the type of device.
- DMR employs a dedicated balloon catheter to induce hydrothermal ablation and regeneration of the duodenal mucosa.
- DMR proved to induce short improvement in glucose homeostasis in patients with poorly controlled T2DM and obesity in the short-term as well as a good safety profile, as reported by well-designed trials.

- DJBL (Endobarrier) proved good results in terms of weight loss and obesity-related comorbidities improvement; nevertheless, it has been retired because of the high rate of SAEs.
- Data the safety and efficacy of other devices are still very limited. Duodenal mucosal regeneration by electroporation therapy (ReCET) seems to be very promising for the treatment of T2DM, as shown by recent interim data.
- As research on the treatment of obesity and metabolic diseases is evolving very rapidly, novel devices and combined strategy will be probably available in the near future.

ACKNOWLEDGMENTS

Thanks to Francesca Benedetta Calabretta for drawing the illustrations (francescacalabretta@icloud.com). The authors from Fondazione Policlinico Universitario Agostino Gemelli IRCCS want to thank Fondazione Roma for their continuous support of the scientific research - FR-CEMAD 21-25 and the Italian Ministry of Health RC 2024".

DISCLOSURES

Ivo Boskoski is a consultant for Apollo Endosurgery, Boston Scientific, Nitinotes, Pentax, Cook Medical, Microtech, ERBE, Siemens, Myka labs, and Endo Tools Therapeutics S.A., conducts sponsored lectures for Apollo Endosurgery, Boston Scientific, Cook Medical, Microtech, is recipient of research grant from Apollo Endosurgery, Endo Tool Therapeutics, and ERBE, and is scientific advisory board member for Nitinotes and Myka labs. The other authors declared no conflict of interest.

REFERENCES

1. Rinella ME, Lazarus JV, Ratziu V, et al. A multisociety Delphi consensus statement on new fatty liver disease nomenclature. Ann Hepatol 2023;29(1):101133.
2. Acosta A, Streett S, Kroh MD, et al. White Paper AGA: POWER - Practice Guide on Obesity and Weight Management, Education, and Resources. Clin Gastroenterol Hepatol Off Clin Pract J Am Gastroenterol Assoc. 2017;15(5):631–49.e10.
3. World Health Organization. Obesity and Overweight. Available at: https://www.who.int/news-room/fact-sheets/detail/obesity-and-overweight. [Accessed 12 September 2023].
4. Angelidi AM, Belanger MJ, Kokkinos A, et al. Novel noninvasive approaches to the treatment of obesity: from pharmacotherapy to gene therapy. Endocr Rev 2022;43(3):507–57.
5. Jacobsen SH, Olesen SC, Dirksen C, et al. Changes in gastrointestinal hormone responses, insulin sensitivity, and beta-cell function within 2 weeks after gastric bypass in non-diabetic subjects. Obes Surg 2012;22(7):1084–96.
6. Mummadi RR, Kasturi KS, Chennareddygari S, et al. Effect of bariatric surgery on nonalcoholic fatty liver disease: systematic review and meta-analysis. Clin Gastroenterol Hepatol Off Clin Pract J Am Gastroenterol Assoc. 2008;6(12): 1396–402.
7. Gniuli D, Calcagno A, Dalla Libera L, et al. High-fat feeding stimulates endocrine, glucose-dependent insulinotropic polypeptide (GIP)-expressing cell hyperplasia in the duodenum of Wistar rats. Diabetologia 2010;53(10):2233–40.
8. Angelini G, Salinari S, Castagneto-Gissey L, et al. Small intestinal metabolism is central to whole-body insulin resistance. Gut 2021;70(6):1098–109.

9. Theodorakis MJ, Carlson O, Michopoulos S, et al. Human duodenal enteroendocrine cells: source of both incretin peptides, GLP-1 and GIP. Am J Physiol Endocrinol Metab 2006;290(3):E550–9.

10. Nguyen NQ, Debreceni TL, Bambrick JE, et al. Accelerated intestinal glucose absorption in morbidly obese humans: relationship to glucose transporters, incretin hormones, and glycemia. J Clin Endocrinol Metab 2015;100(3):968–76.

11. Verdam FJ, Greve JWM, Roosta S, et al. Small intestinal alterations in severely obese hyperglycemic subjects. J Clin Endocrinol Metab 2011;96(2):E379–83.

12. Van Baar ACG, Nieuwdorp M, Holleman F, et al. The duodenum harbors a broad untapped therapeutic potential. Gastroenterology 2018;154(4):773–7.

13. Rubino F, Forgione A, Cummings DE, et al. The mechanism of diabetes control after gastrointestinal bypass surgery reveals a role of the proximal small intestine in the pathophysiology of type 2 diabetes. Ann Surg 2006;244(5):741–9.

14. Arterburn DE, Telem DA, Kushner RF, et al. Benefits and risks of bariatric surgery in adults: a review. JAMA 2020;324(9):879–87.

15. ASGE Bariatric Endoscopy Task Force, Sullivan S, Kumar N, et al. ASGE position statement on endoscopic bariatric therapies in clinical practice. Gastrointest Endosc 2015;82(5):767–72.

16. Cherrington AD, Rajagopalan H, Maggs D, et al. Hydrothermal duodenal mucosal resurfacing. Gastrointest Endosc Clin N Am 2017;27(2):299–311.

17. Haidry RJ, Van Baar AC, Galvao Neto MP, et al. Duodenal mucosal resurfacing: proof-of-concept, procedural development, and initial implementation in the clinical setting. Gastrointest Endosc 2019;90(4):673–81.e2.

18. Rajagopalan H, Cherrington AD, Thompson CC, et al. Endoscopic duodenal mucosal resurfacing for the treatment of type 2 diabetes: 6-month interim analysis from the first-in-human proof-of-concept study. Diabetes Care 2016;39(12):2254–61.

19. Van Baar ACG, Holleman F, Crenier L, et al. Endoscopic duodenal mucosal resurfacing for the treatment of type 2 diabetes mellitus: one year results from the first international, open-label, prospective, multicentre study. Gut 2020;69(2):295–303.

20. Mingrone G, van Baar AC, Devière J, et al. Safety and efficacy of hydrothermal duodenal mucosal resurfacing in patients with type 2 diabetes: the randomised, double-blind, sham-controlled, multicentre REVITA-2 feasibility trial. Gut 2022;71(2):254–64.

21. de Oliveira GHP, de Moura DTH, Funari MP, et al. Metabolic effects of endoscopic duodenal mucosal resurfacing: a systematic review and meta-analysis. Obes Surg 2021;31(3):1304–12.

22. Van Baar ACG, Meiring S, Smeele P, et al. Duodenal mucosal resurfacing combined with glucagon-like peptide-1 receptor agonism to discontinue insulin in type 2 diabetes: a feasibility study. Gastrointest Endosc 2021;94(1):111–20.e3.

23. Van Baar ACG, Beuers U, Wong K, et al. Endoscopic duodenal mucosal resurfacing improves glycaemic and hepatic indices in type 2 diabetes: 6-month multicentre results. JHEP Rep 2019;1(6):429–37.

24. Hadefi A, Verset L, Pezzullo M, et al. Endoscopic duodenal mucosal resurfacing for nonalcoholic steatohepatitis (NASH): a pilot study. Endosc Int Open 2021;09(11):E1792–800.

25. Van Baar ACG, Haidry R, Rodriguez Grunert L, et al. Duodenal mucosal resurfacing: Multicenter experience implementing a minimally invasive endoscopic procedure for treatment of type 2 diabetes mellitus. Endosc Int Open 2020;08(11):E1683–9.

26. Sartoretto A, O'Neal D, Holt B, et al. Duodenal mucosal regeneration induced by endoscopic pulsed electric field treatment improves glycemic control in patients with type ii diabetes - interim results from a first-in-human study. Gastrointest Endosc 2023;97(6):AB11-2.
27. Busch C, Meiring S, Van Baar A, et al. Re-cellularization via electroporation therapy (recet) combined with glp-1ra to replace insulin therapy in patients with type 2 diabetes 6 months results of the eminent study. Gastrointest Endosc 2023; 97(6):AB760.
28. Rodriguez L, Reyes E, Fagalde P, et al. Pilot clinical study of an endoscopic, removable duodenal-jejunal bypass liner for the treatment of type 2 diabetes. Diabetes Technol Ther 2009;11(11):725-32.
29. Ruban A, Miras AD, Glaysher MA, et al. Duodenal-jejunal bypass liner for the management of type 2 diabetes mellitus and obesity: a multicenter randomized controlled trial. Ann Surg 2022;275(3):440-7.
30. Caiazzo R, Branche J, Raverdy V, et al. Efficacy and safety of the duodeno-jejunal bypass liner in patients with metabolic syndrome: a multicenter randomized controlled trial (ENDOMETAB). Ann Surg 2020;272(5):696-702.
31. Koehestanie P, de Jonge C, Berends FJ, et al. The effect of the endoscopic duodenal-jejunal bypass liner on obesity and type 2 diabetes mellitus, a multicenter randomized controlled trial. Ann Surg 2014;260(6):984-92.
32. van Rijn S, Roebroek YGM, de Jonge C, et al. Effect of the endobarrier device: a 4-year follow-up of a multicenter randomized clinical trial. Obes Surg 2019;29(4): 1117-21.
33. Jirapinyo P, Haas AV, Thompson CC. Effect of the duodenal-jejunal bypass liner on glycemic control in patients with type 2 diabetes with obesity: a meta-analysis with secondary analysis on weight loss and hormonal changes. Diabetes Care 2018;41(5):1106-15.
34. Roehlen N, Laubner K, Nicolaus L, et al. Impact of duodenal-jejunal bypass liner (DJBL) on NAFLD in patients with obesity and type 2 diabetes mellitus. Nutr Burbank Los Angel Cty Calif 2022;103-104:111806.
35. Roehlen N, Laubner K, Bettinger D, et al. Duodenal-Jejunal Bypass Liner (DJBL) improves cardiovascular risk biomarkers and predicted 4-year risk of major CV events in patients with type 2 diabetes and metabolic syndrome. Obes Surg 2020;30(4):1200-10.
36. Betzel B, Drenth JPH, Siersema PD. Adverse events of the duodenal-jejunal bypass liner: a systematic review. Obes Surg 2018;28(11):3669-77.
37. Oh JH, Kang D, Kang W, et al. Proton pump inhibitor use increases pyogenic liver abscess risk: a Nationwide Cohort Study. J Neurogastroenterol Motil 2021;27(4): 555-64.
38. Available at: https://clinicaltrials.gov/study/NCT04101669.
39. Ren M, Zhou X, Yu M, et al. Prospective study of a new endoscopic duodenal-jejunal bypass sleeve in obese patients with nonalcoholic fatty liver disease (with video). Dig Endosc Off J Jpn Gastroenterol Endosc Soc. 2023;35(1):58-66.
40. Sandler BJ, Rumbaut R, Swain CP, et al. Human experience with an endoluminal, endoscopic, gastrojejunal bypass sleeve. Surg Endosc 2011;25(9):3028-33.
41. Sandler BJ, Biertho L, Anvari M, et al. Totally endoscopic implant to effect a gastric bypass: 12-month safety and efficacy outcomes. Surg Endosc 2018; 32(11):4436-42.
42. Sandler BJ, Rumbaut R, Swain CP, et al. One-year human experience with a novel endoluminal, endoscopic gastric bypass sleeve for morbid obesity. Surg Endosc 2015;29(11):3298-303.

43. Machytka E, Bužga M, Zonca P, et al. Partial jejunal diversion using an incision-less magnetic anastomosis system: 1-year interim results in patients with obesity and diabetes. Gastrointest Endosc 2017;86(5):904–12.
44. Sauer N, Rösch T, Pezold J, et al. A new endoscopically implantable device (Sati-Sphere) for treatment of obesity–efficacy, safety, and metabolic effects on glucose, insulin, and GLP-1 levels. Obes Surg 2013;23(11):1727–33.
45. Nesargikar PN, Jaunoo SS. Natural orifice translumenal endoscopic surgery (N.O.T.E.S). Int J Surg 2009;7(3):232–6.
46. Simopoulos C, Kouklakis G, Zezos P, et al. Peroral transgastric endoscopic pro-cedures in pigs: feasibility, survival, questionings, and pitfalls. Surg Endosc 2009; 23(2):394–402.
47. Chiu PWY, Wai Ng EK, Teoh AYB, et al. Transgastric endoluminal gastrojejunos-tomy: technical development from bench to animal study (with video). Gastroint-est Endosc 2010;71(2):390–3.
48. Gonzalez JM, Ouazzani S, Monino L, et al. First fully endoscopic metabolic pro-cedure with NOTES gastrojejunostomy, controlled bypass length and duodenal exclusion: a 9-month porcine study. Sci Rep 2022;12(1):21.
49. Jastreboff AM, Kaplan LM, Frías JP, et al. Triple–hormone-receptor agonist reta-trutide for obesity — a phase 2 trial. N Engl J Med 2023;389(6):514–26.
50. Jastreboff AM, Aronne LJ, Ahmad NN, et al. Tirzepatide once weekly for the treat-ment of obesity. N Engl J Med 2022;387(3):205–16.
51. Chakraborti CK. New-found link between microbiota and obesity. World J Gastro-intest Pathophysiol 2015;6(4):110–9.
52. Torres-Fuentes C, Schellekens H, Dinan TG, et al. The microbiota-gut-brain axis in obesity. Lancet Gastroenterol Hepatol 2017;2(10):747–56.
53. Ramadi KB, McRae JC, Selsing G, et al. Bioinspired, ingestible electroceutical capsules for hunger-regulating hormone modulation. Sci Robot 2023;8(77): eade9676.

Novel Devices for Endoscopic Suturing

Past, Present, and Future

Khushboo Gala, MBBS, Vitor Brunaldi, MD, PhD,
Barham K. Abu Dayyeh, MD, MPH*

KEYWORDS

- Endoscopic suturing • Endobariatrics • Gastric remodeling • POSE 2.0 • Endomina
- EndoZip • Endoscopic sleeve gastroplasty

KEY POINTS

- Endoscopic suturing carries multiple applications, including approximation of tissue defects, anchoring stents, hemostasis, and primary and secondary bariatric interventions.
- Currently, the only device with widespread commercial availability in the United States is the OverStitch endoscopic suturing system (Apollo Endosurgery, Austin, TX, USA).
- Novel devices are under study and refinement, including primary obesity surgery endoluminal 2.0 using the incisionless operating platform system (USGI Medical, San Clemente, CA, USA) and E-ESG using the Endomina system (TAPES, Endo Tools Therapeutics SA, Gosselies, Belgium), both of which have Food and Drug Administration clearance in the United States, and EndoZip system (NitiNotes Medical).

 Video content accompanies this article at http://www.giendo.theclinics.com.

INTRODUCTION/HISTORY/BACKGROUND

One of the pivotal advances in endoscopic therapeutic techniques has been endoscopic suturing, which has helped reduce the need for surgical interventions in many situations. It has been successfully described in multiple applications, including the approximation of tissue defects, anchoring stents, hemostasis, and primary and secondary bariatric interventions. Primary endobariatric procedures use endoscopic suturing for gastric remodeling with the intention of weight loss. Endoscopic suturing continues to be explored in newer indications like organ reconstruction postendoscopic and surgical interventions, treatment of gastroesophageal reflux disease (GERD), and facilitation of endoscopic submucosal dissection. It has the potential

Department of Gastroenterology and Hepatology, Mayo Clinic, 200 First Street Southwest, Rochester, MN 55905, USA
* Corresponding author.
E-mail address: abudayyeh.barham@mayo.edu
Twitter: @KhushbooSGala (K.G.); @Vbrunaldi (V.B.); @babudayyeh (B.K.A.D.)

Gastrointest Endoscopy Clin N Am 34 (2024) 733–742
https://doi.org/10.1016/j.giec.2024.06.007
1052-5157/24/© 2024 Elsevier Inc. All rights reserved, including those for text and data mining, AI training, and similar technologies.

advantages of shorter hospital stays, reduced postprocedure pain, faster recovery, and lack of visible scarring compared to surgery.[1]

Endoscopic suturing devices have undergone a significant evolution since the initial conception of the idea. The first device to be developed was the EndoCinch in 1994.[2] It was initially used in the treatment of GERD and further developed for endobariatrics in 2003 by Thompson and colleagues.[3,4] Subsequently, multiple devices were developed, including the NDO Plicator (NDO Surgical, Mansfield, Mass, USA), EsophyX (EndoGastric Solutions, Redmond, Wash, USA), Endoscopic Suturing Device (Wilson Cook, Winston-Salem, NC, USA), g-Prox (USGI, San Clemente, Calif, USA), and Eagle Claw (Olympus Medical Systems Corp, Tokyo, Japan). Unfortunately, all these devices had significant limitations that prevented their widespread use. Currently, the device with widespread commercial availability in the United States is the OverStitch endoscopic suturing system (Apollo Endosurgery, Austin, TX, USA).[5] This had received 510(k) clearance for OverStitch in 2008 and received Food and Drug Administration (FDA) De Novo Marketing Authorization for Apollo endoscopic sleeve gastroplasty (ESG), Apollo ESG SX (ESG with single channel endoscope), Apollo REVISE (transoral outlet reduction [TORe]), and Apollo REVISE SX systems (TORe with single channel endoscope) in July 2022. It has been found to have excellent safety and high technical success rates in both randomized clinical trial and multicenter retrospective analyses.[6,7]

The OverStitch system uses a single-use endoscopic suturing device for the placement of full-thickness sutures. Sutures can be placed in a continuous or interrupted pattern using permanent (2–0 and 3–0 polypropylene) or absorbable (2–0 and 3–0 polydioxanone) sutures. The OverStitch device has been used for gastric remodeling for ESG, a procedure that imbricates the entire greater curvature of the stomach, leading to the creation of a narrow sleeve with a significant reduction in gastric volume. ESG has been found to be safe and effective for weight loss in many prospective and retrospective studies, including a recent multicenter randomized control trial (Multicentre ESG Randomised Interventional Trial - MERIT trial).[8,9] Given the robust data supporting weight loss up to 20% outside of the randomized controlled trial (RCT) and remission of metabolic comorbidities, ESG has gained global popularity and adoption.[10,11] A separate article discusses ESG in detail.

USGI INCISIONLESS OPERATING PLATFORM: PRIMARY OBESITY SURGERY ENDOLUMINAL 2.0

The incisionless operating platform (IOP) is an FDA-cleared device used to perform the primary obesity surgery endoluminal (POSE) and POSE 2.0 procedures. Similar to ESG, this procedure aims to reduce gastric volume; however, this is performed using full-thickness gastric plications (serosa-to-serosa approximation) rather than suturing (mucosa-to-mucosa approximation). The POSE procedure was evaluated in the MILE-POST (Multicenter Study of an Incisionless Operating Platform for Primary Obesity vs. Diet and Exercise) and ESSENTIAL trials. Although differences observed between weight loss in the active and sham groups in the ESSENTIAL were statistically significant (percentage total body weight loss [%TBWL] of $4.95 \pm 7.04\%$ in active and $1.38 \pm 5.58\%$ in sham groups, respectively), the procedure failed to meet the super superiority margin as set forth in the study design.[12,13] A new technique, POSE 2.0, was developed to overcome the limitations of the previous design. This uses the IOP to create plications targeting the reduction of the gastric body and antrum, rather than the fundus.[14] Jirapinyo and colleagues[15] have also described distal POSE using 2 techniques: the single-helix and double-helix plication technique, and shown in a prospective registry study that the double-helix plication technique is superior, with a mean %TBWL of 20.3% ± 8.3% at 1 year.

The IOP (USGI Medical, San Clemente, Calif, USA) has 4 distinct components: (1) transport, (2) g-Lix, (3) g-Prox EZ, and (4) g-Cath EZ (**Fig. 1**).[16]

The transport is a flexible device with a control handle and 2 wheels that can be used to deflect the tip in all 4 directions and 4 working channels to deploy the accessories. There is also an additional side port that may be used for the insertion of an ultrathin upper endoscope.

The g-Lix is a tissue anchor catheter, the g-Prox is an endoscopic grasper, and the g-Cath is a tissue anchor delivery catheter. The g-Lix has a helical design at the distal end used for anchoring and positioning the target tissue inside the g-Prox. The g-Prox is multifunctional and rotatable, with each distal serrated jaw being 3.3 cm in length and capable of capturing a large amount of tissue. The jaws also contain a suture-cutting component to trim the excess g-Cath suture. The g-Cath is a tissue anchor delivery catheter that is preloaded with a dynamic snowshoe suture anchor and has a needle at the distal end. Once the target tissue is mobilized inside g-Prox, the needle penetrates through the tissue and releases the pair of preloaded suture anchors and cinches them to form a plication.

Preoperative/Preprocedure Planning

Contraindications to the procedure include severe systemic illnesses, substance use disorders, uncontrolled eating disorders, psychiatric disorders, pregnancy, and coagulopathy. Endoscopic contraindications are noted during initial diagnostic endoscopy, and include esophageal stricture, esophageal varices, or other anatomy and/or conditions that could preclude passage of endoluminal instruments. Additional exclusions include active gastric or duodenal ulcers, surgically altered gastric anatomy, active gastric inflammation, 1 cm or greater gastric polyps, and greater than 3 cm hiatal hernia.

The preprocedural workup includes

- Laboratories (ie, blood count, platelets, coagulation, and kidney function tests).
- Evaluation for comorbid conditions (ie, lipid panel, liver enzymes, fasting glucose, insulin, and hemoglobin A1c).
- Preanesthetic examinations depending on ASA status (ie, electrocardiogram and chest radiography).

POSE2.0™ incisionless operating platform

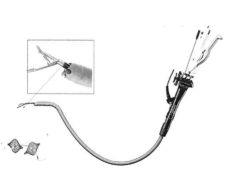
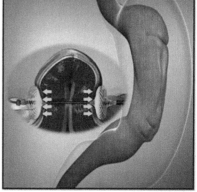

Fig. 1. The POSE 2.0 device platform.

A diagnostic upper endoscopy is also mandatory, but it can be done immediately before the procedure if no contraindication is anticipated.

Recovery and Rehabilitation (Including Postprocedure Care)

Patients should be monitored postprocedure for pain and tolerance of liquids, preferably overnight. They should be discharged with a prescription of analgesics and antiemetics for the management of accommodative symptoms. Similar to other endoscopic gastric remodeling procedures, full-dose proton pump inhibitors (PPIs) for 6 to 12 weeks and sucralfate for 1 week are recommended.

Considering the multifactorial trait of obesity as a disease, a multidisciplinary approach is recommended with close follow-up, on a monthly basis. The postprocedural diet consists of 4 weeks of full liquids transitioned to semisolid and solid according to patients' tolerance. An individualized 30 min/d exercise plan should also be implemented throughout the follow-up.

Outcomes

Lopez-Nava and colleagues[16,17] described a preliminary experience with 73 patients, with a %TBWL of 15.7% at 6 months and no adverse events reported. The study reported technical success rate of 98.7%, and 4 patients had adverse events. Forty-six patients completed 1 year and had a %TBWL of 17.8% ± 9.5. A prospective multicenter trial in 3 centers (HM Sanchinarro University Hospital in Madrid, Spain; Teknon Medical Center in Barcelona, Spain; and the Mayo Clinic in Rochester, Minnesota) described the experience of 44 patients.[14] The procedure was technically successful in all subjects and no serious adverse events were noted. Mean %TBWL at 12 months was 15.7% ± 6.8%, and improvements in lipid profile, liver biochemistries, and hepatic steatosis as well as quality-of-life questionnaires were seen at 6 months. Repeat assessment was performed in 26 patients at 24 months and showed fully intact plications. The first RCT to assess the technical feasibility, safety, efficacy of POSE 2.0 has just concluded, and results are awaited (NCT03837691). Newer techniques to improve the efficacy and efficiency of the procedure are also being developed. We have described the POSE 2.0 Enfolding Technique (POSE 2.0et), which uses a lower number (6–8) of plications staggered in a linear manner along the greater curvature of the stomach[18] (Video 1).

ENDOMINA: ENDOMINA ENDOSCOPIC SLEEVE GASTROPLASTY

The Endomina is another novel gastric remodeling device (TAPES, Endo Tools Therapeutics SA, Gosselies, Belgium) that has been approved by the Conformité Européenne for endoscopic suturing, and it has FDA clearance for tissue approximation. It is a triangulation platform that can be used with any flexible endoscope and a dedicated needle to create gastrointestinal sutures and has been used to perform endoscopic sleeve gastroplasty (E-ESG).

Equipment

The Endomina system is composed of a universal triangulation platform, grasping forceps, and a needle for tissue piercing and approximation (TAPES; **Figs. 2** and **3**). Each TAPES is loaded with 2 anchors connected by sutures, which can be used for the creation of single or double plications. The anchors are then pulled toward each other using a snare until the formation of a tight serosa-to-serosa apposition. The system can be affixed to various standard endoscopes and provides a bendable therapeutic channel that can move independently.

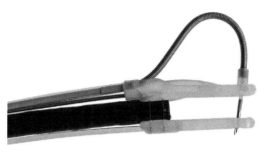

Fig. 2. The Endomina device platform.

A video representation is provided in Video 2.

Recovery and Rehabilitation (Including Postprocedure Care)

Patients should be monitored postprocedure for pain and tolerance of liquids, preferably overnight. They should be discharged with a prescription of analgesics and antiemetics for the management of accommodative symptoms. The recommended dose and duration of proton pump inhibitors is 40 mg once a day for 3 months.

The postprocedural diet consists of 3 days of full liquids transitioned to semisolid and solid hypocaloric diet (1400 kcal) according to patients' tolerance.

Outcomes

The Endomina platform has primarily been studied in Europe. The first experience in human subjects was reported by Huberty and colleagues,[19] in which 11 patients with obesity underwent E-ESG. No severe adverse events were observed. Mean % TBWL was 7.3% at 6 months. This device was studied by the same group in an RCT (2:1 randomization to lifestyle modification plus E-ESG or lifestyle modification alone [control group]), with a follow-up time of 12 months.[20] At 6 months, a crossover to E-ESG was offered to the control group. Mean excess weight loss at 6 months was significantly higher in the treatment than in the control group (38.6%, n = 45 (E-ESG); versus 13.4%, n = 21 [controls]; $P < .001$). At 12 months, the E-ESG group achieved a mean EWL of 45.1% and a %TBWL of 11.8%. No severe adverse events were observed. Another randomized trial by the same group reviewed 3 different suture

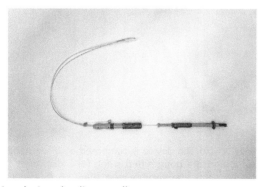

Fig. 3. The Endomina device—loading needle.

patterns for E-ESG and showed comparable efficacy for all patterns, with an overall EWL of greater than 25% and TBWL of greater than 10% at 12 months.[21,22]

Endozip
Equipment

The EndoZip platform (NitiNotes, Caesarea, Israel) is a novel, automated, operator-independent endoscopic suturing device. Its distal part is articulated to allow positioning in any anatomy. Therefore, the gastric restriction with the EndoZip platform has also been called "robotic endoscopic sleeve gastroplasty."[23]

The system is a gastroscope-like device composed of 3 main segments (**Fig. 4**A): the distal bougie, which is responsible for grasping tissue and deploying full-thickness sutures (**Fig. 5**A); the handle, which is the control unit (**Fig. 4**B); and the insertion tube that connects the handle to the bougie and has a channel for a thin gastroscope (5.4 mm), one for CO_2 insufflation, and one for vacuum application (see **Fig. 4**A).

The handle is connected to a reusable power supplier that provides energy for the motor unit to operate. The motor unit is the automated part of the device and receives feedback from 5 sensors to control stitching, tightening, and cinching of the suture wire. Automatic safety mechanisms deploy suturing after it senses the removal of the gastroscope and adequate tissue imbrication into the designated stitching ports. Similarly, there is tracking of the needle passing and sensors to activate wire cutting after the needle has reached its parking area. Besides that, the handle also exhibits a mechanic control that the endoscopist uses to position the distal bougie in the desired location before suturing.

The distal bougie has gaps in specific positions that optimize tissue apprehension by applying negative pressure (see **Fig. 5**A). After activation by the motor unit, a customized, helicoidal needle drives 2-0 polypropylene sutures through the tissue inside the bougie gaps to create anterior-to-posterior apposition (**Fig. 5**B).[24]

Preoperative/Preprocedure Planning

Eligible patients for EndoZip gastroplasty include those with obesity (>30 kg/m²) who are either unfit for or refuse bariatric surgery, with a history of failure to lose weight with

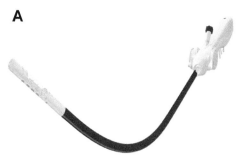
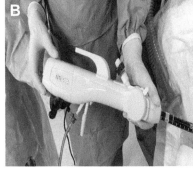

Fig. 4. The EndoZip device. (*A*) The device is composed of 3 segments: the handle (*right side*), the insertion tube, and the bougie (*left side*); (*B*) – details of the handle showing the gastroscope port (*red port*), the vacuum port (*blue port*), and the insufflation port (*white*).

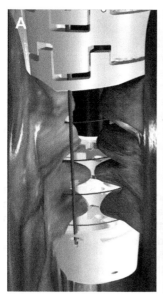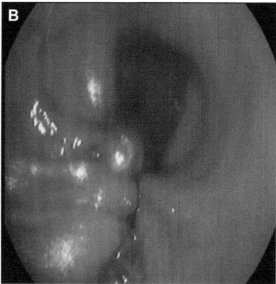

Fig. 5. The robotic endoscopic sleeve gastroplasty. (*A*) Schematics of the bougie gaps showing tissue apprehension through negative pressure; (*B*) final endoscopic view after an EndoZip procedure.

standard medical therapy, and who can understand the risks and give informed consent.

Just like other endoscopic suturing procedures, the EndoZip has a few contraindications. The most common ones are previous gastric or esophageal surgery, severe GERD, gastrointestinal strictures, Zenker's diverticulum, esophageal motility disorders, active peptic ulcer disease, gastrointestinal tumors, esophageal or gastric varices, gastroparesis, poorly controlled systemic diseases, pregnancy, coagulopathy, immunosuppressive therapy, poorly controlled psychiatric disease, chronic drugs or alcohol abuse, or any malignancy.

A video representation is provided in Video 3.

Recovery and Rehabilitation (Including Postprocedure Care)

After the procedure, patients are admitted overnight until they can take oral liquids. Patients are usually discharged within 24 hours or on the same day of the procedure if they had undergone EndoZip in the morning.[24] Around 50% of patients will require oral analgesic to control mild-to-moderate abdominal pain, and a minority of individuals will experience nausea requiring antiemetics. Similar to other endoscopic gastric remodeling procedures, full-dose PPIs for 6 to 12 weeks and sucralfate for 1 week are recommended.[8]

The hypocaloric diet after EndoZip entails 4 weeks of full liquids transitioned to semisolid and solid according to patients' tolerance.

Outcomes

To date, 2 case series[23,24], 1 case video report,[25] and 1 animal study[26] have been published on EndoZip. Lopez Nava and colleagues[24] published the first-in-human study in 2020 reporting outcomes from 11 Spanish patients undergoing EndoZip. The technical success was 100% and the mean duration of the procedure was 54.6 ± 23.9 minutes with a median of 3 sutures per patient. All 11 patients completed the 6 month follow-up and had a mean %TBWL of 16.2 ± 6.0, corresponding to a mean of 54.3 ± 28.4 %EWL. There was one serious adverse event—a respiratory tract infection demanding 48 hour admission and antibiotics.

Shamah recently published an animal study describing the histologic effects related to the sutures delivered with EndoZip compared to the Apollo OverStitch. The Endo-Zip showed consistent tunnelization of the gastric body and a very similar histologic reaction to that elicited with the Apollo OverStitch.

A health economics study and a pilot multicenter study on EndoZip are underway.

FUTURE DIRECTIONS

Newer and better suturing devices are in the pipeline, and clinical care is improving as the comprehension of the physiopathology of obesity also expands.

Each one of the devices and procedures outlined in the present study addresses a different limitation of the current endoscopic gastric reduction method. POSE 2.0 delivers serosa-to-serosa anchors that are exceptionally durable; the Endomina addresses costs and availability; and EndoZip reduces the need for human resources and increases reproducibility by decreasing operator-related variations. In the future, one should expect an endoscopic device/procedure that concentrates all those characteristics in a single platform.

Another expectation for the near future is the rise of combination therapies. One could combine EBTs with different physiologies (ie, gastric reduction with malabsorptive procedures),[27–29] as well as EBTs with medications. Broader approaches could further enhance the efficacy of EBTs, with weight loss outcomes approaching those of bariatric surgery.[30]

SUMMARY

Novel gastric remodeling procedures and devices have demonstrated exciting preliminary results, and their approval by regulatory agencies could help disseminate this minimally invasive and effective technology.

CLINICS CARE POINTS

- POSE 2.0: revised version of the POSE procedure using the IOP system; targets the reduction of the gastric body and antrum, rather than the fundus; creates full-thickness plications.

- Endomina: universal triangulation platform that can be used with any flexible endoscope and a dedicated needle to create full-thickness sutures used to perform endoscopic sleeve gastroplasty (E-ESG).

- EndoZip: automated, single-operator device that deploys full-thickness spiral sutures faster and more reproducible than other gastric remodeling procedures.

DISCLOSURE

B.K. Abu Dayyeh is a consultant for DyaMx, Boston Scientific, USGI Medical, and Endo-TAGSS; gets research support from Boston Scientific, United States, USGI Medical, United States, Apollo Endosurgery, Spatz Medical, GI Dynamics, Cairn

Diagnostics, Aspire Bariatrics, and Medtronic; is a speaker for Johnson and Johnson, Endogastric Solutions, and Olympus. The remaining authors have nothing to disclose.

SUPPLEMENTARY DATA

Supplementary data to this article can be found online at https://doi.org/10.1016/j.giec.2024.06.007.

REFERENCES

1. Law R, Martin JA. Endoscopic stitching: techniques and indications. Curr Opin Gastroenterol 2014;30(5):457–62.
2. Swain P. Endoscopic suturing: now and incoming. Gastrointest Endosc Clin N Am 2007;17(3):505–20, vi.
3. Thompson CC, Slattery J, Bundga ME, et al. Peroral endoscopic reduction of dilated gastrojejunal anastomosis after Roux-en-Y gastric bypass: a possible new option for patients with weight regain. Surg Endosc 2006;20(11):1744–8 [published Online First: 20061005].
4. Schwartz MP, Wellink H, Gooszen HG, et al. Endoscopic gastroplication for the treatment of gastro-oesophageal reflux disease: a randomised, sham-controlled trial. Gut 2007;56(1):20–8 [published Online First: 20060608].
5. Moran EA, Gostout CJ, Bingener J. Preliminary performance of a flexible cap and catheter-based endoscopic suturing system. Gastrointest Endosc 2009;69(7):1375–83.
6. Sharaiha RZ, Kumta NA, DeFilippis EM, et al. A large multicenter experience with endoscopic suturing for management of gastrointestinal defects and stent anchorage in 122 patients: a retrospective review. J Clin Gastroenterol 2016;50(5):388–92.
7. Maselli R, Palma R, Traina M, et al. Endoscopic suturing for GI applications: initial results from a prospective multicenter European registry. Gastrointest Endosc 2022;96(5):780–6 [published Online First: 20220608].
8. Abu Dayyeh BK, Bazerbachi F, Vargas EJ, et al. Endoscopic sleeve gastroplasty for treatment of class 1 and 2 obesity (MERIT): a prospective, multicentre, randomised trial. Lancet 2022;400(10350):441–51 [published Online First: 20220728].
9. Hedjoudje A, Abu Dayyeh BK, Cheskin LJ, et al. Efficacy and safety of endoscopic sleeve gastroplasty: a systematic review and meta-analysis. Clin Gastroenterol Hepatol 2020;18(5):1043–10453 e4 [published Online First: 20190820].
10. Alqahtani AR, Elahmedi M, Aldarwish A, et al. Endoscopic gastroplasty versus laparoscopic sleeve gastrectomy: a noninferiority propensity score-matched comparative study. Gastrointest Endosc 2022;96(1):44–50 [published Online First: 20220303].
11. Popov V, Storm AC. Toward a better understanding of endoscopic bariatric therapies. Clin Gastroenterol Hepatol 2023;21(6):1422–6 [published Online First: 20230405].
12. Miller K, Turro R, Greve JW, et al. MILEPOST multicenter randomized controlled trial: 12-month weight loss and satiety outcomes after pose (SM) vs. medical therapy. Obes Surg 2017;27(2):310–22.
13. Sullivan S, Swain JM, Woodman G, et al. Randomized sham-controlled trial evaluating efficacy and safety of endoscopic gastric plication for primary obesity: The ESSENTIAL trial. Obesity 2017;25(2):294–301 [published Online First: 20161221].
14. Lopez Nava G, Arau RT, Asokkumar R, et al. Prospective multicenter study of the primary obesity surgery endoluminal (POSE 2.0) procedure for treatment of

obesity. Clin Gastroenterol Hepatol 2023;21(1):81–89 e4 [published Online First: 20220506].

15. Jirapinyo P, Thompson CC. Comparison of distal primary obesity surgery endolumenal techniques for the treatment of obesity (with videos). Gastrointest Endosc 2022;96(3):479–86 [published Online First: 20220511].

16. Lopez-Nava G, Asokkumar R, Turro Arau R, et al. Modified primary obesity surgery endoluminal (POSE-2) procedure for the treatment of obesity. VideoGIE 2020;5(3):91–3 [published Online First: 20200117].

17. Lopez Nava G, Asokkumar R, Laster J, et al. Primary obesity surgery endoluminal (POSE-2) procedure for treatment of obesity in clinical practice. Endoscopy 2021;53(11):1169–73 [published Online First: 20210121].

18. Al Khatry M, Abu Dayyeh BK. The primary obesity surgery endoluminal 2.0 enfolding technique (POSE 2.0et): modification to enhance efficiency and increase restriction. Obes Surg 2023;33(6):1953–4 [published Online First: 20230417].

19. Huberty V, Ibrahim M, Hiernaux M, et al. Safety and feasibility of an endoluminal-suturing device for endoscopic gastric reduction (with video). Gastrointest Endosc 2017;85(4):833–7 [published Online First: 20160822].

20. Huberty V, Boskoski I, Bove V, et al. Endoscopic sutured gastroplasty in addition to lifestyle modification: short-term efficacy in a controlled randomised trial. Gut 2020. https://doi.org/10.1136/gutjnl-2020-322026 [published Online First: 20201028].

21. Gkolfakis P, Van Ouytsel P, Mourabit Y, et al. Weight loss after endoscopic sleeve gastroplasty is independent of suture pattern: results from a randomized controlled trial. Endosc Int Open 2022;10(9):E1245–53 [published Online First: 20220914].

22. Wallstabe I, Oberaender N, Weimann A, et al. Endoscopic sleeve gastroplasty using the novel Endomina device for morbidly obese patients. Endoscopy 2018;50(11):E327–8 [published Online First: 20180905].

23. Bove V, Matteo MV, Pontecorvi V, et al. Robotic endoscopic sleeve gastroplasty. Gut 2023;72(1):27–9 [published Online First: 20220712].

24. Lopez-Nava G, Asokkumar R, Rull A, et al. Safety and feasibility of a novel endoscopic suturing device (EndoZip TM) for treatment of obesity: first-in-human study. Obes Surg 2020;30(5):1696–703.

25. Kral J, Selucka J, Waloszkova K, et al. Cutting-edge novel device in the treatment of obesity. Endoscopy 2023;55(S 01):E1124–5 [published Online First: 20231012].

26. Shamah SE. Safety and performance evaluation of the automated helical suturing system system as compared with manual endoscopic suturing platform endoscopic sleeve gastroplasty in porcine model. iGIE 2023. https://doi.org/10.1016/j.igie.2023.10.002.

27. Ghoz H, Jaruvongvanich V, Matar R, et al. A preclinical animal study of combined intragastric balloon and duodenal-jejunal bypass liner for obesity and metabolic disease. Clin Transl Gastroenterol 2020;11(9):e00234.

28. Sartoretto A, Marinos G, Sui Z. Concurrent placements of a duodenal-jejunal bypass liner and an intragastric balloon among severely obese patients: a case series. ACG Case Rep J 2019;6(6):e00101 [published Online First: 20190625].

29. Brunaldi VO, Neto MG. Endoscopic procedures for weight loss. Curr Obes Rep 2021;10(3):290–300 [published Online First: 20210723].

30. Badurdeen D, Hoff AC, Hedjoudje A, et al. Endoscopic sleeve gastroplasty plus liraglutide versus endoscopic sleeve gastroplasty alone for weight loss. Gastrointest Endosc 2021;93(6):1316–13124 e1 [published Online First: 20201017].

Combination Therapies

Anti-Obesity Medications and Endoscopic Bariatric Procedures

Megan E. White, MD[a], Vladimir Kushnir, MD[b],*

KEYWORDS

- Obesity • Pharmacotherapy • Endoscopic bariatric treatment • Combination therapy

KEY POINTS

- Endoscopic bariatric treatment can bridge the gap between pharmacologic and surgical bariatric treatment.
- Combination of pharmacologic and endoscopic treatment options for obesity can provide improved weight loss benefits.
- Life-style interventions are key to long term success with both endoscopic and pharmacologic weight loss interventions.

BACKGROUND

Endoscopic Bariatric Technology (EBT) has rapidly developed over the past 2 decades due to the underutilization of surgery and historically limited effectiveness of pharmacotherapy for obesity and its metabolic complications. EBT relies on minimally invasive endoscopic interventions in the gastrointestinal tract to facilitate weight loss. While EBT provides a lesser degree of weight loss then surgery, it is less invasive, and thus, appealing to a broader patient population. EBT is currently recommended in patients who have tried and failed lifestyle or medical management or require adjunctive therapy to lifestyle or medical management due to comorbidities.[1] With the recent expansion of pharmacologic therapy for overweight and obesity, there is opportunity to combine pharmacologic therapy with endoscopic bariatric therapy to meet patient goals that may not be achieved with EBT alone.

[a] Division of Gastroenterology, Washington University School of Medicine, Washington University/Barnes Jewish Hospital, 660 South Euclid #8124, St Louis, MO 63110, USA; [b] Division of Gastroenterology, Washington University School of Medicine, Washington University, 660 South Euclid #8124, St Louis, MO 63110, USA
* Corresponding author.
E-mail address: Vkushnir@wustl.edu

Gastrointest Endoscopy Clin N Am 34 (2024) 743–756
https://doi.org/10.1016/j.giec.2024.06.003   **giendo.theclinics.com**
1052-5157/24/© 2024 Elsevier Inc. All rights are reserved, including those for text and data mining, AI training, and similar technologies.

OVERVIEW OF ENDOSCOPIC BARIATRIC TECHNOLOGY

Intragastric balloons (IGB) are the oldest EBT and remain a popular choice for patients today. The first IGB prototype was created in 1985 called the Garren-Edwards bubble, which was quickly discontinued due to risk profile.[2] Since then, a multitude of IGBs have been created to improve both safety and efficacy. Most IGBs are placed endoscopically and filled with saline or gas and removed endoscopically after 6 months.[3,4] While placed, they increase satiation, delay gastric emptying, and restrict food ingestion.[3] On average, IGB result in 7% to 15% total body weight loss (TBWL) at 12 months.[5,6] The risk of severe complications is rare and includes migration, obstruction, and gastric perforation. Other side effects include pain, nausea, Gastroesophageal reflux disease and uncommonly gastric ulcers. Studies show positive effect on weight loss up to 12 months after removal. Long-term studies up to 5 years show weight regain 1 to 2 years after procedure with continued weight gain through the 5 year study protocol.[7,8] Both studies showed excess body weight loss (EBWL) of around 9% at 5 years from greater than 20% at time of balloon removal. Please refer to Diogo Turiani Hourneaux de Moura and colleagues' article, "Intragastric Balloons: Practical Considerations," in this issue for more information on intragastric balloons.

Endoscopic sleeve gastroplasty (ESG) is another common EBT that is meant to reduce the volume of the stomach similarly as laparoscopic sleeve gastrectomy (LSG). However, unlikely LSG, ESG slows gastric emptying, which increases the feeling of satiety.[9] The first ESG was conducted in 2013 and the Apollo Overstitch system was Food and Drug Administration (FDA)-approved in 2022 for body mass index (BMI) 30 to 50, based on the outcome of the MERIT study.[10] ESG is a partially reversible endoscopic suturing technique that restricts the stomach approximately 70%.[3,10,11] Patients commonly have abdominal pain and nausea especially in the first week following procedure, which typically improves rapidly thereafter. Severe complications include gastric leak (<1%) and gastric bleeding (<1%). While gastric restriction is the main cause of efficacy in ESG, there is also notable delayed gastric emptying.[12] On a physiologic level, there are some data to suggest a decrease in ghrelin, an orexigenic hormone released in the gastric fundus, after ESG, which may contribute to maintenance of weight loss.[12,13] Studies show TBWL at 12 months post ESG around 15% to 20%.[3,11,14] Five year follow-up data show maintenance of TBWL; however, in one study, 26% of patients were on adjuvant pharmacotherapy due to weight regain after ESG.[15,16] Of note, in large longitudinal studies of ESG, retightening or redo of the ESG for inadequate weight loss or weight regain was needed in up to 26% of patients.[3,10,15] The Primary Obesity Surgical Endoluminal (POSE) and POSE 2.0 system is a gastric plication procedure similar to the ESG but differs in the pattern of endoscopic suturing of the stomach as it specifically targets the fundus as opposed to the greater curvature with fundal sparing seen in ESG suturing technique.[17,18] This is not currently widely commercially available in the United States.

The duodenal bypass liner and duodenal resurfacing techniques were created to mimic gastric bypass surgery. The duodenojejunal bypass liner (DJBL) is a device that is implanted in the proximal small intestine.[19] This device is typically removed after 12 months. The DJBL is not currently FDA-approved in the United States. Duodenal resurfacing uses thermic energy to disrupt the duodenal mucosa. Both procedures block absorption of nutrition in the proximal small intestines and have been shown to improve metabolic diseases such as diabetes.[3,19] TBWL at time or removal was found to be 18.9% in one metanalysis, but 6 to 24 months after removal, that dropped to 7.2% to 12%.[19,20] The aspire system is no long on the market but some patients still have their aspire device. This is a percutaneous gastrostomy tube that allows for drainage of 30% of calories following each meal (**Table 1**).[21]

COMBINATION OF PHARMACOTHERAPY AND ENDOSCOPIC BARIATRIC THERAPY

There are multiple FDA-approved pharmacologic therapies that can be used for obesity management. Most pharmacologic therapies provide between 5% and 10% TBWL. However, the recent introduction of incretin medications has revolutionized pharmacotherapy for obesity, with trials consistently demonstrating TBWL greater than 10% with these agents. Currently, pharmacologic treatment is recommended in patients with BMI greater than or equal to 27 with obesity related comorbidity or BMI greater than or equal to30 and should be continued if it meets appropriate weight loss standards of 5% TBWL at 3 months with tolerable side effect profile.[22] However, the major drawback of all pharmacologic interventions for obesity is rapid weight regain upon discontinuation of medications.[23] Moreover, long-term compliance with pharmacotherapy is poor, with 7% to 18% of patients discontinuing medications within 12 months in clinical trial.[24,25] In a more recent study looking at prescription refills, found that only 19% of patients were taking their anti-obesity medications at 12 months with the highest refill rate for semaglutide at 40% at 12 months.[26] Reasons for discontinuation include side effects, limited effectiveness, cost, and availability.[25,27]

Thus, there has been growing interest in combination of pharmacotherapy with anatomic interventions such as EBT and bariatric surgery. Combination therapy can be used for early inadequate weight loss, as a planned additive therapy to reach the patients goals, which would be otherwise unrealistic with EBT alone, or weight regain following EBT.

Phentermine is the oldest currently approved weight loss medication on the market but is currently only approved for short-term use (3 months). When combined with topiramate can be used long-term with good safety profile. Topiramate is also approved migraines and alcohol abuse making this medication combination especially favorable in these patient populations. There are multiple studies showing efficacy of phentermine

Table 1				
Weight loss and risks of endoscopic bariatric technology				
EBT	**TBWL 6 mns**	**TBWL 12 mns**	**TBWL 5 Year**	**Risks/Side Effects**
IGB[2]	13%	11%		Obstruction (0.8%), perforation (0.1%), pain, nausea, gastric ulcers
ESG[3,11,15]	8%–18%	15–16	15.9%	Gastric leak (0.5%), Gastric bleeding (0.5%), nausea, pain
POSE[17,18]	16%	5%–15%		Gastric bleeding, nausea, vomiting, pain
DBJL[19,20]		14.6%–18.9%	12%[a]	Nausea, vomiting, pain, obstruction, hepatic abscess (rare)
Aspire[21]		12.1%		Bleeding, infection, ulceration, indigestion, nausea, vomiting

[a] n dropped from 44 in original study to 15 at 4 year (2 year post explant).

and phentermine topiramate in bariatric surgery patients.[28–30] It is especially useful in patients with binge eating patterns, which can be common after bariatric surgery and EBT. A prospective study by Zilberstein and colleagues of 16 patients who underwent adjustable gastric banding (AGB) with post-operative binge eating behaviors found increase in EBWL from 20.9% to 34.1% after augmentation with topiramate.[31] A retrospective study by Schwartz colleagues was performed in patients who underwent either Roux-en-Y gastric bypass (RYGB) or LSG with phentermine or phentermine-topiramate lost 12% to 13% of excess body weight after 90 days of use.[30] Lastly, a study of patients undergoing LSG with BMI greater than 50 were assessed to see if peri- and post-operative use of phentermine-topiramate would improve weight loss outcomes. Patients were compared to historic controls. This study showed the mean BMI 2 years after LSG was 33.8 for patients on phentermine-topiramate versus 42 for historic controls.[32]

Orlistat has recently fallen out of favor due to poorer efficacy and malabsorption side effects. However, this medication is cheap and found over the counter so still has some utility for weight loss. It works via inhibition of gastric and pancreatic lipases causing poor fat absorption. This should be used very cautiously for patients at risk for malabsorption such as RYGB. A study by Zoss and colleagues on orlistat in AGB patients showed significant weight loss of 8 kg during an 8 month follow-up.[33]

Naltrexone-bupropion is also approved for weight loss. It is contraindicated in patients with severe hypertension, opioid use, or seizure disorders. Studies show improved inhibition and ability to resist cravings,[34] thus, it is especially good for food cravings and addictive behaviors. There are no studies directly assessing its use in the post-bariatric or EBT patients.

The newest medications to undergo approval are the incretin medications–Glucagon like peptide – 1 receptor agonists (GLP-1) and gastric inhibitory polypeptides (GIPs) receptor agonists. These include liraglutide (GLP-1) specifically at the 3 mg dose, semaglutide (GLP-1) specifically at the 2.4 mg dose and the newest, approved for weight loss November of 2023, is tirzepatide (GLP-1/GIP). While liraglutide has had modest weight loss benefits on par with previously approved anti-obesity medications, semaglutide and tirzepatide show staggering results with TBWL in the 15% to 20% (**Table 2**). The most recent incretin to be studied is Retatrutide, a GLP-1/GIP/Glucagon receptor, which is currently in phase 3 trials for weight loss. Preliminary phase 2 trials are very encouraging with weight loss on par with some bariatric surgeries.

Given the popularity of incretin medications, there have been significant enthusiasm and a growing body of evidence for use of these medications in conjunction with bariatric surgery and EBT. A small study by Caroline Hoff and colleagues of ESG alone or with semaglutide found significantly more weight loss in the semaglutide group that was on par with expected weight loss of an LSG.[39] A retrospective study by Badurdeen and colleagues on liraglutide use starting 5 months after ESG showed significant improvement in TBWL at 1 year after ESG of 20.5% in ESG alone and 24.7% in ESG plus liraglutide group.[13]

More limited data are available on the use of incretin medications in combination with IGB. Mosli and colleagues evaluated the use of liraglutide in patients treated with IGB; liraglutide was started 1 month after to balloon placement and continued until 1 month after balloon removal; they demonstrated improved weight loss with liraglutide plus IGB group over the IGB alone (18.5 vs 10.2 kg). However, after adjusting for cofounders, was no longer significant.[40] Interestingly, there was no increase in patient reported nausea, abdominal pain, heartburn, or early IGB removal in patients on liraglutide. Another study by Jense and colleagues found that 11.3% of patients undergoing IGB selected

Table 2
Summary of incretin medications in weight loss

Study	Medication	Number of Participants	Duration	Weight Loss (% TBWL)	>5% TBWL	>10% TBWL	FDA-Approved For Weight Loss
Pi-Sunyer et al,[35] 2015	Liraglutide 3.0 mg	3731	56 wk	8.0%	62.3%	33.1%	Yes at 3.0 mg
Garvey et al,[36] 2015	Liraglutide 3.0	396	56 wk	5.8%	51.8%	22.8%	Yes at 3.0 mg
Wilding et al,[24] 2021	Semaglutide 2.4 mg	1961	68 wk	14.9%	86.4%	69.1%	Yes at 2.4 mg
Jastreboff et al,[37] 2022	Tirzepatide	2539	72 wk				Yes
	5 mg			15%	85%	68.5%	
	10 mg			19.5%	89%	78.1%	
	15 mg			20.9%	91%	83.5%	
Jastreboff et al,[38] 2023	Retatrutide	338	48 wk				In phase 3 studies
	1 mg			8.7%	92%	75%	
	4 mg			17.1%	100%	91%	
	8 mg			22.8%	100%	93%	
	12 mg			24.2%			

combination therapy with an anti-obesity medication (89% chose liraglutide). Weight loss was found to be 12.6% TBWL at 12 weeks when IGB was combined with medication versus 11.6% TBWL with balloon alone.[41]

A study by Gala and colleagues looked at the real world data of patient prescribed anti-obesity medications (AOM) at any time within a year of their ESG.[42] They stratified by type GLP-1 versus non-GLP-1 AOM. After 24 months, there was no difference in TBWL between no AOM, GLP-1, and other AOMs. However, it is notable that this was a real world study and most patients prescribed AOMs were done due to weight recidivism or failure to lose weight to goal. Thus, this likely represents a positive outcome that patients who did not respond as intended to ESG could achieve intended response with addition of AOMs.

Multiple studies have been conducted on liraglutide post bariatric surgery (most commonly in RYGB or LSG), which show significant improvements in weight with liraglutide as compared with controls.[43–47] Interestingly, when compared to patients taking liraglutide who have not undergone bariatric surgery to patients on liraglutide who have undergone bariatric surgery, there was no difference in gastrointestinal side effects.[46] It is also notable that patients with prior bariatric surgery taking liraglutide versus placebo, there was also no significant increase in gastrointestinal side effects.[45] A study by Lautenbach and colleagues[48] with use of semaglutide in patients with prior RYGB or LSG with inadequate weight loss or weight regain showed 10.3% TBWL 6 months after the initiation of semaglutide. There was no difference in weight loss in patients with inadequate weight loss or weight regain or based on type of bariatric surgery (**Table 3**).

APPROACH TO COMBINATION OF PHARMACOLOGIC AND ENDOSCOPIC THERAPY

The decision to combine pharmacologic and endoscopic therapy for weight loss should be made on an individual basis with communication with the patient. It is important to understand patient goals and medical comorbidities when deciding on the ideal approach. The physician and patient need to be realistic about the expected weight loss with EBTs along with the side effects and indefinite use expected for pharmacologic therapy. Multiple studies have shown the additive effects of medications with bariatric surgery, which can be extrapolated to EBTs, as well as a few studies on the use of pharmacologic agents to augment EBTs. Various degrees of weight loss are associated with improvement in a variety of medical co-morbidities (**Table 4**). Pharmacologic therapy can be added for increased weight loss.

Timing and selection of pharmacologic therapy should be based on patients' comorbidities and desired weight loss. Both the total amount of weight loss and other indications or side effects of medications can be used to determine which medications are best in augmentation for each individual patient (**Table 5**).

If EBT alone is not expected to allow patient to reach desired weight loss, it may be prudent to plan augmentation in the peri-procedure period.[32,40] Alternatively, studies in bariatric surgery patients have found that augmentation at weight plateau led to more successful outcomes then when used after weight recidivism.[61–63] Therefore, it is important to assess patients throughout their weight loss journey and offer pharmacologic therapy at plateau if they have not reached desired weight loss rather than just after weight regain. Medications need to be timed to avoid excessive side effects. The incretin medications are known to cause gastrointestinal side effects and may need to consider holding or not starting these medications until 4 to 6 weeks after EBTs that are also expected to cause negative gastrointestinal side effects.[40] However, overall, these medications appear to be just as well-tolerated in the bariatric surgery

Table 3
Review of studies on pharmacotherapy augmentation after bariatric surgery or endoscopic bariatric procedures

Study	Bariatric Procedure	Medication	Number of Participants	Duration	Additional Weight Loss (kg)	Additional Weight Loss vs TWBL vs EBWL
Schwartz et al,[30] 2016	RYGB or LABG	Phentermine	52	90 d	6.35	12.8%EBWL
		Phentermine-topiramate	13		3.81	12.9% EBWL
Zoss et al,[33] 2002	LABG	Orlistat 120 mg TID	38	8 mn	8	
Wharton et al,[44] 2019	RYGB, LABG, LSG	Liraglutide 3 mg	117	1 year	6.3	5.5% TBWL
Suliman et al,[46] 2019	Any bariatric surgery	Liraglutide	188	16 wk	6	6.1% TBWL
Pajecki et al,[47] 2013	Any Bariatric surgery	Liraglutide	15	8–28 wk	7.5	
Gazda et al,[49] 2021	Any bariatric surgery	Any GLP-1	207	9 mn		6.9% TBWL
Jensen et al,[50] 2023	Any bariatric surgery	Liraglutide	50	6 mn		7.3% TBWL
		Semaglutide				9.8% TBWL
Lautenbach et al,[48] 2022	RYGB or LSG	Semaglutide	44	6 mn		10.3% TBWL
Mosli et al,[40] 2017	IGB	Liraglutide	108	12 mn	8 kg[a]	
Mehta et al,[51] 2023	IGB	Any anti-obesity medication (AOM)	102	12		2.9% TBWL
Badurdeen et al,[13] 2021	ESG	Liraglutide	52	12 mn		4% TBWL
Gala et al,[42] 2024	ESG	Any AOM	1506	24 mn		No difference

[a] After look at cofounding variables, no difference in mean weight loss between participants who used liraglutide.

Table 4	
Weight loss required for disease remission or clinically significant improvement[52–55]	
Disease	**%TBWL**
Diabetes prevention	2%–5%
Hypertriglyceridemia	2%–5%
Elevated systolic blood pressure	2%–5%
Polycystic ovarian syndrome	2%–10%
Metabolic Associated Steatotic Liver Disease	5%
Established diabetes	5%–10%
Elevated diastolic blood pressure	5%–10%
Hyperlipidemia	5%–10%
Urinary incontinence	5%–10%
Sexual dysfunction	5%–10%
Obstructive sleep apnea	10%
Metabolic liver disease – fibrosis regression	10%
Knee osteoarthritis	10%–20%

population as the non-bariatric surgery population.[45,46] Further, the specific class of medications should be picked based on patient comorbidities, eating patterns, and side effect profile. Overall, the combination of pharmacologic and endoscopic treatment for obesity can be very successful and provide not only desired weight loss for patients but also improve or ameliorate medical co-morbidities.

Multiple pharmacologic agents are available for diabetes including both FDA and non-FDA approved medications for weight loss. Combining a pharmacologic therapy for diabetes that also causes weight loss is a widely accepted augmentation strategy to both bariatric surgeries and EBTs.[13,63] GLP-1 agonists Liraglutide and Semaglutide are both approved for weight loss and diabetes although at different doses. However, weight loss is seen even at the approved diabetic doses to a lesser extent.[22] Tirzepatide is now approved in both diabetes and obesity. Other diabetic medications are available that are not FDA-approved for obesity but show modest weight loss. Both metformin and sodium-glucose co-transporter 2 (SGLT-2) inhibitors lead to very modest weight loss but are approved for diabetes. SGLT-2 inhibitors are also approved for cardiovascular disease.[64–66] While these medications have less weight loss efficacy, their price and side effect profile may be ideal for some patients.

Naltrexone-bupropion can be used in patients with mild depression, binge eating disorder, and alcohol and nicotine abuse. Its weight loss mechanism is thought to be due to decreasing food cravings.[67] This can be especially helpful in patients with high oral intake due to cravings, which can cause failure of adequate weight loss in ESG, sleeve gastrectomy, and gastric bypass due to dilation of the gastric sleeve or pouch. Naltrexone is an opioid receptor antagonist and should not be used in the direct peri-procedural period if opioids are expected to be needed for pain control.

Phentermine-topiramate can be used for patients with headaches but also the topiramate component has been shown to be helpful in binge eating disorder.[68] Topiramate; however, is not FDA-approved for binge eating disorder, and use with this indication would be considered off-label. Studies in sleeve gastrectomy have shown that patients with binge eating disorders or loss of control of eating often do worse post operation including less weight loss.[69] This can be extrapolated to patients with EBTs such as ESG. Another study of topiramate use in patient is laparoscopic

Table 5
Review of currently Food and Drug Administration-approved medications for weight loss

	% TBWL	% Achieving 5% TWBL[56]	% Achieving 10% TBWL[56]	Approved Conditions Other than Obesity	Side Effects	Contraindications
Phentermine[57]	7.4	96[a]	63[a]		Tachycardia, hypertension, tremor, anxiety, dry mouth, constipation	Cardiovascular disease, hyperthyroidism, Gluacoma
Phentermine-Topiramate[58]	9.8	67–70	47–48	Migraines, alcohol abuse	As above + insomnia, cognitive side effects	As above + nephrolithiasis, pregnancy
Orlistat[59]	9.6[b]	44–51	14–29		Abdominal pain, steatorrhea	Malabsorptive conditions
Naltrexone-buproprion[60]	6.1	45–51	19–28	Alcohol use disorder, nicotine use, mild depression	Headache, nausea, vomiting, constipation	Use of opioid narcotics, seizures (and conditions that lower seizure threshold)
Liraglutide (3 mg)[35,36,56]	8.4	50–73	25–37	Diabetes, cardiovascular risk reduction	Nausea, vomiting, diarrhea, constipation, abdominal pain	MEN-2, medullary thyroid cancer, pancreatitis, gastroparesis
Semaglutide (2.4 mg)	14.9	86.4	69.1	As above	As above	As above
Tirzepatide (15 mg)[37]	20.9	91	83.9	Diabetes	Nausea, vomiting, constipation, abdominal pain	MEN-2, medullary thyroid cancer

[a] High placebo weight loss in this study as well with > 20% with 5% or more TBWL.
[b] Only 3% TBWL in placebo controlled trials.

AGB with inadequate weight loss and binge eating patterns that were prescribed topiramate had improved EBWL from 20.9% to 34.1%.[31] Patients should be screened for eating disorders such as binge eating disorders prior to EBT but even in patients who have already undergone EBT, ongoing screening for eating disorders should be done and treated if appropriate.

SUMMARY

EBT has now been firmly established as a safe and effective treatment for patients with obesity. While EBT still lag surgery with regard to weight loss efficacy the combination of EBT with AOMs holds significant promise for obtaining weight loss comparably to that seen with weight loss surgery and can be used for patients with inadequate weight loss after EBT or weight regain after EBT. Moreover, EBT may help to reduce the typical weight regain, which occurs in patients who have lost weight with AOMs and wish to wean off medications.

CLINICS CARE POINTS

- The combination of endoscopic and pharmacologic interventions for obesity can provide greater weight loss then ether intervention alone, providing weight loss on par with surgical interventions.
- Understanding the pharmacology and side effect profile of anti-obesity medications is critical to maximizing effectiveness, minimize side effects and avoiding premature discontinuation.

DISCLOSURE

The authors have nothing to disclosures.

REFERENCES

1. ASGE Bariatric Endoscopy Task Force, Sullivan S, Kumar N, et al. ASGE position statement on endoscopic bariatric therapies in clinical practice. Gastrointest Endosc 2015;82(5):767–72.
2. Ibrahim Mohamed BK, Barajas-Gamboa JS, Rodriguez J. Endoscopic Bariatric Therapies: Current Status and Future Perspectives. Jsls 2022;26(1).
3. Goyal H, Kopel J, Perisetti A, et al. Endobariatric procedures for obesity: clinical indications and available options. Therapeutic Advances in Gastrointestinal Endoscopy 2021;14. 2631774520984627.
4. Kim SH, Chun HJ, Choi HS, et al. Current status of intragastric balloon for obesity treatment. World J Gastroenterol 2016;22(24):5495–504.
5. Kozłowska-Petriczko K, Pawlak KM, Wojciechowska K, et al. The Efficacy Comparison of Endoscopic Bariatric Therapies: 6-Month Versus 12-Month Intragastric Balloon Versus Endoscopic Sleeve Gastroplasty. Obes Surg 2023;33(2):498–505.
6. Shah R, Davitkov P, Abu Dayyeh BK, et al. AGA Technical Review on Intragastric Balloons in the Management of Obesity. Gastroenterology 2021;160(5):1811–30.
7. Ashrafian H, Monnich M, Braby TS, et al. Intragastric balloon outcomes in super-obesity: a 16-year city center hospital series. Surg Obes Relat Dis 2018;14(11):1691–9.
8. Kotzampassi K, Grosomanidis V, Papakostas P, et al. 500 intragastric balloons: what happens 5 years thereafter? Obes Surg 2012;22(6):896–903.

9. Abu Dayyeh BK, Acosta A, Camilleri M, et al. Endoscopic Sleeve Gastroplasty Alters Gastric Physiology and Induces Loss of Body Weight in Obese Individuals. Clin Gastroenterol Hepatol 2017;15(1):37–43.e1.

10. Abu Dayyeh BK, Bazerbachi F, Vargas EJ, et al. Endoscopic sleeve gastroplasty for treatment of class 1 and 2 obesity (MERIT): a prospective, multicentre, randomised trial. Lancet 2022;400(10350):441–51.

11. Hedjoudje A, Abu Dayyeh BK, Cheskin LJ, et al. Efficacy and Safety of Endoscopic Sleeve Gastroplasty: A Systematic Review and Meta-Analysis. Clin Gastroenterol Hepatol 2020;18(5):1043–53.e4.

12. Abu Dayyeh BK, Acosta A, Camilleri M, et al. Endoscopic Sleeve Gastroplasty Alters Gastric Physiology and Induces Loss of Body Weight in Obese Individuals. Clin Gastroenterol Hepatol 2017;15(1):37–43.e1.

13. Badurdeen D, Hoff AC, Hedjoudje A, et al. Endoscopic sleeve gastroplasty plus liraglutide versus endoscopic sleeve gastroplasty alone for weight loss. Gastrointest Endosc 2021;93(6):1316–24.e1.

14. Storm AC, Abu Dayyeh BK, Topazian M. Endobariatrics: A Primer. Clin Gastroenterol Hepatol 2018;16(11):1701–4.

15. Sharaiha RZ, Hajifathalian K, Kumar R, et al. Five-Year Outcomes of Endoscopic Sleeve Gastroplasty for the Treatment of Obesity. Clin Gastroenterol Hepatol 2021;19(5):1051–7.e2.

16. Bhandari M, Kosta S, Reddy M, et al. Four-year outcomes for endoscopic sleeve gastroplasty from a single centre in India. J Minim Access Surg 2023;19(1):101–6.

17. Sullivan S, Swain JM, Woodman G, et al. Randomized sham-controlled trial evaluating efficacy and safety of endoscopic gastric plication for primary obesity: The ESSENTIAL trial. Obesity (Silver Spring) 2017;25(2):294–301.

18. Lopez-Nava G, Asokkumar R, Turró Arau R, et al. Modified primary obesity surgery endoluminal (POSE-2) procedure for the treatment of obesity. VideoGIE 2020;5(3):91–3.

19. Betzel B, Cooiman MI, Aarts EO, et al. Clinical follow-up on weight loss, glycemic control, and safety aspects of 24 months of duodenal-jejunal bypass liner implantation. Surg Endosc 2020;34(1):209–15.

20. Jirapinyo P, Haas AV, Thompson CC. Effect of the Duodenal-Jejunal Bypass Liner on Glycemic Control in Patients With Type 2 Diabetes With Obesity: A Meta-analysis With Secondary Analysis on Weight Loss and Hormonal Changes. Diabetes Care 2018;41(5):1106–15.

21. Thompson CC, Abu Dayyeh BK, Kushner R, et al. Percutaneous Gastrostomy Device for the Treatment of Class II and Class III Obesity: Results of a Randomized Controlled Trial. Am J Gastroenterol 2017;112(3):447–57.

22. Apovian CM, Aronne LJ, Bessesen DH, et al. Pharmacological Management of Obesity: An Endocrine Society Clinical Practice Guideline. J Clin Endocrinol Metabol 2015;100(2):342–62.

23. Wilding JPH, Batterham RL, Davies M, et al. Weight regain and cardiometabolic effects after withdrawal of semaglutide: The STEP 1 trial extension. Diabetes Obes Metabol 2022;24(8):1553–64.

24. Wilding JPH, Batterham RL, Calanna S, et al. Once-Weekly Semaglutide in Adults with Overweight or Obesity. N Engl J Med 2021;384(11):989–1002.

25. Khera R, Murad MH, Chandar AK, et al. Association of Pharmacological Treatments for Obesity With Weight Loss and Adverse Events: A Systematic Review and Meta-analysis. JAMA 2016;315(22):2424–34.

26. Gasoyan H, Pfoh ER, Schulte R, et al. Early- and later-stage persistence with antiobesity medications: A retrospective cohort study. Obesity 2024;32(3):486–93.

27. Chakhtoura M, Haber R, Ghezzawi M, et al. Pharmacotherapy of obesity: an update on the available medications and drugs under investigation. eClinicalMedicine 2023;58.

28. Lucas E, Simmons O, Tchang B, et al. Pharmacologic management of weight regain following bariatric surgery. Front Endocrinol (Lausanne) 2022;13:1043595.

29. Edgerton C, Mehta M, Mou D, et al. Patterns of Weight Loss Medication Utilization and Outcomes Following Bariatric Surgery. J Gastrointest Surg 2021;25(2): 369–77.

30. Schwartz J, Chaudhry UI, Suzo A, et al. Pharmacotherapy in Conjunction with a Diet and Exercise Program for the Treatment of Weight Recidivism or Weight Loss Plateau Post-bariatric Surgery: a Retrospective Review. Obes Surg 2016;26(2): 452–8.

31. Zilberstein B, Pajecki D, Garcia de Brito AC, et al. Topiramate after adjustable gastric banding in patients with binge eating and difficulty losing weight. Obes Surg 2004;14(6):802–5.

32. Ard JD, Beavers DP, Hale E, et al. Use of phentermine-topiramate extended release in combination with sleeve gastrectomy in patients with BMI 50 kg/m(2) or more. Surg Obes Relat Dis 2019;15(7):1039–43.

33. Zoss I, Piec G, Horber FF. Impact of orlistat therapy on weight reduction in morbidly obese patients after implantation of the Swedish adjustable gastric band. Obes Surg 2002;12(1):113–7.

34. Roberts CA, Christiansen P, Halford JCG. Pharmaceutical approaches to weight management: behavioural mechanisms of action. Current Opinion in Physiology 2019;12:26–32.

35. Pi-Sunyer X, Astrup A, Fujioka K, et al. A randomized, controlled trial of 3.0 mg of liraglutide in weight management. N Engl J Med 2015;373(1):11–22.

36. Garvey WT, Birkenfeld AL, Dicker D, et al. Efficacy and safety of Liraglutide 3.0 mg in individuals with overweight or obesity and type 2 diabetes treated with basal insulin: the SCALE insulin randomized controlled trial. Diabetes Care 2020;43(5):1085–93.

37. Jastreboff AM, Aronne LJ, Ahmad NN, et al. Tirzepatide Once Weekly for the Treatment of Obesity. N Engl J Med 2022;387(3):205–16.

38. Jastreboff AM, Kaplan LM, Frías JP, et al. Triple–Hormone-Receptor Agonist Retatrutide for Obesity — A Phase 2 Trial. N Engl J Med 2023;389(6):514–26.

39. Carolina Hoff A, Barrichello S, Badurdeen D, et al. ID: 3492486 Semaglutide in association to endoscopic sleeve gastroplasty: taking endoscopic batriatric procedures outcomes to the next level. Gastrointest Endosc 2021;93(6):AB6–7.

40. Mosli MM, Elyas M. *Does combining liraglutide with intragastric balloon insertion improve sustained weight reduction?* Saudi. J Gastroenterol 2017;23(2):117–22.

41. Jense MTF, Palm-Meinders IH, Sanders B, et al. The Swallowable Intragastric Balloon Combined with Lifestyle Coaching: Short-Term Results of a Safe and Effective Weight Loss Treatment for People Living with Overweight and Obesity. Obes Surg 2023;33(6):1668–75.

42. Gala K, Ghusn W, Brunaldi V, et al. Outcomes of concomitant antiobesity medication use with endoscopic sleeve gastroplasty in clinical US settings. Obesity Pillars 2024;11:100112.

43. Miras AD, Pérez-Pevida B, Aldhwayan M, et al. Adjunctive liraglutide treatment in patients with persistent or recurrent type 2 diabetes after metabolic surgery

(GRAVITAS): a randomised, double-blind, placebo-controlled trial. Lancet Diabetes Endocrinol 2019;7(7):549–59.

44. Wharton S, Kuk JL, Luszczynski M, et al. Liraglutide 3.0 mg for the management of insufficient weight loss or excessive weight regain post-bariatric surgery. Clin Obes 2019;9(4):e12323.

45. Thakur U, Bhansali A, Gupta R, et al. Liraglutide Augments Weight Loss After Laparoscopic Sleeve Gastrectomy: a Randomised, Double-Blind, Placebo-Control Study. Obes Surg 2021;31(1):84–92.

46. Suliman M, Buckley A, Al Tikriti A, et al. Routine clinical use of liraglutide 3 mg for the treatment of obesity: Outcomes in non-surgical and bariatric surgery patients. Diabetes Obes Metabol 2019;21(6):1498–501.

47. Pajecki D, Halpern A, Cercato C, et al. Short-term use of liraglutide in the management of patients with weight regain after bariatric surgery. Rev Col Bras Cir 2013;40(3):191–5.

48. Lautenbach A, Wernecke M, Huber TB, et al. The Potential of Semaglutide Once-Weekly in Patients Without Type 2 Diabetes with Weight Regain or Insufficient Weight Loss After Bariatric Surgery-a Retrospective Analysis. Obes Surg 2022; 32(10):3280–8.

49. Gazda CL, Clark JD, Lingvay I, et al. Pharmacotherapies for Post-Bariatric Weight Regain: Real-World Comparative Outcomes. Obesity (Silver Spring) 2021;29(5): 829–36.

50. Jensen AB, Renström F, Aczél S, et al. Efficacy of the Glucagon-Like Peptide-1 Receptor Agonists Liraglutide and Semaglutide for the Treatment of Weight Regain After Bariatric surgery: a Retrospective Observational Study. Obes Surg 2023;33(4):1017–25.

51. Mehta A, Shah S, Dawod E, et al. Impact of Adjunctive Pharmacotherapy With Intragastric Balloons for the Treatment of Obesity. The American Surgeon™ 2023; 89(4):707–13.

52. Ryan DH, Yockey SR. Weight Loss and Improvement in Comorbidity: Differences at 5%, 10%, 15%, and Over. Curr Obes Rep 2017;6(2):187–94.

53. Wing RR, Lang W, Wadden TA, et al. Benefits of modest weight loss in improving cardiovascular risk factors in overweight and obese individuals with type 2 diabetes. Diabetes Care 2011;34(7):1481–6.

54. Glass LM, Dickson RC, Anderson JC, et al. Total body weight loss of $\geq$ 10 % is associated with improved hepatic fibrosis in patients with nonalcoholic steatohepatitis. Dig Dis Sci 2015;60(4):1024–30.

55. Messier SP, Resnik AE, Beavers DP, et al. Intentional Weight Loss in Overweight and Obese Patients With Knee Osteoarthritis: Is More Better? Arthritis Care Res (Hoboken) 2018;70(11):1569–75.

56. Ard J, Fitch A, Fruh S, et al. Weight Loss and Maintenance Related to the Mechanism of Action of Glucagon-Like Peptide 1 Receptor Agonists. Adv Ther 2021; 38(6):2821–39.

57. Li Z, Hong K, Yip I, et al. Body weight loss with phentermine alone versus phentermine and fenfluramine with very-low-calorie diet in an outpatient obesity management program: a retrospective study. Curr Ther Res Clin Exp 2003;64(7): 447–60.

58. Allison DB, Gadde KM, Garvey WT, et al. Controlled-release phentermine/topiramate in severely obese adults: a randomized controlled trial (EQUIP). Obesity (Silver Spring) 2012;20(2):330–42.

59. Drew BS, Dixon AF, Dixon JB. Obesity management: update on orlistat. Vasc Health Risk Manag 2007;3(6):817–21.

60. Greenway F, Fujioka K, Plodkowski RA, et al. Effect of naltrexone plus bupropion on weight loss in overweight and obese adults (COR-I): A multicentre, randomised, double-blind, placebo-controlled, phase 3 trial. Lancet 2010;376:595–605.

61. Toth AT, Gomez G, Shukla AP, et al. Weight Loss Medications in Young Adults after Bariatric Surgery for Weight Regain or Inadequate Weight Loss: A Multi-Center Study. Children (Basel) 2018;5(9).

62. Stanford FC, Toth AT, Shukla AP, et al. Weight Loss Medications in Older Adults After Bariatric Surgery for Weight Regain or Inadequate Weight Loss: A Multicenter Study. Bariatr Surg Pract Patient Care 2018;13(4):171–8.

63. Stanford FC, Alfaris N, Gomez G, et al. The utility of weight loss medications after bariatric surgery for weight regain or inadequate weight loss: A multi-center study. Surg Obes Relat Dis 2017;13(3):491–500.

64. Pereira MJ, Eriksson JW. Emerging Role of SGLT-2 Inhibitors for the Treatment of Obesity. Drugs 2019;79(3):219–30.

65. Heidenreich PA, Bozkurt B, Aguilar D, et al. 2022 AHA/ACC/HFSA Guideline for the Management of Heart Failure: A Report of the American College of Cardiology/American Heart Association Joint Committee on Clinical Practice Guidelines. Circulation 2022;145(18):e895–1032.

66. Yerevanian A, Soukas AA. Metformin: Mechanisms in Human Obesity and Weight Loss. Curr Obes Rep 2019;8(2):156–64.

67. Wang GJ, Zhao J, Tomasi D, et al. Effect of combined naltrexone and bupropion therapy on the brain's functional connectivity. Int J Obes (Lond) 2018;42(11):1890–9.

68. Guerdjikova AI, Williams S, Blom TJ, et al. Combination Phentermine-Topiramate Extended Release for the Treatment of Binge Eating Disorder: An Open-Label, Prospective Study. Innov Clin Neurosci 2018;15(5–6):17–21.

69. Anbara T. The impacts of eating disorders on sleeve gastrectomy outcomes. Surgery in Practice and Science 2023;13:100165.

How to Build an Endobariatric Practice
Set Up, Branding, and Marketing

Janese Laster, MD[a],*, Marianna Papademetriou, MD[b]

KEYWORDS

- Endobariatric practice • Bariatric endoscopy • Obesity • Nutrition • Branding
- Marketing

KEY POINTS

Beginning a practice in endobariatrics can be a challenging undertaking. Here, the authors outline the important steps to transitioning into a practice in endobariatrics geared towards gastroenterologists interested in weight management.

- This article discusses how to obtain adequate training in both technical skills and post-procedure management.
- This article also discusses how to research targeted patient demographics.
- The authors explain how to brand, market, and advertise.
- It highlights the importance of building a network of advisors.

INTRODUCTION

In the United States, the prevalence of obesity has increased from 30.5% in 1999 to 2000 to 41.7% in 2017 to 2020 according to National Health and Nutrition Examination Survey data.[1] Proportionally, there has been a rise in obesity-related comorbidities including diabetes, hypertension, and hyperlipidemia.[2] Obesity is a complex disease with layered signaling pathways for appetite stimulation and satiation and increased or decreased energy expenditure. Most experts agree obesity is caused by an interplay of environmental factors, food availability, increased processed food intake, genetics and epigenetics, physical activity, cultural cues, medication side effects, psychological stress, and other factors. For decades, the mainstay for treatment has been limited to diet, exercise, and lifestyle changes. Bariatric surgery has become a crucial element in obesity management; however, the uptake has stagnated in the last 20 years.[3] Over the same time frame, endoscopic bariatric and metabolic therapies (EBMTs), which offer a less invasive approach than bariatric surgery, have gained

[a] Georgetown University Medical Center; Gut Theory Total Digestive Care, 1712 North Street Northwest Suite 101, Washington, DC 20036, USA; [b] Georgetown University Medical Center, Washington DC VA Medical Center, 50 Irving Street Northwest, Washington, DC 20422, USA
* Corresponding author.
E-mail address: jlaster@guttheoryhealth.com

Gastrointest Endoscopy Clin N Am 34 (2024) 757–763
https://doi.org/10.1016/j.giec.2024.04.003
1052-5157/24/© 2024 Elsevier Inc. All rights reserved.

steady momentum in research and commercial domains. EBMTs which in the United States currently includes, intragastric balloons and endoscopic sleeve gastroplasty (ESG), have been shown to be safe and effective for weight loss and reversing obesity-related comorbidities.[4,5] The gastric balloon is indicated for those with a body mass index (BMI) greater than 30 to 40 kg/m^2 and ESG for those with a BMI greater than 30 to 50 kg/m^2, in addition to diet and lifestyle changes. Unfortunately, many gastroenterologists lack exposure to endobariatric procedures during their standard fellowship training. Furthermore, practical skills including business strategy, marketing, and economic planning are not part of a standard fellowship curriculum. Physicians with an interest in bariatric endoscopy need additional resources to facilitate a successful practice that includes EBMTs. Ultimately, increasing the number of gastreonterologists trained in EBMTs will improve access to these important therapeutics for patients.

How to Transition to Endobariatrics

There are multiple preliminary factors to consider prior to starting an endobariatrics practice.[6] Many of the initial decisions depend on the desired practice setting. This may be within an academic center, group practice, or as a solo practitioner. Each practice space has its own unique start up challenges (**Fig. 1**).

The following background steps are necessary considerations.

1. Obtain adequate technical procedural training and knowledge in postop care management.
2. Research the patient population to ensure there is a reasonable market for out-of-pocket procedures and utilize this to build a business plan.
3. Market and advertise new procedures and services to patients and referring physicians.
4. Build a network of mentors to advise.

In the following sections, we explore some of these important decisions in more detail.

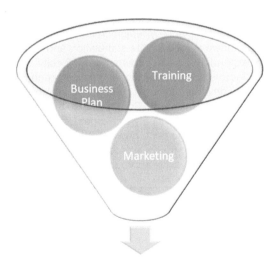

Endobariatrics Practice

Fig. 1. Necessary components to build a endobariatrics practice.

Obtaining Exposure, Mentorship, and Training

Access to training in bariatric endoscopy can prove difficult within the confines of a designated 3-year gastroenterology fellowship. Therefore, many physicians will need supplemental exposure opportunities during or after fellowship training. A traditional structured advanced fellowship in an institution with an endobariatrics program is ideal; however, limited opportunities are available. Many physicians obtain training after fellowship through alternative means. As newer technologies emerge, practicing physicians will need to seek ongoing training experiences to learn newer or more advanced techniques beyond fellowship training. Additionally, training opportunities with international experts are available abroad, although these are often self-funded. Device manufacturers also offer hands-on training courses and may offer proctorship arrangements with experts at high-volume centers. Additionally, the Association of Bariatric Endoscopy, a subdivision of the American Society of Gastroenterology Endoscopy,[7] offers a hands-on training course that allows the participant to encounter proctoring and obtain certification in advanced bariatric procedures, including suturing.

Training in nutrition and weight management is also limited during fellowship years. An understanding of nutrition, obesity management, and obesity pharmacologic therapy is important for optimal patient outcomes. This training may be obtained through formal dedicated nutrition, obesity medicine, or endobariatric fellowships or by attending courses, lectures, workshops, and procedural proctoring by mentors. There are board certifications for nutrition through the National Board of Physician Nutrition, certification examination for nutrition Specialist; or obesity medicine through the American Board of Obesity Medicine and the American College of Lifestyle Medicine. In addition to providing necessary background knowledge for appropriate patient care, these board certifications may also help with marketing one's unique skill set.

For the physician who has already completed fellowship or a fellow who is unable to train within one of these programs, consider the following options: (a) contact those programs to set up shadowing experiences, (b) attend hands-on courses, (c) attend lectures both virtually and in person to learn risks, benefits, new techniques, data, and complications from experts, and (d) research regional device representatives for local mobile laboratories that offer hands-on experiences. Representatives can also provide information on how to become certified to obtain equipment, and on being proctored or assisted during live cases for experience.

Research Your Patient Population and Create a Business Plan

In all practice settings, start by considering the patient population in the location of practice. Use the electronic medical record data to determine the proportion of patients with weight-related medical comorbidities and those that may benefit from EBMTs. Research publicly available city and neighborhood data on obesity prevalence rates to determine the potential patient pool. Evaluate for local competing practices in the private and academic sector and potential referral pool for each site. Seek out the local small business association (SBA) office to obtain free data on local marketing trends. Use these data to create a business plan based on the population's needs. A business plan template can be found online (eg, Liveplan. com) to provide a step-by-step guide to incorporate the necessary information. This typically includes sections on opportunity, patient population, target market, competitors, practice advantage/solution, marketing, advertising and sales plan, operations, key metrics and milestones, and financial forecasts. This business plan will provide a financial outlook when presenting for approval from an academic center or group practice, or to obtain financing from banking institutions for a solo practice.

Getting Started in Different Practice Settings

Solo practice

The first step is often finding the ideal practice location. The target municipality's SBA can be an invaluable resource. There, utilize statistics for each neighborhood to consider the ideal location of the future practice to include demographics such as education, income, marital status, and so forth. Research the region's prevalence of obesity and overweight populations. The summary of this information can be utilized to determine the best practice location.

The SBA can also provide information on how to create a business plan, best modes of marketing in the area, and how to think about obtaining funding that may be location specific. Next, it is prudent to identify market competitors in the area such as weight loss clinics, bariatric surgeons, and other endobariatric practices. Research potential referral physician groups in the area which may include plastic surgeons, gynecologist, fertility specialist, hepatologist, orthopedic surgeons, and primary care physicians. Choosing to partner with a local bariatric surgeon may be mutually beneficial for referrals and comprehensive care.

A health care law firm may file appropriate documents for a medical practice and provide legal advice and assistance in the formation of legal entities. They will help with applying for the name of your practice and determining the most appropriate legal entity type. Other document requirements will vary by state.

Work with an insurance broker for both malpractice and personal liability insurance quotes to compare and pick the best coverage for the practice area. Work with device representatives for information on equipment pricing, certification, and sample start up documents for pre-procedure and post-procedure care.

Research local ambulatory centers to apply for privileges to complete endobariatric procedures. Although most procedures are done on an outpatient basis, it is also important to identify a local hospital to obtain privileges as well to admit patients if needed in the future.

Private practice

In a private practice setting, many of the aforementioned steps for initial set up are already completed. Here, the initial step is to audit the current patient population for those that would be potential candidates for this service. This information can be used as a needs assessment for a business plan. Create a full business plan to include costs of equipment, cost of procedure, overall revenue for practice, and plan for follow-up, including the use of additional support services such as dieticians. Each practice may differ in the process for device approval; therefore, inquire with the office manager for the steps of approval. Keep in mind that the lead time for device acquisition may be considerable. This wait time can be utilized efficiently for patient recruitment and workup. Discuss with the office manager about changes in schedule timing for these patients and possible insurance reimbursement codes for visits versus cash—pay bundle.

Hospital-based or academic center

Joining an established bariatric center and academic practice involves different steps than solo practice. Having the support of the division/department chairs in gastroenterology and surgery is optimal for moving forward toward a common goal. Assuming that the center already has an established bariatric surgery program, the business plan will allow for demonstration as to how new services will fit optimally to provide access to novel techniques and services. Other important stakeholders are dieticians, psychologists, endoscopy techs, other gastroenterologists, anesthesiologists, coders/billers, and administrators, all of whom are already employed by the institution. Each discipline will need a new process for how to assess and accommodate additional patient referrals. Some specialists may not be familiar with EBMTs, and an introduction to the procedures, outcomes, and appropriate patients may also be needed.

Key items of discussion include block time for a dedicated clinic, endoscopy time utilization, and administrative time for necessary start-up meetings. Support staff asssitance may also be crucial to handle patient questions, symptom management, and follow-up. It should be noted that procedures may take longer earlier on in the endoscopist's practice and this may need to be accommodated in calculations for endoscopy time utilization. Since many private insurance companies do not cover endoscopic bariatric procedures, a fee structure will need to be established. Additionally, support from institutional billers and administrative staff can be utilized to provide patient letters and communicate with peer reviewers to obtain prior authorizations.[7]

A reasonable approach to establishing presence within a medical center community is to begin with referrals for endoscopic revisions. These patients are at higher risk for surgical interventions when compared to risks associated to primary bariatric surgery. Therefore, endoscopic revisions often offer lower risk for the patient.[8] Certain patients who qualify for primary obesity surgery likewise may elect to avoid surgery. Surgical colleagues may provide a significant patient referral base once appropriate patient characteristics are established.

Lastly, utilize the available infrastructure of the academic institution to increase referrals. This may include grand rounds presentations to share information about EBMTs with other subspecialties, and increase awareness of your expertise and novel techniques. New consults can also be created in the electronic medical record that include patient selection criteria to streamline referrals.

Branding

Branding is not often a focus during training for the new physician. Nevertheless, branding is crucial for recognition and can play an important role in the success of a practice.[9–11] For a new solo practice, the first step is to work with an agency that helps with building a brand personality. The agency should assist with selection of color palette, brand characteristics, logo, and tagline development, in addition to research of competitor palettes. Brand esthetics should suit the clinician and practice owner as well as appeal to the targeted patient population. Many details may be outside the typical repertoire of the practicing physician but are critically important to consider. For example, understanding the significance of color choices and the responses they evoke. Examples used by design firms include choosing red for power, love, excitement, and strength or black for elegance, luxury, classic, and sophistication. Additionally, the logo and font used both add to the brand characteristic to attract the targeted demographic. Examples include choices that lean more mature or youthful, masculine or feminine, and traditional or modern. An agency will help to consider the intended emotional response and the message conveyed through advertising to potential patients. Ultimately, the brand should tell the story of the practice.

If within a private practice or academic center, it will be crucial to meet with the marketing and branding team to understand the current brand guidelines. University or practice reputation locally and more broadly can greatly impact marketing of services.

Marketing/Advertising

For solo practice, use information from the SBA to understand the demographic of the target patient population and advertising and conversion data to determine best marketing mediums. Examples include radio, television, Web site banners and ads, social media–sponsored ads, podcasts, Google paid ads, local newspaper and magazine ads, local newsletters, local email lists, patient discussion board advertising, popular blog advertisements, and physician list servs. It remains important to calculate the cost of each modality of advertisement and to keep track of the analytics to determine the best return on investment for your specific area and practice. It takes time to collect data to assess the number of leads to conversion to patients. This will allow for fine tuning in real time on a monthly or quarterly basis.

In a private practice and academic center, adequate department support is needed to advocate for receiving the appropriate advertising budget to attract new patients. There may be restrictions on the types of marketing available due to hospital and practice regulations. Utilize the established university or practice group reputation in marketing strategies as name recognition can facilitate patient selection and may inform patient preferences.

A practical way to build a referral base is to provide informational and educational didactics to primary care, endocrinology, gynecology, and other relevant groups. This can be in the setting of a grand rounds or lunchtime lectures. Consider patient referrals both within the established center from other physicians or clinicians in your group, and from affiliated, or outside, networks. Establish clear criteria for patient selection to facilitate referrals and provide educational materials to outpatient clinics to streamline these referrals.

Build a Network

Technological advances will continue throughout an endoscopist's career, and it is important to continue to build one's repertoire of skills. As such, building and maintaining a network of like-minded physicians in the field of endobariatrics can be invaluable. Those who proctor procedures may likewise continue to offer opinions and expertise for challenging cases. Joining local and virtual continuing medical education events may provide additional insights from various practices. Device manufacturers often provide additional training opportunities for new technologies. Finally, society conferences are available for additional skill building and can provide opportunity for questions and answers.

SUMMARY

Bariatric endoscopy is both an exciting and rapidly expanding field in the treatment algorithm for obesity and metabolic disease management. For the aspiring bariatric endoscopist, training and practice initiation requires diligence and creativity. Important considerations for a new practice include business plan development, market research, branding, and advertising. Endoscopic bariatric and metabolic therapies will continue to evolve as demand increases and training experiences broaden.

DISCLOSURE

The authors have no financial disclosures.

REFERENCES

1. Hales CM, Carroll MD, Fryar CD, et al. Prevelance of obesity and severe obesity amont adults: United States, 2017-2018. NCHS Data Brief, no 360. Hyattsville, MD: National Center for Health Statistics; 2020.

2. Han T, Lean M. A clinical perspective of obesity, metabolic, syndrome, and cardiovascular disease. JRSM Cardiovasc Dis 2016;5:2048004016633371. https://doi.org/10.1177/2048004016633371.

3. Thompson C, Jirapinyo P, Ryan MB, et al. History of bariatric endoscopy: celebrating 20 years of bariatric endoscopy and 10 years since the first endoscopic sleeve gastroplasty. iGIE 2022;1(1):91–103.

4. Abu Dayyeh BK, Bazernachi F, Vargas EJ, et al. Endoscopic sleeve gastroplasty for treatment of class 1 and 2 obesity (MERIT): a prospective, multicentre, randomised trial. Lancet 2022;400(10350):441–51.

5. Sharaiha RZ, Hajifathalian K, Kumar R, et al. Five-Year Outcomes of Endoscopic Sleeve Gastroplasty for the Treatment of Obesity. Clin Gastroenterol Hepatol 2021;19(5):1051–7.

6. ASGE Star Certificate Programs, ASGE, 2024. Available at: https://www.asge.org/home/education/advanced-education-training/star-certificate-programs.

7. Shah SL, Aronne LJ, Sharaiha RZ. Setting up an Endobariatric Weight Loss Program. Am J Gastroenterol 2018;113(11):1567–9.

8. Jirapinyo P, Kumar N, AlSamman MA, et al. Five-year outcomes of transoral outlet reduction for the treatment of weight regain after Rot Lux-en-Y gastric bypass. Gastrointest Endosc 2020;91(5):1067–73.

9. Dahl OJ. Think business! Medical practice Quality,Efficiency, profits. Phoenix, MD: Greenhouse Publishing; 2017.

10. Schwab EF. Surviving and Thriving your First Year in Private Practice. Semin Hear 2016;37(4):293–300.

11. Maley C, Baum N. Branding your medical practice. J Med Pract Manag 2010; 25(6):379–82.

Precision Medicine in Bariatric Procedures

Khushboo Gala, MBBS[a], Wissam Ghusn, MD[a,b],
Andres Acosta, MD, PhD[a,*]

KEYWORDS

- Precision medicine • Bariatric surgery • Bariatric endoscopy • Genetics
- Epigenetics • Obesity

KEY POINTS

- Precision medicine uses a variety of factors including deep phenotyping, omics assays, and environmental factors to devise practices that are individualized to subsets of patients.
- There are wide variations in clinical response to bariatric procedures, and hence individualized approaches to treatment and prediction of outcomes are very pragmatic.
- Precision approaches to bariatric procedures developed thus far include genetic, epigenetic, metabolomic, microbiomic, clinical quantitative traits, and energy balance phenotypes.

INTRODUCTION

The prevalence of obesity in the United States is greater than 40% currently and is estimated to reach nearly 50% by 2030.[1,2] This enormous burden of the disease leads to a heavy strain on the health care system, with $172.74 billion of annual expenditures relating to obesity and related comorbidities in the United States.[3] Obesity has a multifactorial and complex pathophysiology, including environmental factors, genetic and epigenetic factors, microbiome-related disruption, and socioeconomic factors.[4,5] Management options for obesity are evolving, and include lifestyle and behavioral modifications, antiobesity medications, and bariatric procedures (metabolic and bariatric surgery [MBS] and endoscopic bariatric therapies [EBT]).

Bariatric procedures cause significant and sustained weight loss and are the most effective therapeutic option for obesity. Additionally, there are ample data showing

[a] Precision Medicine for Obesity Program, Division of Gastroenterology and Hepatology, Department of Medicine, Mayo Clinic, 200 First Street Southwest, Rochester, MN 55902, USA; [b] Department of Internal Medicine, Boston University Medical Center, Harrison Avenue, Boston, MA 02111, USA
* Corresponding author.
E-mail address: acosta.andres@mayo.edu
Twitter: @KhushbooSGala (K.G.); @Wissam_Ghusn (W.G.); @dr_aac (A.A.)

Gastrointest Endoscopy Clin N Am 34 (2024) 765–779
https://doi.org/10.1016/j.giec.2024.03.004
1052-5157/24/© 2024 Elsevier Inc. All rights reserved.

significant improvement of obesity-related co-morbidities and overall mortality with MBS.[6–8] Contemporary techniques of MBS include laparoscopic sleeve gastrectomy (LSG), Roux-en-Y gastric bypass (RYGB), and adjustable gastric banding. RYGB is considered the most effective option, albeit with the highest rate of major adverse events.[9] Recent years have seen the evolution of EBT, with procedures like intragastric balloons (IGB) and endoscopic sleeve gastroplasty (ESG) gaining global popularity and FDA approval. Overall, bariatric procedures are getting increasingly popular, although they faced a small dip during the coronavirus disease 2019 pandemic. The American Society for Metabolic and Bariatric Surgery estimates close to 200,000 bariatric procedures are performed annually in the United States.[8,9]

Obesity mediates tissue injury in various ways. Excessive lipid accumulation in obesity overwhelms the body's lipid metabolism pathways. This leads to malfunctions in the endoplasmic reticulum and mitochondria, increasing levels of reactive oxidative species, free fatty acids, and intermediates like ceramide. These free fatty acid intermediates trigger various proinflammatory kinases, leading to an increase in inflammatory adipokines and infiltration by immune cells like macrophages and type 1 T helper (TH1). Additionally, these intermediates and the ensuing inflammatory environment activate nuclear factor κB, altering gene transcription. These alterations impact insulin signaling in several ways, including changes in insulin receptor phosphorylation and function, and cause tissue damage, especially when ectopic fat accumulates in the liver and vascular structures. These various changes are likely contributors to both localized and systemic inflammation[5] (**Fig. 1**).

Precision medicine is a practice wherein prevention and treatment strategies take individual variability into account.[10] Most current prevention and treatment approaches are formulated and based on the average patient, and hence less than optimal for many patients. Precision medicine steps away from this one-size-fits-all approach. It involves using a variety of factors including deep phenotyping using clinical, physiologic, and behavioral characteristics, omics assays (eg, genomics,

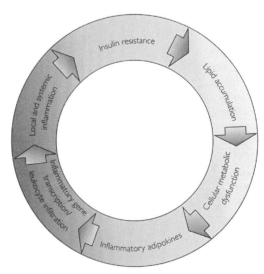

Fig. 1. Obesity-related tissue dysfunction. (*Reproduced from* Busebee B, Ghusn W, Cifuentes L, Acosta A. Obesity: A Review of Pathophysiology and Classification. Mayo Clin Proc. 2023;98(12):1842-57.)

epigenomics, transcriptomics, and microbiomics among others), and environmental factors to devise practices that are individualized to subsets of patients.[11] The Precision Medicine Initiative started in the United States in 2015 generated much excitement in the medical community and has been driving impetus for research and development in this arena.[12] Although much of this focus has been in the realm of oncology, precision medicine is increasingly being considered for the management of other chronic diseases like obesity.

Precision medicine for obesity is an evolving field. Obesity is a multi-factorial disease that is influenced by genetic, epigenetic, and environmental factors. Hence, incorporating elements like omics assays and clinical phenotyping can help with the clinical stratification of patients with obesity based on the underlying pathophysiology. In turn, this may help treat patients in an individualized and targeted manner. This is crucially important to optimize outcomes in bariatric surgery. It is well known that despite the efficacy of bariatric surgery and EBT, these procedures have a heterogenous response among patients. A study using the Longitudinal Assessment of Bariatric Surgery (LABS) database showed that there are distinct trajectories of weight loss among different patients in both the initial and long-term follow-up.[10] Even controlling for follow-up and patient compliance, the authors see variations in clinical response to bariatric procedures. Personalizing the therapeutic modality to the individual can lead to enhanced effectiveness and tolerability. Hence, precision medicine has untapped potential and enormous implications for use in bariatric procedures. The authors review advances in precision medicine made in the field of bariatrics and discuss future avenues and challenges.

GENETICS

Genes play an important role in obesity, with genetic factors accounting for 40% to 70% of an individual's predisposition to obesity.[13] Large genome-wide association studies have identified more than 300 loci in which single nucleotide polymorphisms (SNPs) are associated with development of obesity.[13] Simulation studies have shown that currently known SNPs do not account for more than 20% of variance in body mass index (BMI). However, there are likely many SNPs influencing obesity yet to be described. Polygenic risk scores have been developed that have the ability to predict BMI and obesity-related comorbidities with good accuracy.[14,15] Monogenic obesity (developed due to mutations or deficiencies in a single gene) and syndromic obesity (severe obesity associated with additional phenotypes and other organ abnormalities) are relatively uncommon, accounting for less than 5% of all severe obesity. Several genes and mechanistic pathways have been implicated in monogenic obesity, including the leptin-melanocortin pathway (LMP) and syndromes such as Bardet-Biedl syndrome, Alstrom syndrome, and Carpenter syndrome.[16]

As described previously, weight loss after bariatric procedures is extremely varied. Data suggest that a component of this variability may be attributed to strong genetic determinants. A study evaluating heritability of weight loss to RYGB showed that first-degree relative pairs had a similar response to surgery, which was not seen with cohabitating or unrelated individuals.[17,18] These genetic determinants seem to play a more dominant role in combination restrictive/malabsorptive procedures, rather than purely restrictive procedures like gastric banding.[19] Different weight-loss trajectories have been ascribed to genetic markers in 4 obesity genes: the mass and obesity-associated (FTO), insulin-induced gene 2 (INSIG2), melanocortin 4 receptor (MC4R), and proprotein convertase subtilisin/kexin type 1 (PCSK1) genes.[20] A recent systematic review and meta-analysis on this topic demonstrated that uncoupling protein (UCP) variant rs660339 and FKBP5 have been consistently associated with greater and lesser weight loss after bariatric surgery, respectively.[19] It did note that studies evaluating other genes like FTO and MC4R have been inconsistent with their association with outcomes after bariatric surgery. However, multiple studies have shown that in the short term, weight loss outcomes after bariatric surgery have been found to be similar in patients with and without variants in LMP.[21,22] Patients with variants in LMP have been found to have progressive and significant weight regain in the mid term and long term after RYGB.[23] This has been attributed to initial strong changes in neuroenteric hormone signaling being able to work through an impaired LMP and produce an effective short-term weight loss, but not being able to sustain this in the long term. Through a study of the Mayo Clinic biobank, the authors have also shown that patients with variants in LMP have weight recurrence after endoscopic transoral outlet reduction for RYGB[24] (**Fig. 2**).

Heritability of obesity traits is complemented by the interaction of genes and the environment, including unfavorable dietary, activity, and lifestyle factors. Keeping this in mind, multiple genetic risk scores have been developed, which incorporate SNPs along with variations in multiple anthropometric traits based on demographic and environmental characteristics. Several studies have evaluated several genetic risk scores examining weight loss from 12 to 96 months after bariatric surgery and found them to be predictive of outcomes.[24–26] With further development, longer study periods, and external validation, these risk scores may be a valuable tool in our armamentarium of predicting outcomes after surgery and personalizing therapeutic modalities.

Therapeutic opportunities are being explored for patients with known genetic predisposition to obesity. Setmelanotide is an MC4 receptor agonist developed for the treatment of obesity arising from proopiomelanocortin, PCSK1, or leptin receptor deficiency.[25,26] Use of phentermine-topiramate extended release in patients with a "hungry brain" phenotype, which may include patients with variants in the LMP, has been shown to superior results compared to usual care.[27]

Overall, genetic profiling of patients prior to bariatric procedures presents an exciting avenue to influence outcomes. Firstly, if preoperative evaluation reveals a high genetic score for obesity, they may benefit from a lower criteria threshold for receiving procedures, and may benefit from more aggressive, combination

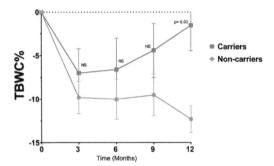

Fig. 2. Effects of heterozygous variants in the leptin-melanocortin pathway on transoral outlet reduction after roux-en-Y gastric bypass: a case–control study and review of literature. (Gala, K., Ghusn, W., Fansa, S. et al. Effects of Heterozygous Variants in the Leptin-Melanocortin Pathway on Transoral Outlet Reduction After Roux-en-Y Gastric Bypass: A Case–Control Study and Review of Literature. OBES SURG 33, 1284–1288 (2023). https://doi.org/10.1007/s11695-023-06462-0.)

restrictive/malabsorptive procedures. Secondly, genetic risk scoring can help with predicting outcomes. Lastly, using a combination of appropriate pharmacotherapy may help patients with high genetic risk achieve optimal weight loss outcomes after bariatric procedures.

EPIGENETICS

Epigenetic changes interact with the DNA or transcript without changes to the nucleotide sequence and alter gene expression.[28] The epigenome can be altered by the effect of external environmental factors, providing a dynamic response by the organism in a short time. Distinct epigenetic patterns have been identified in patients with obesity and metabolic diseases. Additionally, there is a growing body of literature that suggests that epigenetic modifications could be involved in the mechanisms underlying the response to bariatric surgery. It is well known that bariatric surgery has several effects on metabolism apart from weight loss, including improved insulin sensitivity, improved risk of cardiovascular disease and cancer, and resolution of the chronic inflammatory state induced by obesity.[29] It is hypothesized that bariatric surgery could influence epigenetic changes and gene expression, leading to these improvements in metabolism.[30] These modifications are best evaluated using epigenetic markers, which include DNA methylation, histone post-translational modification (PTM), and non-coding RNAs (ncRNAs) including microRNAs (miRNAs) and long non-coding RNAs (lncRNAs).[31]

DNA methylation is the most widely studied epigenetic marker in relation with obesity. Large, epigenome-wide association studies have showed the correlation between changes in DNA methylation and excess adiposity.[32,33] Changes induced by bariatric surgery have been shown to be different, and generally more prominent, compared to those induced by diet/lifestyle modifications.[31] These changes are so significant that a study showed durable and detectable changes even in the subsequent offspring methylome and transcriptome of a mother who underwent RYGB.[34] Data suggest that bariatric surgery modifies the DNA methylation profile of the specific genes, measured in both specific tissues like liver, adipose tissue, and skeletal muscle as well as peripheral blood.[35] Changes in methylation of specific genes have been demonstrated, including PGC1A, PDK4, and SORBS3.[36] Analysis of skeletal muscle has shown that bariatric surgery leads to hypermethylation at CpG shores and exonic regions close to transcription start sites, hence potentially influencing the epigenome.[37] Additionally, there are changes reported in the methylation of specific genes belonging to inflammatory pathways, such as SERPINE-1, interleukin (IL)-6, tumor necrosis factor-alpha (TNF-A), IL-1B, and polycystic kidney disease-4 (PKD4).[38] Studies have shown changes in methylation patterns can be predictive of weight outcomes; for instance, a study demonstrated that patients with greater weight loss after RYGB had lower SERPINE-1 methylation levels 6 months after surgery.[39]

Other epigenetic changes and markers after bariatric surgery are being investigated. A recent study showed pilot data on the use of microRNA (miRNA) to predict weight loss outcomes after bariatric surgery. They reported 6 different miRNA that had previously been implicated in regulation of fatty acid biosynthesis, adipocyte proliferation, type 2 diabetes, and obesity that had the potential for discriminating between the high and low weight loss groups after surgery.[26] Liu and colleagues studied differentially expressed genes for subcutaneous adipose tissue after bariatric surgery and used integrated bioinformatics analyses to identify hub genes and associated pathways affected after bariatric surgery.[24] Several animal models have studied changes in the expression of lncRNAs after bariatric surgery, and have identified potential targets for prediction of outcomes after surgery.[30]

The next steps in this field need to be made in establishing the clinical significance of methylation and other epigenetic variations. Defining these changes in the epigenome can help prognosticate and even serve as therapeutic targets for the weight-loss and metabolic outcomes to bariatric surgery.

METABOLOMICS

Metabolomics represents the systematic identification and quantification of metabolites in a target organism or sample. It signifies a global metabolic profiling of organisms in relation to other variables including genetic variation or external stimuli.[40] Metabolites constitute of intermediate or end-product of metabolism low-molecular weight molecules (<1 kD).[41]

MBS and EBT contribute to a decreased body weight, with a significant effect on glycemic control,[42] cardiovascular disease risk,[43] and other metabolic parameters.[44,45] To better understand this metabolic effect, a significant effort was put to study metabolomics in patients after bariatric procedures. Importantly, MBS alters metabolic profiles compared to non-surgical procedures, when controlling for same weight loss outcomes.[46,47] Hence, MBS has a distinctive metabolic signature that might play a critical role in weight loss and associated improvement in metabolic comorbidities. Although there still have not been reliable preoperative models to predict weight loss, metabolomic analyses can aid in detecting biomarkers that reflect precise preoperative prediction of metabolic and surgical outcome after bariatric procedures.[48]

The most studied procedures in the metabolic field are RYGB (54%) and LSG (29%), followed by other less commonly explored procedures (eg, duodenal-jejunal endoluminal bypass, laparoscopic gastric banding, IGB, ESG).[49] Multiple metabolic pathways are altered after bariatric procedures. These pathways include the amino acids derivatives, bile acids, endocannabinoids, TCA cycle-related metabolites, lipid derivatives, microbiota-related metabolites, and other pathways.[48]

Amino Acids Derivatives

Branched chain amino acids (BCAAs) (ie, valine, leucine, and isoleucine) are known to be upregulated in obesity and type-2 diabetes mellitus (T2DM).[50] This might be due to regulation of BCAA aminotransferase, elevated gut microbiome BCAA synthesis,[51] and/or decreased microbial BCAA uptake and catabolism.[52] In fact, elevated BCAAs reflect a strong biomarker for insulin resistance. Similarly, aromatic amino acids (ie, phenylalanine, tyrosine, and tryptophan) are also upregulated in diseases such as obesity and T2DM. The rise in phenylalanine and tyrosine is attributed to a decrease in tyrosine aminotransferase function caused by insulin resistance and elevated specific metabolites including cysteine and alpha-hydroxybutyrate.[50] As for tryptophan, its metabolic pathways are altered in patients with obesity which is correlated with obesity-related systemic inflammation.[53]

Bariatric surgeries have been demonstrated to decrease the levels of BCAAs and aromatic amino acids in multiple studies.[54,55] These changes might enhance and explain the improvement in metabolic pathways and disease after bariatric surgeries. However, Kramer and colleagues showed that blocking the surgical effect on BCAAs does not alter the potent effects of bariatric surgeries on weight loss and glucose tolerance.[56]

LSG was shown to increase the serum concentration of serine and glycine.[57] Circulating levels of glutamate were also shown to decrease.

Lipid Derivatives and Bile Acids

Among the lipid derivatives, several metabolites were thoroughly studied in patients who underwent bariatric procedures. These include free fatty acids, acylcarnitines (AC), bile acids, and phospholipids. Studies have shown that short-chain AC derived from BCAA decrease after MBS,[47,58] while other short-chain AC increase rapidly and remain elevated for 6 to 12 months.[59,60] Long-chain ACs transiently increase before decreasing in the long term.[59,61]

Unsaturated, long-chain saturated, and non-esterified fatty acids demonstrate a decrease after bariatric surgery in most studies.[59,62] However, medium-chain saturated fatty acids increase after these bariatric surgeries.[63,64] Regarding phospholipids, most sphingomyelins decreased biliopancreatic diversion.[65] However, in RYGB, saturated sphingomyelins decrease while unsaturated increase.[66,67] As for bile acids, bariatric procedures with malabsorption component (eg, RYGB) seem to increase fasting and secondary circulating bile acids[65,68] while restrictive procedures resulted in inconsistent results in the literature.[69]

MICROBIOME

The human microbiota is made up of the 10 to 100 trillion symbiotic microbial cells harbored primarily in the gut of all humans; the human microbiome consists of the genetic material harbored by these cells. Changes in microbiota content are significantly associated with acute and chronic diseases, like obesity, type 2 diabetes, atopic diseases, inflammatory bowel disease, and atherosclerosis.[70]

The gut microbiota of obese patients has significant changes, including an increased Firmicutes/Bacteroidetes ratio at the phylum level, and decrease in Christensenellaceae and the genera Methanobacteriales, Lactobacillus, Bifidobacteria, and Akkermansia.[71] In essence, the gut microbiota regulates energy absorption, central appetite, fat storage, chronic inflammation, and circadian rhythms. It is thus not surprising that there are significant changes in the gut microbioata after MBS. Mechanisms driving these changes include malabsorption status, changes in the metabolism of bile acids, changes in gastric pH, and changes in the metabolism of hormones.[72] There are significant taxonomic changes after surgery, with reports demonstrating an increase in bacterial species richness after surgery, relating to an improved host metabolic profile.[73] There are also data suggesting an increase in functional annotations associated with amino acid utilization, sugar metabolism, and fatty acid utilization after bariatric surgery.[74,75] These changes are likely a major contributor to weight loss and improvements in glycemic and metabolic control. Hence, many new molecular targets and small molecules of microbial origin in the host may be used for prognostication of outcomes, as well as targets for obesity treatment. Although the translation of these findings is in its infancy, the microbiota represents an exciting opportunity for precision medicine in the realm of bariatric procedures.

CLINICAL QUANTITATIVE TRAITS AND PREDICTIVE MODELS

Several clinical tools have been developed to help guide the use of bariatric procedures in patients with obesity. Some scores have been built to predict diabetes remission in patients with T2DM.[76] Other clinical classifications have also demonstrated a possible utility in MBS and EBT.[77,78] Such clinical measurements are of significant importance for physicians treating patients with obesity and related comorbidities (eg, T2DM).

T2DM is one of the major comorbidities that is associated with obesity. In fact, obesity represents the most common risk factor for T2DM.[79] Around 80% to 90% of patients with T2DM have overweight or obesity.[80] Importantly, patients with T2DM are associated with higher all-cause mortality rates related to multiple complications of this disease including cardiovascular disease, respiratory diseases, cerebrovascular disease, cancer, kidney diseases, specific infectious diseases, and other diseases.[81] T2DM was reported to be among the top 10 causes of death in 2019.[82] In addition, its economic burden continues to be rising to reach $245 billion in 2012[83] and $327 billion in 2017.[84] Bariatric surgeries have been shown to be effective in achieving T2DM remission. However, there is a notable heterogeneity in disease remission in patients with T2DM, ranging between 24% and 84%.[76] This wide difference can be attributed to various factors including type of procedure, baseline metabolic parameters, T2DM remission definition, and other contributors. Hence, multiple predictive models have been validated to help evaluate disease remission in patients with T2DM.

One of the most widely used and validated metrics for T2DM remission is the Individualized Metabolic Surgery (IMS) Score constructed by Aminian and colleagues. This is an evidence-based scoring system to select MBS (ie, RYGB and LSG) depending on T2DM severity, predicting disease remission.[85] In a cohort of 659 patients and an external validation cohort of 241 patients, patients were categorized into 3 stages of diabetes severities based on 4 different parameters. This score is based on preoperative variables like number of diabetes medications, insulin use, duration of diabetes (years), and glycemic control (HbA1c <7%). Depending on the score, patients can be classified either into the mild category: score 0 to 25; moderate category: 25< Score ≤95; and severe category: greater than 95. Patients with mild and severe scores may benefit equally from RYGB and SG in terms of T2DM remission. In fact, both procedures significantly improve T2DM for patients in mild category. However, a severe score, which reflects a limited functional β-cell reserve, denotes a similar low efficacy in both procedures for T2DM remission. As for the moderate severity, RYGB demonstrated better remission rates compared to SG, attributing to a more pronounced neurohormonal effect. Hence, this score provides an applicable model to help select bariatric procedures. Although more recent studies show similar efficacy of RYGB and SG in the intermediate group, there remains a clear trend in higher remission rates with lower IMS scores.[86–88]

Another score that was created by Robert and colleagues included multiple predictive factors of T2DM remission at 1 year after MBS. In this cohort, there was no significant difference in T2DM remission between RYGB, SG, and LAGB, with a trend of better outcomes in patients who have undergone RYGB (RYGB: 74%; SG: 50%; LAGB: 50%). Patients with higher scores have a higher chance of T2DM.[89]

The DiaRem score represents an algorithm that predicts T2DM remission rates over 5 years.[90] Based on this score, patients are divided into 5 groups representing different T2DM remission ranges. The Ad-DiaRem score is another model used to predict T2DM remission after RYGB surgeries. It was created with a test cohort of 213 patients and validated in 2 independent cohorts in France (n = 134) and Israel (n = 99). A higher score represents a lower T2DM remission rate after bariatric surgery.[91] Lastly, the ABCD score was initially developed in an Asian population of patients with T2DM (N = 63) who had undergone RYGB and has been validated in a prospectively collected cohort of 176 patients. With the increase in this score, the higher remission rate is expected.[92]

ENERGY BALANCE AND OBESITY PHENOTYPES

Emerging studies highlight the importance of individual variations in energy intake and expenditure in obesity pathophysiology and management plan.[5,27] Energy intake is influenced by both homeostatic mechanisms, which regulate hunger and fullness, and hedonic factors, which are influenced by emotional states. Quantifiable traits such as satiation and satiety, assessed through calorie consumption and gastric emptying rates, respectively, are linked to obesity and can shed light on individual differences in weight gain.[27] In addition, energy expenditure can decrease in response to calorie restriction or weight loss, and this reduction can predict future weight gain. A persistent decline in energy expenditure can even continue years after initial weight loss.[5,93]

A new classification system based on phenotypes related to eating behaviors and energy expenditure seeks to stratify obesity more precisely. This system identifies 4 phenotypes: abnormal satiation, abnormal satiety, emotional eating behavior, and abnormal resting energy expenditure.[27,94] Treatments tailored to these phenotypes have shown better weight loss outcomes than non-specific approaches.[5,27,95] Medications like phentermine-topiramate and GLP-1 agonists have been effective in managing specific phenotypes by reducing energy intake and modulating gastric emptying.[27] Further work in this arena may provide insights into the application of bariatric surgery and EBTs, indicating a promising direction for individualized obesity management.

PRECISION MEDICINE IN ENDOSCOPIC BARIATRIC THERAPIES

Endoscopic bariatric therapies (EBTs) are minimally invasive alternatives to bariatric surgery that have emerged over the past few years. These include space-occupying devices like IGBs and TransPyloric Shuttle, and gastric remodeling techniques, such as ESG and primary obesity surgery endoluminal 2.0 (POSE 2.0).[96] Research on precision medicine and omics in these modalities is lacking.

Moreover, the authors' group has explored the use of physiologic predictors of outcomes after EBTs. In a prospective feasibility study, 32 patients who underwent placement of IGBs had their gastric emptying time measured at baseline and 3 months following the procedure.[97] Patients who had a delay in gastric emptying had significantly higher weight loss compared to those who had no change in their gastric emptying. A meta-analysis also showed that IGBs cause delayed gastric emptying, correlating to weight loss.[98] One study showed that IGBs cause a delay in emptying of solid foods only.[99] This has also been explored in patients undergoing ESG, who also experienced delayed gastric emptying, correlating with short-term weight loss, as well as changes in gastric accommodation.[78] When comparing modalities, it has been shown that IGBs cause more significant delay in gastric emptying compared to ESG, with these changes having a greater effect on weight loss.[77] Overall, these differences in physiologic responses have been predictive of response to therapy, and could be used to select interventions.

SUMMARY

Precision medicine-based studies are paving the way for personalized treatment of obesity and outcomes after bariatric procedures. The traditional approach of "one size fits all" does not take into account the remarkable heterogeneity of obesity while positioning treatments for patients, and hence results in underwhelming responses to therapies. This includes bariatric procedures, which have a high rate for reversal of obesity and metabolic syndrome if used in the right patient. Using personalized approaches with high-resolution technologies based on "omics profiling" will help optimize treatment approaches and outcomes. Although in early stages, precision medicine has a tremendous potential in the management of obesity and related diseases.

CLINICS CARE POINTS

- Precision medicine is a practice in which prevention and treatment strategies take individual variability into account.
- Significant data in the realm of genetics shows that response to MBS is affected by underlying genetic determinants.
- Areas like epigenetics and metabolomics are in their infancy for use in bariatric procedures.
- Clinical quantitive tools and predictive models for prediction of outcomes after bariatric procedures are evolving.

DISCLOSURES

A. Acosta and Mayo Clinic hold equity in Phenomix Sciences Inc. and are inventors of intellectual property licensed to Phenomix Sciences Inc. A. Acosta served as a consultant for Rhythm Pharmaceuticals, General Mills, Amgen, Bausch Health, RareStone; has contracts with Vivus Inc, Satiogen Pharmaceutical, and Rhythm pharmaceutical. The remaining authors have nothing to disclose.

REFERENCES

1. Ward ZJ, Bleich SN, Cradock AL, et al. Projected U.S. State-Level Prevalence of Adult Obesity and Severe Obesity. N Engl J Med 2019;381(25):2440–50.
2. National Health and Nutrition Examination Survey 2017–March 2020 Prepandemic Data Files Development of Files and Prevalence Estimates for Selected Health Outcomes, (2021).
3. Ward ZJ, Bleich SN, Long MW, et al. Association of body mass index with health care expenditures in the United States by age and sex. PLoS One 2021;16(3): e0247307.
4. Lin X, Li H. Obesity: Epidemiology, Pathophysiology, and Therapeutics. Front Endocrinol 2021;12:706978.
5. Busebee B, Ghusn W, Cifuentes L, et al. Obesity: a review of pathophysiology and classification. Mayo Clin Proc 2023;98(12):1842–57.
6. O'Brien PE, Hindle A, Brennan L, et al. Long-Term Outcomes After Bariatric Surgery: a Systematic Review and Meta-analysis of Weight Loss at 10 or More Years for All Bariatric Procedures and a Single-Centre Review of 20-Year Outcomes After Adjustable Gastric Banding. Obes Surg 2019;29(1):3–14.
7. Carlsson LMS, Sjoholm K, Jacobson P, et al. Life Expectancy after Bariatric Surgery in the Swedish Obese Subjects Study. N Engl J Med 2020;383(16): 1535–43.
8. Sjostrom L. Review of the key results from the Swedish Obese Subjects (SOS) trial - a prospective controlled intervention study of bariatric surgery. J Intern Med 2013;273(3):219–34.
9. Arterburn D, Wellman R, Emiliano A, et al, PCORnet Bariatric Study Collaborative. Comparative Effectiveness and Safety of Bariatric Procedures for Weight Loss: A PCORnet Cohort Study. Ann Intern Med 2018;169(11):741–50.
10. Collins FS, Varmus H. A new initiative on precision medicine. N Engl J Med 2015; 372(9):793–5.
11. Ramaswami R, Bayer R, Galea S. Precision Medicine from a Public Health Perspective. Annu Rev Publ Health 2018;39:153–68.

12. Ashley EA. The precision medicine initiative: a new national effort. JAMA 2015; 313(21):2119–20.
13. Barsh GS, Farooqi IS, O'Rahilly S. Genetics of body-weight regulation. Nature 2000;404(6778):644–51.
14. Khera AV, Chaffin M, Wade KH, et al. Polygenic Prediction of Weight and Obesity Trajectories from Birth to Adulthood. Cell 2019;177(3):587–596 e9.
15. Seral-Cortes M, Sabroso-Lasa S, De Miguel-Etayo P, et al. Development of a Genetic Risk Score to predict the risk of overweight and obesity in European adolescents from the HELENA study. Sci Rep 2021;11(1):3067.
16. Ranadive SA, Vaisse C. Lessons from extreme human obesity: monogenic disorders. Endocrinol Metab Clin N Am 2008;37(3):733–51.
17. Hatoum IJ, Greenawalt DM, Cotsapas C, et al. Heritability of the weight loss response to gastric bypass surgery. J Clin Endocrinol Metab 2011;96(10): E1630–3.
18. Sarzynski MA, Jacobson P, Rankinen T, et al. Associations of markers in 11 obesity candidate genes with maximal weight loss and weight regain in the SOS bariatric surgery cases. Int J Obes 2011;35(5):676–83.
19. Hagedorn JC, Morton JM. Nature versus nurture: identical twins and bariatric surgery. Obes Surg 2007;17(6):728–31.
20. Still CD, Wood GC, Chu X, et al. High allelic burden of four obesity SNPs is associated with poorer weight loss outcomes following gastric bypass surgery. Obesity 2011;19(8):1676–83.
21. Cooiman MI, Kleinendorst L, Aarts EO, et al. Genetic Obesity and Bariatric Surgery Outcome in 1014 Patients with Morbid Obesity. Obes Surg 2020;30(2): 470–7.
22. Aslan IR, Campos GM, Calton MA, et al. Weight loss after Roux-en-Y gastric bypass in obese patients heterozygous for MC4R mutations. Obes Surg 2011; 21(7):930–4.
23. Campos A, Cifuentes L, Hashem A, et al. Effects of Heterozygous Variants in the Leptin-Melanocortin Pathway on Roux-en-Y Gastric Bypass Outcomes: a 15-Year Case-Control Study. Obes Surg 2022;32(8):2632–40.
24. Gala K, Ghusn W, Fansa S, et al. Effects of Heterozygous Variants in the Leptin-Melanocortin Pathway on Transoral Outlet Reduction After Roux-en-Y Gastric Bypass: A Case-Control Study and Review of Literature. Obes Surg 2023; 33(4):1284–8.
25. Markham A. Setmelanotide: First Approval. Drugs 2021;81(3):397–403.
26. Clement K, van den Akker E, Argente J, et al. Setmelanotide POMC and LEPR Phase 3 Trial Investigators. Efficacy and safety of setmelanotide, an MC4R agonist, in individuals with severe obesity due to LEPR or POMC deficiency: single-arm, open-label, multicentre, phase 3 trials. Lancet Diabetes Endocrinol 2020;8(12):960–70.
27. Acosta A, Camilleri M, Abu Dayyeh B, et al. Selection of Antiobesity Medications Based on Phenotypes Enhances Weight Loss: A Pragmatic Trial in an Obesity Clinic. Obesity 2021;29(4):662–71.
28. Wu C, Morris JR. Genes, genetics, and epigenetics: a correspondence. Science 2001;293(5532):1103–5.
29. Cornejo-Pareja I, Clemente-Postigo M, Tinahones FJ. Metabolic and Endocrine Consequences of Bariatric Surgery. Front Endocrinol 2019;10:626.
30. Izquierdo AG, Crujeiras AB. Obesity-Related Epigenetic Changes After Bariatric Surgery. Front Endocrinol 2019;10:232.

31. Aronica L, Levine AJ, Brennan K, et al. A systematic review of studies of DNA methylation in the context of a weight loss intervention. Epigenomics 2017;9(5): 769–87.
32. Dick KJ, Nelson CP, Tsaprouni L, et al. DNA methylation and body-mass index: a genome-wide analysis. Lancet 2014;383(9933):1990–8.
33. Wahl S, Drong A, Lehne B, et al. Epigenome-wide association study of body mass index, and the adverse outcomes of adiposity. Nature 2017; 541(7635):81–6.
34. Guenard F, Deshaies Y, Cianflone K, et al. Differential methylation in glucoregulatory genes of offspring born before vs. after maternal gastrointestinal bypass surgery. Proc Natl Acad Sci U S A 2013;110(28):11439–44.
35. Morcillo S, Macias-Gonzalez M, Tinahones FJ. The Effect of Metabolic and Bariatric Surgery on DNA Methylation Patterns. Curr Atherosclerosis Rep 2017; 19(10):40.
36. Day SE, Garcia LA, Coletta RL, et al. Alterations of sorbin and SH3 domain containing 3 (SORBS3) in human skeletal muscle following Roux-en-Y gastric bypass surgery. Clin Epigenet 2017;9:96.
37. Barres R, Kirchner H, Rasmussen M, et al. Weight loss after gastric bypass surgery in human obesity remodels promoter methylation. Cell Rep 2013;3(4): 1020–7.
38. Kirchner H, Nylen C, Laber S, et al. Altered promoter methylation of PDK4, IL1 B, IL6, and TNF after Roux-en Y gastric bypass. Surg Obes Relat Dis 2014;10(4): 671–8.
39. Nicoletti CF, Nonino CB, de Oliveira BA, et al. DNA Methylation and Hydroxymethylation Levels in Relation to Two Weight Loss Strategies: Energy-Restricted Diet or Bariatric Surgery. Obes Surg 2016;26(3):603–11.
40. Idle JR, Gonzalez FJ. Metabolomics. Cell Metab 2007;6(5):348–51.
41. Pantelis AG. Metabolomics in Bariatric and Metabolic Surgery Research and the Potential of Deep Learning in Bridging the Gap. Metabolites 2022;12(5):458.
42. Mingrone G, Panunzi S, De Gaetano A, et al. Bariatric–metabolic surgery versus conventional medical treatment in obese patients with type 2 diabetes: 5 year follow-up of an open-label, single-centre, randomised controlled trial. Lancet 2015;386(9997):964–73.
43. Doumouras AG, Wong JA, Paterson JM, et al. Bariatric Surgery and Cardiovascular Outcomes in Patients With Obesity and Cardiovascular Disease. Circulation 2021;143(15):1468–80.
44. Skubleny D, Switzer NJ, Gill RS, et al. The impact of bariatric surgery on polycystic ovary syndrome: a systematic review and meta-analysis. Obes Surg 2016;26: 169–76.
45. Cohen RV, Pereira TV, Aboud CM, et al. Effect of gastric bypass vs best medical treatment on early-stage chronic kidney disease in patients with type 2 diabetes and obesity: a randomized clinical trial. JAMA surgery 2020;155(8):e200420.
46. Tulipani S, Griffin J, Palau-Rodriguez M, et al. Metabolomics guided insights on bariatric surgery versus behavioral interventions for weight loss. Obesity 2016; 24(12):2451–66.
47. Khoo CM, Muehlbauer MJ, Stevens RD, et al. Postprandial metabolite profiles reveal differential nutrient handling after bariatric surgery compared to matched caloric restriction. Ann Surg 2014;259(4):687.
48. Ha J, Kwon Y, Park S. Metabolomics in Bariatric Surgery: Towards Identification of Mechanisms and Biomarkers of Metabolic Outcomes. Obes Surg 2021;31(10): 4564–74.

49. Samczuk P, Ciborowski M, Kretowski A. Application of Metabolomics to Study Effects of Bariatric Surgery. J Diabetes Res 2018;2018:6270875.

50. Adams SH. Emerging perspectives on essential amino acid metabolism in obesity and the insulin-resistant state. Adv Nutr 2011;2(6):445–56.

51. Holeček M. Why are branched-chain amino acids increased in starvation and diabetes? Nutrients 2020;12(10):3087.

52. Pedersen HK, Gudmundsdottir V, Nielsen HB, Hyotylainen T, Nielsen T, Jensen BA, Forslund K, Hildebrand F, Prifti E, Falony G, Le Chatelier E, Levenez F, Doré J, Mattila I, Plichta DR, Pöhö P, Hellgren LI, Arumugam M, Sunagawa S, Vieira-Silva S, Jørgensen T, Holm JB, Trošt K, MetaHIT Consortium, Kristiansen K, Brix S, Raes J, Wang J, Hansen T, Bork P, Brunak S, Oresic M, Ehrlich SD, Pedersen O. Human gut microbes impact host serum metabolome and insulin sensitivity. Nature 2016;535(7612):376–81.

53. Cussotto S, Delgado I, Anesi A, et al. Tryptophan Metabolic Pathways Are Altered in Obesity and Are Associated With Systemic Inflammation. Front Immunol 2020; 11:557.

54. Modesitt SC, Hallowell PT, Slack-Davis JK, et al. Women at extreme risk for obesity-related carcinogenesis: Baseline endometrial pathology and impact of bariatric surgery on weight, metabolic profiles and quality of life. Gynecol Oncol 2015;138(2):238–45.

55. Tan HC, Hsu JW, Kovalik J-P, et al. Branched-chain amino acid oxidation is elevated in adults with morbid obesity and decreases significantly after sleeve gastrectomy. J Nutr 2020;150(12):3180–9.

56. Bozadjieva Kramer N, Evers SS, Shin JH, et al. The Role of Elevated Branched-Chain Amino Acids in the Effects of Vertical Sleeve Gastrectomy to Reduce Weight and Improve Glucose Regulation. Cell Rep 2020;33(2):108239.

57. Liu Y, Jin J, Chen Y, et al. Integrative analyses of biomarkers and pathways for adipose tissue after bariatric surgery. Adipocyte 2020;9(1):384–400.

58. Magkos F, Bradley D, Schweitzer GG, et al. Effect of Roux-en-Y gastric bypass and laparoscopic adjustable gastric banding on branched-chain amino acid metabolism. Diabetes 2013;62(8):2757–61.

59. Luo P, Yu H, Zhao X, et al. Metabolomics Study of Roux-en-Y Gastric Bypass Surgery (RYGB) to Treat Type 2 Diabetes Patients Based on Ultraperformance Liquid Chromatography-Mass Spectrometry. J Proteome Res 2016;15(4):1288–99.

60. Samczuk P, Luba M, Godzien J, et al. Gear mechanism" of bariatric interventions revealed by untargeted metabolomics. J Pharm Biomed Anal 2018;151:219–26.

61. Oberbach A, Bluher M, Wirth H, et al. Combined proteomic and metabolomic profiling of serum reveals association of the complement system with obesity and identifies novel markers of body fat mass changes. J Proteome Res 2011; 10(10):4769–88.

62. Lopes TI, Geloneze B, Pareja JC, et al. Blood Metabolome Changes Before and After Bariatric Surgery: A (1)H NMR-Based Clinical Investigation. OMICS 2015; 19(5):318–27.

63. Wijayatunga NN, Sams VG, Dawson JA, et al. Roux-en-Y gastric bypass surgery alters serum metabolites and fatty acids in patients with morbid obesity. Diabetes Metab Res Rev 2018;34(8):e3045.

64. Narath SH, Mautner SI, Svehlikova E, et al. An Untargeted Metabolomics Approach to Characterize Short-Term and Long-Term Metabolic Changes after Bariatric Surgery. PLoS One 2016;11(9):e0161425.

65. Ramos-Molina B, Castellano-Castillo D, Alcaide-Torres J, et al. Differential effects of restrictive and malabsorptive bariatric surgery procedures on the serum lipidome in obese subjects. J Clin Lipidol 2018;12(6):1502–12.

66. Herzog K, Berggren J, Al Majdoub M, et al. Metabolic Effects of Gastric Bypass Surgery: Is It All About Calories? Diabetes 2020;69(9):2027–35.

67. Kayser BD, Lhomme M, Dao MC, et al. Serum lipidomics reveals early differential effects of gastric bypass compared with banding on phospholipids and sphingolipids independent of differences in weight loss. Int J Obes 2017;41(6):917–25.

68. Fiamoncini J, Fernandes Barbosa C, Arnoni Junior JR, et al. Roux-en-Y Gastric Bypass Surgery Induces Distinct but Frequently Transient Effects on Acylcarnitine, Bile Acid and Phospholipid Levels. Metabolites 2018;8(4).

69. Vaz M, Pereira SS, Monteiro MP. Metabolomic signatures after bariatric surgery - a systematic review. Rev Endocr Metab Disord 2022;23(3):503–19.

70. Ursell LK, Metcalf JL, Parfrey LW, et al. Defining the human microbiome. Nutr Rev 2012;70(Suppl 1):S38–44.

71. Liu BN, Liu XT, Liang ZH, et al. Gut microbiota in obesity. World J Gastroenterol 2021;27(25):3837–50.

72. Ulker I, Yildiran H. The effects of bariatric surgery on gut microbiota in patients with obesity: a review of the literature. Biosci Microbiota Food Health 2019; 38(1):3–9.

73. Palleja A, Kashani A, Allin KH, et al. Roux-en-Y gastric bypass surgery of morbidly obese patients induces swift and persistent changes of the individual gut microbiota. Genome Med 2016;8(1):67.

74. Tremaroli V, Karlsson F, Werling M, et al. Roux-en-Y Gastric Bypass and Vertical Banded Gastroplasty Induce Long-Term Changes on the Human Gut Microbiome Contributing to Fat Mass Regulation. Cell Metabol 2015;22(2):228–38.

75. Graessler J, Qin Y, Zhong H, et al. Metagenomic sequencing of the human gut microbiome before and after bariatric surgery in obese patients with type 2 diabetes: correlation with inflammatory and metabolic parameters. Pharmacogenomics J 2013;13(6):514–22.

76. Park JY. Prediction of Type 2 Diabetes Remission after Bariatric or Metabolic Surgery. J Obes Metab Syndr 2018;27(4):213–22.

77. Rapaka B, Maselli DB, Lopez-Nava G, et al. Effects on physiologic measures of appetite from intragastric balloon and endoscopic sleeve gastroplasty: results of a prospective study. Chin Med J (Engl) 2022;135(10):1234–41.

78. Vargas EJ, Rizk M, Gomez-Villa J, et al. Effect of endoscopic sleeve gastroplasty on gastric emptying, motility and hormones: a comparative prospective study. Gut 2022.

79. Leitner DR, Frühbeck G, Yumuk V, et al. Obesity and Type 2 Diabetes: Two Diseases with a Need for Combined Treatment Strategies - EASO Can Lead the Way. Obes Facts 2017;10(5):483–92.

80. Nianogo RA, Arah OA. Forecasting Obesity and Type 2 Diabetes Incidence and Burden: The ViLA-Obesity Simulation Model. Front Public Health 2022;10: 818816.

81. Li S, Wang J, Zhang B, et al. Diabetes Mellitus and Cause-Specific Mortality: A Population-Based Study. Diabetes Metab J 2019;43(3):319–41.

82. Xu J, Murphy SL, Kochanek KD, Arias E. Deaths: Final data for 2019. 2021.

83. Nianogo RA, Arah OA. Forecasting Obesity and Type 2 Diabetes Incidence and Burden: The ViLA-Obesity Simulation Model. Front Public Health 2022;10: 818816.

84. Association AD. Economic costs of diabetes in the US in 2017. Diabetes Care 2018;41(5):917–28.
85. Aminian A, Brethauer SA, Andalib A, et al. Individualized Metabolic Surgery Score: Procedure Selection Based on Diabetes Severity. Ann Surg 2017;266(4): 650–7.
86. Saarinen I, Grönroos S, Hurme S, et al. Validation of the individualized metabolic surgery score for bariatric procedure selection in the merged data of two randomized clinical trials (SLEEVEPASS and SM-BOSS). Surg Obes Relat Dis 2022.
87. Ghusn W, Ma P, Ikemiya K, et al. The role of diabetes severity scores in predicting disease remission in patients with BMI > 50 kg/m2 undergoing Roux-En-Y gastric bypass and sleeve gastrectomy: a multi-centered study. Surg Endosc 2023; 37(9):7114–20.
88. Ghusn W, Hage K, Vierkant RA, et al. Type-2 diabetes mellitus remission prediction models after Roux-En-Y gastric bypass and sleeve gastrectomy based on disease severity scores. Diabetes Res Clin Pract 2024;208:111091.
89. Robert M, Ferrand-Gaillard C, Disse E, et al. Predictive factors of type 2 diabetes remission 1 year after bariatric surgery: impact of surgical techniques. Obes Surg 2013;23(6):770–5.
90. Still CD, Wood GC, Benotti P, et al. Preoperative prediction of type 2 diabetes remission after Roux-en-Y gastric bypass surgery: a retrospective cohort study. Lancet Diabetes Endocrinol 2014;2(1):38–45.
91. Aron-Wisnewsky J, Sokolovska N, Liu Y, et al. The advanced-DiaRem score improves prediction of diabetes remission 1 year post-Roux-en-Y gastric bypass. Diabetologia 2017;60(10):1892–902.
92. Lee W-J, Hur KY, Lakadawala M, et al. Predicting success of metabolic surgery: age, body mass index, C-peptide, and duration score. Surg Obes Relat Dis 2013; 9(3):379–84.
93. Fothergill E, Guo J, Howard L, et al. Persistent metabolic adaptation 6 years after "The Biggest Loser" competition. Obesity 2016;24(8):1612–9.
94. Ghusn W, Cifuentes L, Campos A, et al. Association Between Food Intake and Gastrointestinal Symptoms in Patients With Obesity. Gastro Hep Adv 2023;2(1): 121–8.
95. Cifuentes L, Ghusn W, Feris F, et al. Phenotype tailored lifestyle intervention on weight loss and cardiometabolic risk factors in adults with obesity: a single-centre, non-randomised, proof-of-concept study. EClinicalMedicine 2023;58: 101923.
96. Popov V, Storm AC. Toward a Better Understanding of Endoscopic Bariatric Therapies. Clin Gastroenterol Hepatol 2023;21(6):1422–6.
97. Lopez-Nava G, Jaruvongvanich V, Storm AC, et al. Personalization of Endoscopic Bariatric and Metabolic Therapies Based on Physiology: a Prospective Feasibility Study with a Single Fluid-Filled Intragastric Balloon. Obes Surg 2020;30(9): 3347–53.
98. Vargas EJ, Bazerbachi F, Calderon G, et al. Changes in time of gastric emptying after surgical and endoscopic bariatrics and weight loss: a systematic review and meta-analysis. Clin Gastroenterol Hepatol 2020;18(1):57–68. e5.
99. Barrichello S, Badurdeen D, Hedjoudje A, et al. The Effect of the Intra-gastric Balloon on Gastric Emptying and the DeMeester Score. Obes Surg 2020;30(1): 38–45.

Approach to the Treatment of Children and Adolescents with Obesity

Elizabeth Hegedus, BS[a], Alaina P. Vidmar, MD[a],*,
Madeline Mayer, BS[a], Roshni Kohli[a], Rohit Kohli, MBBS, MS[b]

KEYWORDS

- Pediatric obesity • Obesity pharmacotherapy • Metabolic and bariatric surgery
- Intensive health and behavior lifestyle modification

KEY POINTS

- Pediatric obesity remains a major public health concern that results in life-limiting complications if left untreated.
- The 2023 American Academy of Pediatric clinical practice guidelines emphasize that pediatric obesity is a complex, multifactorial, chronic disease and requires a comprehensive treatment approach.
- The treatment approach should incorporate intensive health and behavioral lifestyle modifications with concurrent use of obesity pharmacotherapy and bariatric surgery based on the severity of the disease at presentation.
- Life-limiting complications, such as type 2 diabetes and metabolism-associated steatotic liver disease, must be screened for routinely to ensure treatment is initiated early.
- The current evidence supports that obesity treatment is safe and effective. There is no evidence that the watchful waiting approach is appropriate.

INTRODUCTION

Pediatric obesity continues to be an omnipresent disease, 1 in 5 children and adolescents have obesity in the United States.[1,2] In pediatric cohorts, obesity is defined as a body mass index (BMI) greater than the 95th percentile for age and sex.[2,3] Increases in

Funding source: (1) K23DK134801 NIH, United States, NIDDK, United States, (2) Sacchi Foundation Research Scientist, (3) ISCT American Diabetes Association 11-22-ICTSN-32, and (4) The Southern California Center for Latino Health Pilot Award 2022.
[a] Department of Pediatrics, Children's Hospital Los Angeles and Keck School of Medicine of USC, Center for Endocrinology, Diabetes and Metabolism, 4650 Sunset Boulevard, Los Angeles, CA 90027, USA; [b] Department of Pediatrics, Division of Gastroenterology, Children's Hospital Los Angeles and Keck School of Medicine of USC, 4650 Sunset Boulevard, Los Angeles, CA 90027, USA
* Corresponding author.
E-mail address: avidmar@chla.usc.edu

Gastrointest Endoscopy Clin N Am 34 (2024) 781–804
https://doi.org/10.1016/j.giec.2024.06.004
1052-5157/24/© 2024 Elsevier Inc. All rights reserved, including those for text and data mining, AI training, and similar technologies.

pediatric obesity have been accompanied with a rising incidence of youth-onset life-limiting comorbidities, such as type 2 diabetes, metabolism-associated steatotic liver disease (MASLD), and sleep apnea.[4] Pediatric obesity has a higher incidence in Latino and Black youth, as well as low-income and middle-income groups.[4,5] Acknowledging the increasing prevalence of pediatric obesity, the American Association of Pediatrics (AAP) produced new guidelines in January 2023 for the care of children and adolescents with obesity.[6]

The AAP recommends proactive and intentional screening of all pediatric patients, using BMI to screen and diagnose for overweight and obesity and systematic screening of risk factors such as family history, racial identity, adverse childhood experiences, and income status. This proactive screening is intended to provide early intervention and support for families. This recommendation is a deviation from the early "watch and wait" recommendations that arose out of the previous clinical practice guidelines published in 2007.[6–8] At yearly well-child examinations, pediatricians are encouraged to provide lifestyle modification recommendations such as screen time recommendations, nutrition, and physical activity advice.[6] At minimum, the AAP recommends screening for comorbidities associated with obesity and providing guidance on the risks associated with these comorbidities and living with elevated BMI throughout childhood with the goals of early diagnosis and intervention not being a certain number on the scale or size of one's body but reduction of life-limiting complications over time.[6,8]

There are multiple potential interventions for those patients identified with obesity.[6] The AAP recommends a comprehensive treatment approach in which intensive lifestyle modification, obesity pharmacotherapy, and bariatric surgery are offered concurrently as warranted by the severity of the presentation.[6,9,10] The current evidence suggests that the most effective intensive health behavior and lifestyle treatment (IHBLT) programs offer family-centered interventions with multidisciplinary counseling on nutrition and physical activity over a 3 to 12 month period.[11,12] There is growing evidence that virtual interventions are equally effective.[13–15] The impact of these interventions reflects a dose-dependent relationship between number of contact hours and treatment effectiveness.[6] Patients should be referred to IHBLT as soon as possible, once a patient has been diagnosed with obesity, as early intervention is essential to prevent youth-onset comorbidities. When referring patients to IHBLT, physicians should use motivational interviewing and a patient-centered, nonjudgmental approach.[16] The AAP emphasizes that while a comprehensive IHBLT approach is the gold standard, clinicians should be empowered to utilize whatever time and resources they have available, to deliver health education to their patients regardless of if they are able to meet the moderate-intensity to high-intensity contact hours recommended.[6] Studies have shown that repeat small doses of nutrition education, such as education on reduction of sugar-sweetened beverages, delivered at routine well-child visits, can lead to sustained behavior change and thus should be incorporated as well.[17–21]

The AAP consensus statement suggests that pediatricians and other pediatric health care providers should offer adolescents aged 12 years and older with obesity, weight loss pharmacotherapy, according to medication indications, risks, and benefits, as an adjunct to health behavior and lifestyle treatment.[6,22–27] In addition, the statement reports that pharmacotherapy may also be appropriate to children aged 8 to 11 years with more severe or life-threatening comorbidities. For youth aged 13 years and older with class II obesity, defined as a BMI 120% or greater of 95th percentile and an obesity-related comorbidity, or class III obesity, defined as a BMI 140% or greater of 95th percentile, without a comorbidity, bariatric surgery may be an appropriate recommendation.[6,28–30]

The comorbidities associated with youth-onset obesity tend to have a more severe disease progression in youth compared to their adult counterparts with the same obesity-related condition.[31–33] A comorbidity of focus in this study is MASLD, formerly called as nonalcoholic fatty liver disease. MASLD occurs in association with increased adiposity and insulin resistance and has rapidly evolved into the most common liver disease seen in the pediatric population.[34] MASLD has the highest prevalence in Hispanic children and a lower prevalence in black children. Growing evidence suggests that pediatric MASLD is a more severe disease than adult onset given the earlier age of disease of development and is believed to be the most common reason for liver transplant in the United States. Screening for MASLD should begin at the age of 10 years for patients with obesity by obtaining a lipid panel, fasting glucose, alanine aminotransferase, and aspartate aminotransferase every 2 years.[34] There is a direct association between the treatment of MASLD and the treatment of pediatric obesity. Best practices in the management of pediatric MASLD are not clearly defined, and thus, there is much to incorporate from the new AAP guidelines regarding how to best treat youth with obesity and MASLD. Currently, the first-line intervention for MASLD focuses on lifestyle modifications with a particular focus on the reduction of added sugars and increase in daily physical activity.[34] Children should avoid sugar-sweetened beverages, limit screen time to less than 2 hours per day, and exercise for 60 minutes per day. To date, there are no pharmacotherapies specifically Food and Drug Administration (FDA) approved for the treatment of MASLD in youth.

REVIEW OF DIETARY INTERVENTIONS FOR PEDIATRIC OBESITY MANAGEMENT

Behavioral interventions are the cornerstone for the management of obesity. The following section will summarize the major dietary interventions recommended for children with obesity. The overarching theme of these interventions is to reduce daily caloric intake, optimize healthful food consumption, and reduce BMI to, in turn, help decrease the risk of developing obesity-related comorbidities like MASLD. Increasing evidence suggests that the nutrition approach that results in the greatest reduction in BMI is that for which the family can adhere consistently. Sustained engagement with a nutrition approach is multifactorial; however, multiple studies have shown that families prefer nutrition approaches that allow for flexibility with daily schedules, availability of low-cost options, and are delivered in association with education to inform youth and families how these nutritional changes are resulting in improved health and wellness.[35–37]

Reduction in Added Sugar

The reduction of added sugar has been utilized as a dietary approach in the treatment of MASLD in youth.[38] Previous data have linked high intake of added sugars with severity of MASLD due to increased hepatic lipid accumulation. The AAP clinical practice guidelines highlighted education to reduce the intake of sugar-sweetened beverages as one of the best starting places for general pediatricians to target who have limited time and resources in patients with obesity.[6,34] Several clinical studies have investigated the association between reduction of dietary added sugar intake and alanine aminotransferase (ALT) levels in cohorts of youth with obesity compared to healthy control youth. Schwarz and colleagues[39] conducted a study in Latino and Black children aged 9 to 18 years with obesity with history of high added sugar intake (>50 g per day) and showed that by restricting their fructose intake to 4% of the participants daily energy intake for 10 days, there was an associated reduction in hepatic fat, de novo lipogenesis, and visceral fat. Schwimmer and colleagues[38] conducted a randomized controlled trial investigating a low added sugar nutrition approach in youth with obesity and MASLD in 40 adolescent male individuals who were randomized to either control or a low-sugar approach with less than 3% of daily intake of sugar. At week 8, youth in the low-sugar group had a significant reduction in hepatic steatosis compared to control.

Carbohydrate Restrictions

A carbohydrate (CHO) restriction regimen restricts CHO consumption by limiting foods high in CHOs and replacing them with foods containing a higher percentage of fat and protein. Though there can be variability in specific dietary recommendations, the consensus is to limit CHOs from 20 to 50 g of total CHOs per day. CHO restriction interventions have been shown to decrease BMI compared to baseline and had a greater reduction in BMI compared to low-fat diets. Though the research is limited, some results have shown CHO restriction is associated with significant reduction in hepatic de novo lipogenesis, hepatic fat, and fasting insulin.[40–45] Goss and colleagues[46] investigated reducing daily CHO intake, by providing prepared meals to families of youth with obesity and MASLD for 8 weeks and reported at the end of the study that there was a significant reduction in hepatic lipid content in the CHO-restricted group compared to control.

Calorie Restriction

A calorie restriction nutrition intervention consists of daily caloric intake under the recommend intake for weight maintenance. To determine the weight maintenance recommendation, the resting energy expenditure (REE) and active energy expenditure (AEE) must be determined. There are many proposed predictive equations to determine the REE. Systematic reviews have found the Molnár formula to be most predictive for children with obesity.[47]

Molnar formula

Female individuals: REE $= 0.046 \times$ weight $- 4.492 \times 1/\text{height}^2 - 0.151 \times$ race $+ 5.841$ ($R^2 = 0.824$)

Male individuals: REE $= 0.037 \times$ weight $- 4.67 \times 1/\text{height}^2 - 0.159 \times$ race $+ 6.792$ ($R^2 = 0.884$)

To determine the AEE, the REE will be adjusted by a multiplier based off the patient's activity level. The multipliers based off the exercise levels as followed sedentary (little to no exercise) $= 1.2$, lightly active (light exercise/sports 1–3 d/wk) $= 1.375$, moderately active (moderate activity/sports 3–5 d/wk) $= 1.555$, very active (hard activity/sports 6–7 d/wk) $= 1.725$. Calorie restriction nutrition interventions have consistently shown reduction in weight or BMI in pediatric populations with obesity. When combined with an exercise regimen, weight reduction is even greater.

Dietary Approach to Stop Hypertension

The Dietary Approach to Stop Hypertension (DASH) recommends a higher intake of fruits, vegetables, and whole foods with a decreased intake of processed foods, salt, and refined sugar as a means to decrease the risk of developing hypertension.[48] The recommendations include 6 to 8 servings of whole grains, 6 or less servings of protein, 4 to 5 servings of fruit, 4 to 5 servings of vegetables, 2 to 3 servings of low-fat dairy products, and less than 2300 mg of sodium per day with an ideal goal of less than 1500 mg.[48–50] To quantify dietary adherence, the DASH score was created. A higher DASH score indicates greater adherence to the diet. There are conflicting results regarding the relationship between DASH score and change in BMI.[48,50]

Currently, there are no trials investigating the use of the DASH diet to treat MASLD in youth. However, several trials in adult cohorts have suggested that when compared to control, the DASH diet results in significant reductions in weight, waist circumference, serum ALT, triglycerides, and C-reactive protein levels.[51-53] These findings suggest that the DASH diet may provide metabolic improvement in the underlying etiology of MASLD in youth and may, therefore, be an appropriate approach.

Time-Restricted Eating

A time-restricted eating (TRE) diet confines all dietary and caloric beverage intake to a predefined window of time, typically to 8 hours per day.[54] There has been limited research evaluating the impact of TRE on BMI in pediatric cohorts. A case study of 4 pediatric patients with obesity showed a decrease in body mass index z-score (zBMI) after 4 months of TRE.[55] Vidmar and colleagues[56] demonstrated that 12 weeks of 8 hour TRE with a self-selected eating window resulted in a 3% reduction in weight in excess of the 95th percentile. In adult cohorts, TRE combined with an exercise program has been shown to decrease fat mass, reduce liver enzymes, and improve insulin sensitivity in adults with obesity, with and without diabetes.[57-59]

Mediterranean Diet

The Mediterranean (MED) diet is the traditional diet of those in MED countries and is characterized by a high consumption of vegetables and olive oil, a moderate consumption of lean protein and fish, and a minimal consumption of highly processed food. Adherence to the MED diet is associated with a decrease in BMI. In addition, higher adherence to the MED diet is inversely associated with the development of MASLD/metabolic associated steatohepatitis (MASH).[60-63] A meta-analysis assessing the MED diet as an intervention in adult patients with MASLD showed significant improvements in ALT and hepatic steatosis.[51,64] Akbulut and colleagues conducted a trial of MED diet versus low-fat diet in youth with obesity and non-alcoholic fatty liver disease (NAFLD) and found that 12 weeks of MED diet resulted in similar reduction in hepatic steatosis and liver stiffness as those in the low-fat diet group and both groups had a normalization of their ALT levels. However, children in the MED diet intervention group demonstrated more significant reductions in a total insulin levels, fasting blood glucose, and hemoglobin A1c.

How to Implement Dietary Interventions

When considering recommendation of a dietary intervention in youth, it is important to consider the financial and cultural background of the family. There are many possible dietary interventions, the intervention that is most feasible for the family should be recommended first as that is what is most likely to be effective and sustainable. Parents and caregivers play a crucial role in pediatric obesity interventions. Pediatric patients are more likely to achieve BMI reduction if the dietary changes are incorporated into the whole family. Additionally, it is important to promote intrinsic motivation and self-efficacy through motivational interviewing and patient/caregiver empowerment.

REVIEW OF NONDIETARY BEHAVIORAL INTERVENTIONS

Behavior modification is a foundational aspect of weight management in patients in conjunction with dietary and pharmacotherapy interventions.[65-67] The focus of behavioral intervention for weight management is to decrease sedentary behaviors and increase active time throughout the day.[68-70] Studies have shown that there is an inverse relationship between sedentary behavior and activity, such that an increase in time spent doing physical activity is related to a decreased in sedentary time throughout the day.[70–74] Additionally, an increase in physical activity is associated with lower consumption of energy-dense food, higher consumption of fruits and vegetables and a lower BMI.[74]

Common approaches to behavior modification include stimulus control, self-monitoring, reinforcement, and modeling.[75–77] Family-based programs are recommended for children aged 5 to 12 years, with studies showing that parent adoption of healthy behaviors is associated with healthy behaviors in children.[78–82] Furthermore, parental weight loss is associated with weight loss in the child.[83–85] School-based programs have also been found to be an effective approach. A multifactorial approach with behavior modification combined with dietary intervention has been shown to be more effective in weight management when compared to diet or behavior modification alone.[6,7,11]

Cognitive behavioral therapy (CBT) is an additional approach to weight management that aims to identify triggers behind unhealthy eating habits. Patients who received CBT as part of a weight management regimen showed decreased rates of binge eating behaviors and sustained weight loss at 6 months follow-up.

Of note, the average total contact hours for behavioral modification programs in pediatric weight management is 27.7 hours over 6 months.[6] However, there is no statistical correlation between contact hours and treatment outcomes.[86] In a review of intervention efficacy, several intervention types were examined for their ability to achieve treatment goal. Interventions aimed at either increasing physical activity or decreasing sedentary time showed small, significant increase in activity and decreased sedentary behavior, respectively. The review also found that interventions aimed at increasing healthy eating behaviors showed statistical significance in trials that used reinforcement. Additionally, trials that aimed at reducing unhealthy eating behaviors were significantly more effective when treatment lasted longer than 6 months.[87]

REVIEW OF PHARMACOTHERAPY INTERVENTIONS

Pharmacotherapy may be a powerful tool to consider in patients who have not reached weight normality with dietary interventions alone.[22,24,88] The AAP consensus statement states that pediatricians and other pediatric health care providers should offer adolescents aged 12 years and older with obesity weight loss pharmacotherapy, according to medication indications, risks, and benefits, as an adjunct to health behavior and lifestyle treatment.[6,22–27] In addition, the statement reports that pharmacotherapy may also be appropriate for ages 8 to 11 years for patients with more severe or life-threatening comorbidities.[6] The overarching theme of these interventions is to reduce BMI to, in turn, help decrease the risk of developing or progression of obesity-related comorbidities like MASLD. **Tables 1** and **2** summarized the available pediatric obesity pharmacotherapies.

Glucagon-Like-Peptide-1 Receptor Agonist

Glucagon-like-peptide-1 (GLP-1) receptor agonists decrease hunger by slowing gastric emptying and acting on the central nervous system.[89–91] Depending on the medication, it is formulated as a daily oral medication or daily or weekly subcutaneous injection.[90] Exenatide is currently approved in children aged 10 to 17 years with type-2 diabetes.[92] Liraglutide is currently approved for long-term weight management in children aged 12 years or older.[93] Adverse effects include nausea, vomiting, diarrhea, and injection site reaction. Rare complications include pancreatitis, gallbladder disease,

Table 1
Summary of trials of obesity pharmacotherapy in pediatrics

Study	Design	Sample Size (n)	Age (y)	Main Inclusion Criteria	Dose	Duration	Efficacy	Safety	Quality of Evidence
Phentermine									
Lorber et al,[131] 1966	3 parallel-arm (phenmetrazine vs phentermine vs placebo) RCT Outcome measure: weight change (kg)	68	3–15	BMI >95th%	Phenmetrazine 12.5 mg daily Phentermine 15 mg daily	12 wk	Phentermine vs placebo: 0.1 kg	Phentermine arm: insomnia (n = 1)	Low
Rauh et al,[132] 1968	2 parallel-arm (chlorphentermine vs placebo) RCT Outcome measure: weight change (kg)	30	12–18	BMI >95th%	Chlorphentermine 65 mg daily	12 wk	Phentermine vs placebo: 6.7 kg	No SAEs	Low
Ryder et al,[97] 2017	Retrospective chart review Outcome measure: %BMI change	25	12–18	BMI >95th%	Phentermine 15 mg/d	24 wk	Phentermine vs placebo: 4.1% BMI	Phentermine arm: increased blood pressure, heart rate	Moderate
Ali Ibrahim et al,[133] 2022	Retrospective chart review Outcome measure: %BMIp95 change	30	12–18	BMI >95th%	Phentermine 8–37.5 mg/d	24 mo	Youth taking phentermine had mean reduction in %BMIp95 of −15%	AE (n = 6): agitation, sleep disturbances, increased blood pressure, anxiety, photophobia, and dehydration	Low
Topiramate									
Fox et al,[101] 2015	Retrospective chart review Outcome measure: %BMI change	28	14–18	BMI >95th%	Topiramate 25–125 mg/d	24 wk	Topiramate vs lifestyle modification: 4.9% BMI	No SAEs	Low
Fox et al,[134] 2016	2 parallel-arm (topiramate + meal replacement vs placebo) RCT Outcome measure: %BMI change	21	14–18	BMI >120% of the 95th%	Topiramate 75 mg/d	24 wk	Topiramate vs placebo: 1.9% BMI	No SAEs	Low
Consoli et al,[135] 2019	2 parallel-arm (topiramate vs placebo) RCT Outcome measure: %BMI change	62	15–45	Prader–Willi syndrome Youth: BMI >95th% Adult: BMI >30 kg/m²	Topiramate 50–200 mg/d	8 wk	%BMI Change: Topiramate vs placebo: no difference Hyperphagia scores: Topiramate vs placebo: significant reduction in topiramate group	No SAEs	Low

(continued on next page)

Table 1
(continued)

Study	Design	Sample Size (n)	Age (y)	Main Inclusion Criteria	Dose	Duration	Efficacy	Safety	Quality of Evidence
Berman et al,[102] 2023	Case series Outcome measure: %BMIp95 change	5	8–12	BMI >95th% Developmental delay	Topiramate 100 mg/d	16 wk	Topiramate group mean reduction in %BMIp95 −12%	4/5 No SAEs 1/5 drowsiness	Low
PHEN/TPM									
Kelly et al,[105] 2022	3 parallel-arm (PHEN/TPM 7.5 mg/46 mg, vs PHEN/TPM 15 mg/92 mg vs Placebo) RCT Outcome measure: %BMI change	223	14–18	BMI >95th%	PHEN/TPM 7.5 mg/46 mg PHEN/TPM 15 mg/92 mg	56 wk	High-dose PHEN/TPM: 10.44 % BMI vs Low dose PHEN/TPM: 8.11% vs +0.1% Placebo	3 SAEs: bile duct stone, depression, suicidal ideation	High
Liraglutide									
Kelly et al,[136] 2020	RCT	251	12–17	BMI ≥95th%, did not exclude if T2D	3.0 mg daily	56 wk + 26 wk follow-up	zBMI change (SD): ETD of −0.22, favoring intervention ($P = .002$) Reduction in BMI of ≥5%: 43.3% of intervention vs 18.7% of placebo Reduction in BMI of ≥10%: 26.1% of intervention vs 8.1% of placebo	GI AEs more frequent in intervention (64.8% vs 36.5%) AEs leading to discontinuation more frequently in intervention (10.4% vs 0%) Few SAEs (2.4% vs 4.0%)	High
Bensignor et al,[137] 2021	RCT	134	10–16	BMI ≥85th% and T2D	0.6 mg daily 1.2 mg daily 1.8 mg daily	52 wk	BMI change (kg/m²): ETD of −0.89, favoring intervention ($P=.036$) % change in BMI (%): ETF of −2.73, favoring intervention ($P=.028$) %BMIp95 change (%): ETD of −4.42, favoring intervention ($P=.038$) Findings are significant at 52 wk, not at 26 wk	Not evaluated	High

Exenatide

Study	Design	N	Age	Inclusion	Dose	Duration	Outcomes	Adverse events	Quality
Kelly et al,[138] 2012	Randomized, open-label, crossover	12	9–16	BMI ≥1.2 times the 95th%, or BMI ≥35 kg/m²	10 μg twice daily DE: 5 μg twice daily, 10 μg twice daily	6 mo	BMI change (kg/m²): ETD of −1.71, favoring intervention (P=.01) % change in BMI (%): ETD of −4.92, favoring intervention (P=.009) Total body weight change (kg): ETD of −3.9, favoring intervention (P=.02) Insulin-related findings: Fasting insulin change (mU/L): ETD of −7.5, favoring intervention (P=.02) Insulin sensitivity: ETD of +6.1, favoring intervention (P=.02) β-cell function: ETD of +17.97, favoring intervention (P=.03)	Mild nausea in 36%, vomiting in 27%, headache in 27%, abdominal pain in 27%, injection site bruising in 9% (1 participant). No hypoglycemia or pancreatitis	High
Fox et al,[139] 2022	RCT	100	12–18	BMI ≥1.2 times the 95th%	2.0 mg extended release, weekly	52 wk	% change in BMI (%): ETD of −4.1, favoring intervention, did not reach significance (P =.078) Cardiometabolic findings: TG/HDL ratio: ETD of −0.61, favoring intervention (P = .05)	AE frequency similar between groups (96.9% of intervention vs 90.9% of placebo) GI AEs more common in intervention No serious adverse event directly related to the study drug	High
Semaglutide									
Weghuber et al,[94] 2022	RCT	201	12–17	BMI ≥95th% or BMI ≥85th% + weight-related coexisting condition	2.4 mg weekly	68 wk	BMI change from baseline ETD of −16.7, favoring intervention group (P ≤.001) Weight loss of ≥5%: 73% of intervention vs 18% of placebo. Cardiometabolic findings: Improved waist circumference, HbA1c, lipids, AST were greater in intervention	GI AEs greater (62% of intervention vs 42% of placebo) 4% with cholestasis in intervention SAEs in 11% of intervention vs 9% of placebo	High

Abbreviations: %BMIp95, BMI in excess of the 95th percentile; AE, adverse event; BMI, body mass index; BMI >95th%, body mass index greater than the 95th percentile; ETD, estimated treatment difference; GI, gastrointestinal; HbA1c, hemoglobin A1c; LDL, low-density lipoprotein; PHEN/TPM, phentermine/topiramate extended release product; RCT, randomized controlled trial; SAE, serious adverse event; TG, triglycerides.

Table 2
Overview of obesity pharmacotherapy in pediatrics

Agent	Phentermine	Topiramate	PHEN/TPM	Metformin	Liraglutide	Semaglutide	Orlistat	Setmenalotide	Naltrexone/Bupropion
FDA Status	Yes ≥16yo for short-term use	No ≥2 year old for seizures ≥12 year old for migraine prophylaxis	Yes ≥12 year old	No	Yes ≥12 year old	Yes ≥12 year old	Yes ≥12 year old	Yes ≥6 year old with BBS, POMC, LEPR, PCSK1	No
Weight Loss Mechanism of Action	Norepinephrine (NE) reuptake inhibition Increases the release of NE in the central nervous system by releasing NE from presynaptic vesicles. Stimulates release of serotonin and dopamine, from nerve terminals Monoamine oxidase and serotonin reuptake inhibitor	Modulation of GABA Antagonizesalpha-amino-3-hydroxyl-4-isoxazole-propionic acid kainite receptors Carbonic-anhydrase inhibition	Phen + TPM	Decreases hepatic glucose production. Increases insulin sensitivity by increasing peripheral glucose uptake and utilization. Inhibits mitochondrial complex I activity	Glucagon-like peptide-1 receptor agonists (GLP1RA) augment glucose-dependent insulin release and reduce glucagon secretion and gastric emptying Decrease food intake through central modulation of appetite control		Inhibits gastric and pancreatic lipases	melanocortin-4 receptor agonist	Bupropion is a reuptake inhibitor and releasing agent of both norepinephrine and dopamine, and a nicotinic acetylcholine receptor antagonist, and it activates proopiomelanocortin (POMC) neurons. Naltrexone is a pure opioid antagonist
Mode of Administration and Dose	Oral 8 mg, 15 mg, 30 mg, 37.5 mg Daily in morning	Oral Up to 200 mg twice daily (obesity dosing varies widely); extended release formulation	Oral Mid-dose (phentermine7.5 mg/ topiramate extended release 46 mg) High-dose (phentermine15 mg/ topiramate extended release 92 mg) Once daily in the morning	Oral 1000 mg twice daily	3 mg daily	2.4 mg weekly	160 mg TID	3 mg SQ	extended-release tablet contains naltrexone 8 mg/bupropion 90 mg to max of naltrexone 32 mg/bupropion 360 mg
Controlled Substance	Yes Schedule IV	No	Yes Schedule IV	No	No	No	No	No	No

Profile	Tachycardia Palpitations Pulmonary hypertension Agitation Restlessness Insomnia Anxiety Euphoria Tremor	Paresthesia Dizziness Dysgeusia Cognitive Impairment Dry mouth Diarrhea Constipation Fetal toxicity Decreased visual acuity Worsening depression or suicidal thoughts Metabolic acidosis Elevation of creatinine,		Vomiting Diarrhea Lactic acidosis	fatigue, headache, hypoglycemia, mood changes	Steatosis Diarrhea Nausea Bloating	Injection site reaction Headache, Fatigue Nausea Vomiting Diarrhea Spontaneous penile erection	Constipation Dizziness Insomnia Nausea Vomiting Diarrhea Dream disorder Headache disorder Symptoms of anxiety Tinnitus Hypertension Pruritus of skin Urticaria Arthralgia Myalgia Hyperhidrosis Tremor Dysgeusia Skin rash
Contraindications	History of CVD or drug use; MAOI use; hyperthyroidism; glaucoma; agitated states; pregnancy	Pregnancy, glaucoma,	Same contraindications for phentermine and topiramate monotherapy	Renal failure; lactic acidosis	Family history of medullary thyroid carcinoma; pregnancy; breastfeeding	None	pregnancy; breastfeeding	
Use Cautions	High blood pressure, congenital heart disease, use of SSRIs, SNRIs, insulin, or valproic acid, renal disease, metabolic acidosis, history of kidney stones, depression, suicidal ideation, high risk for pregnancy	Kidney stones, glaucoma, high risk for pregnancy due to fetal toxicity, metabolic acidosis, active suicidal ideation, poor cognitive function, and academic struggles	Same use cautions recommended for phentermine and topiramate monotherapy	NA	Pancreatitis	Pancreatitis	None	High blood pressure Congestive heart failure/recent myocardial infarction Bipolar disorder/thoughts of suicide Current or recent use morphine/methadone/buprenorphine Kidney disease Cirrhosis Glaucoma Use/abuse of drugs/alcohol Seizures

(continued on next page)

Table 2
(continued)

Agent	Phentermine	Topiramate	PHEN/TPM	Metformin	Liraglutide	Semaglutide	Orlistat	Setmenalotide	Naltrexone/Bupropion
Cost	Low	Low	Moderate	Low	High		Low	High	Moderate
Patient Selection	Strong hunger; low energy	Poor satiety, food cravings, symptoms of binge eating disorder, migraine, headaches, night eating, seizures	Dual therapy Insurance Coverage Desire for synergist effect with daily dosing	Insulin resistance; concomitant use of anti-psychotic medications	Insulin resistance, type 2 diabetes, polycystic ovarian syndrome; poor satiety; food cravings			Monogenic obesity	Concomitant mood disorder; poor satiety; binge eating disorder

Abbreviations: %BMIp95, BMI in excess of the 95th percentile; %BMIp95, BMI greater than 95th%, body mass index greater than the 95th percentile; CVD, cardiovascular disease; GI, gastrointestinal; AE, adverse event; BMI, body mass index; BMI greater than 95th%, body mass index greater than the 95th percentile; CVD, cardiovascular disease; GI, gastrointestinal; HbA1c, hemoglobin A1c; LDL, low density lipoprotein; MAOI, monoamine oxidase inhibitors; PHEN/TPM, Phentermine/topiramate extended release product; RCT, randomized controlled trial; SAE, serious adverse event; SNRIs, Serotonin–norepinephrine reuptake inhibitors; SSRIs, selective serotonin reuptake inhibitors; TG, triglycerides.

and renal impairment. Liraglutide dosing at starts 0.6 mg up to 3 mg per day. Sema-glutide 2.4 mg weekly was recently FDA approved for the treatment of pediatric obesity in youth aged 12 years and older. The seminal trialed showed a mean BMI reduction of 16% in more than 70% of participants.[94] Semaglutide dosing starts 0.25 mg up to 2.4 mg per week, dosed weekly.[93] These medications have been shown to be the most effective pharmacotherapy with the highest mean reduction in BMI and least amount of heterogeneity in response, unlike many of the other available pharma-cotherapies that have significant heterogeneity in efficacy across individual response rates.[94] **Table 1** summarized pediatric efficacy data of GLP-1 agonists for obesity management.

Phentermine

Phentermine is an indirect sympathomimetic that increases the availability of norepi-nephrine, serotonin, and dopamine and reduces appetite.[95,96] Phentermine is FDA approved for weight loss as short course therapy (3 months or less) in adolescents aged 16 years or older.[97,98] Adverse effects include tachycardia, palpitations, hyper-tension, anxiety, dizziness, insomnia, headache, dry mouth, and gastrointestinal (GI) upset and are dose dependent. Dosing starts at 7.5 mg up to 37.5 mg per day. The weight loss benefit of phentermine is not always increased with increased dose.

Topiramate

Topiramate is an anticonvulsant and gamma-aminobutyric acid (GABA) receptor mod-ifier, causing glutamate inhibition and increased dopamine release and is formulated as a daily oral medication.[98–101] Topiramate is not FDA approved for weight loss in adults or children and is used off-label. Adverse effects include paresthesia, sedation, mood disturbance, visual disturbance, GI upset, and migraine.[99,101,102] These adverse effects are typically dose dependent. Dosing starts at 25 mg to 100 mg daily in twice daily dosing. In youth with obesity, topiramate in combination with lifestyle modifica-tion is effective for decreasing BMI.[101,102]

Phentermine/Topiramate Combination

The phentermine/topiramate combination is a one capsule combination daily pill that is FDA approved for weight loss in youth aged 12 years and older with obesity.[103–105] The safety and efficacy of combining the 2 individual agents together has not yet been determined but is often done off-label to decrease patient financial burden. The phen-termine/topiramate combination includes an immediate release of phentermine with an extended release of topiramate. This combination allows for a decrease in the in-dividual dose of both drugs to decrease occurrence of adverse events. This combina-tion is not recommended for anyone with cardiovascular disease due to rare but significant risk of cardiovascular ischemic events.[103,106] Adverse effects include dry mouth, constipation, paresthesia, sedation, mood disturbance, and visual distur-bance.[107] These adverse effects are typically dose dependent. Dosing starts at 3.75 mg phentermine/23 mg topiramate up to 15 mg phentermine/92 mg topiramate daily. In adolescents with obesity, the combination therapy has been shown to provide significant reduction in BMI with the effects being dose dependent.[108–110]

Orlistat

Orlistat is a gastric lipase inhibitor, decreasing the gastric absorption of dietary fat and is formulated as a daily oral medication. Orlistat is currently FDA approved for long-term weight loss in adolescents and adults. Adverse effects include steatorrhea, fecal urgency, and flatulence, and fat-soluble vitamin deficiency and are not always dose dependent. Dosing starts at is typically 120 mg, 3 times per day. The adverse effects limit the tolerability, and because of this, orlistat is rarely used in pediatric cohorts. Studies show orlistat produces a small decrease in liver enzymes in adolescents as well as a reduction in cholesterol, low-density lipoprotein, fasting glucose, insulin, and blood pressure.[111–115]

Bupropion/Naltrexone Combination

Bupropion is a dopamine-reuptake inhibitor. Naltrexone is an opioid receptor antagonist.[115] The combination is proposed to have a synergistic effect at reducing food intake and is formulated as a daily oral medication. Bupropion/naltrexone is FDA approved for weight loss in adults. There are currently no randomized controlled trials evaluating the impact on weight loss in pediatric cohorts. Adverse effects include nausea, headache, constipation, insomnia, dry mouth, and dizziness. Dosing starts at 8 mg naltrexone/90 mg bupropion up to 32 mg naltrexone/360 mg bupropion daily. Bupropion also has an FDA warning for increasing suicidal ideation in young adults.[110,113,114]

Metformin

Metformin is a biguanide drug that reduces glucose production in the liver, decreases intestinal absorption, and increases insulin sensitivity and is formulated as a daily oral medication.[116] Metformin is only FDA approved for the management of type 2 diabetes. Adverse effects are dose dependent and include bloating, nausea, flatulence, and diarrhea. Lactic acidosis is a rare but potentially fatal complication.[116] Metformin dosing is dependent on the indication and patient comorbidities. Metformin has been shown to result in modest reduction in BMI in pediatric cohorts; however, there is limited evidence to support its use as an obesity pharmacotherapy. Metformin has been shown to support weight reduction in youth taking weight gain promoting antipsychotic agents such as risperidone. In addition, for some adolescent female individuals with polycystic ovarian syndrome, metformin has been shown to be useful in combination with oral contraceptive agents to promote restoration of normal menstrual cycles and improve insulin sensitivity.

Setmelanotide

Setmelanotide is a melanocortin-4 receptor agonist developed for the treatment of obesity arising from proopiomelanocortin (POMC), proprotein convertase subtilisin/kexin type 1 (PCSK1), or leptin receptor (LEPR) deficiency. The drug has received FDA approval for chronic weight management in youth aged 6 years and older with obesity caused by POMC, PCSK1, and LEPR deficiency and those with Bardet–Biedl syndrome. Setmelanotide is administered as a daily subcutaneous injection. The side effect profile includes hyperpigmentation, nausea, vomiting, headaches, spontaneous penile erection, and injection site reactions. The seminal trials have demonstrated significant reduction in BMI and improvement in hunger scores when compared to placebo.[117–119]

SURGICAL INTERVENTIONS

Several surgical procedures exist that are used to augment weight loss in patients with obesity. The AAP recommends bariatric surgery as a treatment option for those with either class 2 obesity with comorbidities or class 3 obesity with or without comorbidities. The AAP recommends bariatric surgery for youth aged 13 years and older who meet the above criteria. The American Society for Metabolic and Bariatric Surgery agrees with the recommendations of the AAP regarding bariatric surgery for pediatric weight management.[1,29,120]

There are multiple bariatric procedures that can be performed; however, sleeve gastrectomy remains the most commonly completed surgery in youth with obesity. *Gastric bypass:* Gastric bypass surgery is characterized by the creation of a small pouch at the top of the stomach and bypassing a portion of the small intestine. This restricts the amount of food one can eat and decreased calorie absorption. *Sleeve gastrectomy:* A larger portion of the stomach is removed, leaving a small, sleeve-shaped pouch. Similar to gastric bypass, this limits the volume of food that can be consumed and also decreases the level of hunger-stimulating hormones that are released. This is the most common surgical procedure performed in pediatric weight management. *Vertical banded gastroplasty:* The stomach is stapled to create a small pouch, while a band is placed around the stomach to restrict the size of the gastric outlet.[28,121,122]

Several studies exist that examine the safety and efficacy of bariatric surgery in pediatric weight management. The Teen-LABS project is a prospective observational study of 242 adolescents as well as two 47 year outcome studies, which provide sufficient data to conclude that bariatric surgery in adolescents is as safe and effective as bariatric surgery in adults. Additionally, a review performed in 2021 supports the conclusions of the Teen-LABS project. Another review performed in 2021 found that early referral for bariatric surgery improves the quality of life in children with obesity.

ENDOSCOPIC THERAPIES

There is growing evidence exploring the use of endoscopic therapies for the treatment of pediatric obesity.[123–127] Several device-based endoscopic treatments have been utilized in adult cohorts with obesity including but not limited to the endoscopic sleeve gastroplasty, endoluminal procedure, and the transoral anterior-to-posterior greater curvature plication procedure.[128] There is a paucity of literature on these techniques in pediatrics cohorts despite the potential as an adjunct therapy to the comprehensive obesity care model.[126,127,129] Several studies have examined the use of the space-occupying intragastric balloon (IGB) in pediatric cohorts with severe obesity.[125–127,130] In pediatric patients, a retrospective study of 27 adolescents with a nonadjustable IGB showed a total body weight loss of 16.35% without any serious adverse events.[130] In addition, a recent study of a swallowable IGB showed an estimate weight loss of 20.1% in 16 children with obesity without any complications.[128] No pediatric studies have evaluated the IGB for MASLD. The most well-studied endobariatric treatment is the endoscopic sleeve gastroplasty (ESG). ESG is an endoscopic procedure that uses full-thickness sutures to plicate the greater curvature of the stomach, creating a tubular sleeve-like configuration. Alqahtani and colleagues[128] presented the first series of youth with obesity (n = 109) undergoing ESG and reported a mean total body weight loss of 16.2% at 12 months, 15.4% at 18 months, and 13.7% at 24 months. All obesity comorbidities were in complete remission from 3 months through the end of the study.[128]

DISCUSSION

Pediatric obesity remains a major public health concern that results in life-limiting complications if left untreated. The 2023 American Academy of Pediatric clinical practice guidelines emphasize that pediatric obesity is a complex, multifactorial, chronic disease and requires a comprehensive treatment approach.[6] The treatment approach should incorporate intensive health and behavioral lifestyles modifications with concurrent use of obesity pharmacotherapy and bariatric surgery based on the severity of the disease at presentation.[6] The evaluation of pediatric obesity requires a thorough medical, medication and social history, screening for social determinants of health, assessment of mental health, detection of disordered eating concerns, and determination of readiness for change as well as physical examination. Life-limiting complications, such as type 2 diabetes and MASLD must be screened for routinely to ensure treatment is initiated early. The current evidence supports that obesity treatment is safe and effective. There is no evidence that the watchful waiting approach is appropriate. Pediatricians and other pediatric health care professionals should offer treatment options early and at the highest available intensity available. The clinical practice guidelines recommend using the framework of a medical home and the chronic care model with a motivational interviewing approach.[6] The goal of treatment is not the number on the scale but the prevention of life-limiting complications that can significantly impact the health of these youth over time.[131–139]

CLINICS CARE POINTS

- The evaluation of pediatric obesity requires a thorough medical, medication and social history, screening for social determinants of health, assessment of mental health, detection of disordered eating concerns and determination of readiness for change as well as physical examination.

- Pediatricians and other pediatric health care professionals should offer treatment options early and at the highest available intensity available.

- The clinical practice guidelines recommend using the framework of a medical home and the chronic care model with a motivational interviewing approach.

- The goal of treatment is not the number on the scale but the prevention of life-limiting complications that can significantly impact the health of these youth over time.

DISCLOSURE

The authors have no financial relationships or conflict of interest relevant to this article to disclose. Conflict of interest: The authors have no financial relationships or conflict of interest relevant to this article to disclose.

REFERENCES

1. Ogden CL, Martin CB, Freedman DS, et al. Trends in obesity disparities during childhood. Pediatrics 2022;150(2). https://doi.org/10.1542/PEDS.2022-056547.
2. Hales CM, Fryar CD, Carroll MD, et al. Trends in obesity and severe obesity prevalence in us youth and adults by sex and age, 2007-2008 to 2015-2016. JAMA 2018;319(16):1723–5.
3. DS F, NF B, EM T, et al. BMI z-Scores are a poor indicator of adiposity among 2- to 19-year-olds with very high BMIs, NHANES 1999-2000 to 2013-2014. Obesity 2017;25(4):739–46.
4. Ogden CL, Fryar CD, Martin CB, et al. Trends in obesity prevalence by race and hispanic origin - 1999-2000 to 2017-2018. JAMA, J Am Med Assoc 2020; 324(12):1208–10.
5. Ogden CL, Fryar CD, Hales CM, et al. Differences in obesity prevalence by demographics and urbanization in US Children and Adolescents, 2013-2016. JAMA 2018;319(23):2410–8.

6. Hampl SE, Hassink SG, Skinner AC, et al. Clinical practice guideline for the evaluation and treatment of children and adolescents with obesity. Pediatrics 2023; 151(2). https://doi.org/10.1542/PEDS.2022-060640.

7. SE B. Expert committee recommendations regarding the prevention, assessment, and treatment of child and adolescent overweight and obesity: summary report. Pediatrics 2007;120(Suppl 4).

8. Kelly AS, Barlow SE, Rao G, et al. Severe obesity in children and adolescents: identification, associated health risks, and treatment approaches: a scientific statement from the American Heart Association. Circulation 2013;128(15): 1689–712.

9. Salam RA, Padhani ZA, Das JK, et al. Effects of lifestyle modification interventions to prevent and manage child and adolescent obesity: a systematic review and meta-analysis. Nutrients 2020;12(8):1–23.

10. Cho K, Park S, Koyanagi A, et al. The effect of pharmacological treatment and lifestyle modification in patients with nonalcoholic fatty liver disease: An umbrella review of meta-analyses of randomized controlled trials. Obes Rev 2022;23(9). https://doi.org/10.1111/OBR.13464.

11. Styne DM, Arslanian SA, Connor EL, et al. Pediatric obesity-assessment, treatment, and prevention: an endocrine society clinical practice guideline. J Clin Endocrinol Metab 2017;102(3):709–57.

12. August GP, Caprio S, Fennoy I, et al. Prevention and treatment of pediatric obesity: An Endocrine Society clinical practice guideline based on expert opinion. J Clin Endocrinol Metab 2008;93(12). https://doi.org/10.1210/jc.2007-2458.

13. Cueto V, Sanders LM. Telehealth Opportunities and Challenges for Managing Pediatric Obesity. Pediatr Clin North Am 2020;67(4):647–54.

14. Calcaterra V, Verduci E, Vandoni M, et al. Telehealth: a useful tool for the management of nutrition and exercise programs in pediatric obesity in the COVID-19 Era. Nutrients 2021;13(11). https://doi.org/10.3390/NU13113689.

15. Shaikh U, Nettiksimmons J, Romano P. Pediatric obesity management in rural clinics in California and the role of telehealth in distance education. J Rural Health 2011;27(3):263–9.

16. Woolford SJ, Resnicow K, Davis MM, et al. Cost-effectiveness of a motivational interviewing obesity intervention versus usual care in pediatric primary care offices. Obesity 2022;30(11):2265–74.

17. Momin SR, Wood AC. Sugar-sweetened beverages and child health: implications for policy. Curr Nutr Rep 2018;7(4):286–93.

18. Nezami BT, Ward DS, Lytle LA, et al. A mHealth randomized controlled trial to reduce sugar-sweetened beverage intake in preschool-aged children. Pediatr Obes 2018;13(11):668–76.

19. Laverty AA, Magee L, Monteiro CA, et al. Sugar and artificially sweetened beverage consumption and adiposity changes: National longitudinal study. Int J Behav Nutr Phys Activ 2015;12(1). https://doi.org/10.1186/s12966-015-0297-y.

20. Copperstone C, Mcneill G, Aucott L, et al. A pilot study to improve sugar and water consumption in Maltese school children. Int J Adolesc Med Health 2019;33(2). https://doi.org/10.1515/IJAMH-2018-0134.

21. Seferidi P, Millett C, Laverty AA. Sweetened beverage intake in association to energy and sugar consumption and cardiometabolic markers in children. Pediatr Obes 2018;13(4):195–203.

22. Kelly AS, Fox CK, Rudser KD, et al. Pediatric obesity pharmacotherapy: current state of the field, review of the literature and clinical trial considerations. Int J Obes 2016;40(7):1043–50.

23. Ioannides-Demos LL, Proietto J, McNeil JJ. Pharmacotherapy for obesity. Drugs 2005;65(10):1391–418.

24. Kühnen P, Biedermann H, Wiegand S. Pharmacotherapy in childhood obesity. Horm Res Paediatr 2022;95(2). https://doi.org/10.1159/000518432.

25. Kelly AS, Fox CK. Pharmacotherapy in the management of pediatric obesity. Curr Diab Rep 2017;17(8). https://doi.org/10.1007/S11892-017-0886-Z.

26. Singhal V, Sella AC, Malhotra S. Pharmacotherapy in pediatric obesity: current evidence and landscape. Curr Opin Endocrinol Diabetes Obes 2021;28(1): 55–63.

27. C B, E K, CK F, et al. Trends in prescribing anti-obesity pharmacotherapy for paediatric weight management: Data from the POWER Work Group. Pediatr Obes 2021;16(1). https://doi.org/10.1111/IJPO.12701.

28. Armstrong SC, Bolling CF, Michalsky MP, et al. Pediatric Metabolic and Bariatric Surgery: Evidence, Barriers, and Best Practices. Pediatrics 2019;144(6). https://doi.org/10.1542/PEDS.2019-3223.

29. JSA P, A B, NT B, et al. ASMBS pediatric metabolic and bariatric surgery guidelines, 2018. Surg Obes Relat Dis 2018;14(7):882–901.

30. Aikenhead A, Knai C, Lobstein T. Effectiveness and cost-effectiveness of paediatric bariatric surgery: a systematic review. Clin Obes 2011;1(1):12–25.

31. Tryggestad JB, Willi SM. Complications and comorbidities of T2DM in adolescents: Findings from the TODAY clinical trial. J Diabet Complicat 2015;29(2).

32. Kumar S, Kelly AS. Review of childhood obesity: from epidemiology, etiology, and comorbidities to clinical assessment and treatment. Mayo Clin Proc 2017; 92(2):251–65.

33. F B, P C, RL G, et al. Racial and ethnic disparities in comorbidities in youth with type 2 diabetes in the pediatric diabetes consortium (PDC). Diabetes Care 2021;44(10):2245–51.

34. Vos MB, Abrams SH, Barlow SE, et al. NASPGHAN Clinical Practice Guideline for the Diagnosis and Treatment of Nonalcoholic Fatty Liver Disease in Children: Recommendations from the Expert Committee on NAFLD (ECON) and the North American Society of Pediatric Gastroenterology, Hepatology and Nutrition (NASPGHAN). J Pediatr Gastroenterol Nutr 2017;64(2):319–34.

35. Johnston CA, Moreno JP, Hernandez DC, et al. Levels of adherence needed to achieve significant weight loss. Int J Obes 2019;43(1):125–31.

36. Jelalian E, Foster GD, Sato AF, et al. Treatment adherence and facilitator characteristics in a community based pediatric weight control intervention. Int J Behav Nutr Phys Act 2014;11(1).

37. Berkowitz RI, Marcus MD, Anderson BJ, et al. Adherence to a lifestyle program for youth with type 2 diabetes and its association with treatment outcome in the TODAY clinical trial. Pediatr Diabetes 2018;19(2):191–8.

38. Schwimmer JB, Ugalde-Nicalo P, Welsh JA, et al. Effect of a low free sugar diet vs usual diet on nonalcoholic fatty liver disease in adolescent boys: a randomized clinical trial. JAMA 2019;321(3):256–65.

39. Schwarz JM, Noworolski SM, Wen MJ, et al. Effect of a high-fructose weight-maintaining diet on lipogenesis and liver fat. J Clin Endocrinol Metab 2015; 100(6):2434–42.

40. Skytte MJ, Samkani A, Petersen AD, et al. A carbohydrate-reduced high-protein diet improves HbA1c and liver fat content in weight stable participants with type 2 diabetes: a randomised controlled trial. Diabetologia 2019;62(11):2066–78.

41. Tay J, Thompson CH, Luscombe-Marsh ND, et al. Effects of an energy-restricted low-carbohydrate, high unsaturated fat/low saturated fat diet versus a high-carbohydrate, low-fat diet in type 2 diabetes: A 2-year randomized clinical trial. Diabetes Obes Metabol 2018;20(4):858–71.

42. Jenkins DJA, Wolever TMS, Taylor RH, et al. Glycemic index of foods: a physiological basis for carbohydrate exchange. Am J Clin Nutr 1981;34(3):362–6.

43. Jansen LT, Yang N, Wong JMW, et al. Prolonged glycemic adaptation following transition from a low- to high-carbohydrate diet: a randomized controlled feeding trial. Diabetes Care 2022. https://doi.org/10.2337/DC21-1970.

44. He M, Wang J, Liang Q, et al. Time-restricted eating with or without low-carbohydrate diet reduces visceral fat and improves metabolic syndrome: A randomized trial. Cell Rep Med 2022;3(10). https://doi.org/10.1016/J.XCRM.2022.100777.

45. Rasmussen L, Christensen ML, Poulsen CW, et al. Effect of high versus low carbohydrate intake in the morning on glycemic variability and glycemic control measured by continuous blood glucose monitoring in women with gestational diabetes mellitus-a randomized crossover study. Nutrients 2020;12(2).

46. Goss AM, Dowla S, Pendergrass M, et al. Effects of a carbohydrate-restricted diet on hepatic lipid content in adolescents with non-alcoholic fatty liver disease: A pilot, randomized trial. Pediatr Obes 2020;15(7).

47. Fuentes-Servín J, Avila-Nava A, González-Salazar LE, et al. Resting energy expenditure prediction equations in the pediatric population: a systematic review. Front Pediatr 2021;9:795364.

48. Bricarello LP, de Moura Souza A, de Almeida Alves M, et al. Association between DASH diet (Dietary Approaches to Stop Hypertension) and hypertension in adolescents: A cross-sectional school-based study. Clin Nutr ESPEN 2020;36:69–75.

49. Dashti HS, Gómez-Abellán P, Qian J, et al. Late eating is associated with cardiometabolic risk traits, obesogenic behaviors, and impaired weight loss. Am J Clin Nutr 2020;113(1):154–61.

50. Garaulet M, Lopez-Minguez J, Dashti HS, et al. Interplay of dinner timing and MTNR1B type 2 diabetes risk variant on glucose tolerance and insulin secretion: a randomized crossover trial. Diabetes Care 2022;45(3):512–9.

51. Paula Bricarello L, Poltronieri F, Fernandes R, et al. Effects of the Dietary Approach to Stop Hypertension (DASH) diet on blood pressure, overweight and obesity in adolescents: A systematic review. Clin Nutr ESPEN 2018;28:1–11.

52. Costello E, Goodrich J, Patterson WB, et al. Diet quality is associated with glucose regulation in a cohort of young adults. Nutrients 2022;14(18).

53. Razavi Zade M, Telkabadi MH, Bahmani F, et al. The effects of DASH diet on weight loss and metabolic status in adults with non-alcoholic fatty liver disease: a randomized clinical trial. Liver Int 2016;36(4):563–71.

54. Fanti M, Mishra A, Longo VD, et al. Time-restricted eating, intermittent fasting, and fasting-mimicking diets in weight loss. Curr Obes Rep 2021;10(2):70–80.

55. AP V, MI G, JK R. Time-limited eating in pediatric patients with obesity-a case series. J Food Sci Nutr Res 2020;02(03).

56. Vidmar Alaina P. NMRJK, SSJHEWCPGMI. Time-limited eating and continuous glucose monitoring in adolescents with obesity: a pilot study. Nutrients 2021; 13(11):3697–712.

57. Manoogian ENC, Chow LS, Taub PR, et al. Time-restricted eating for the prevention and management of metabolic diseases. Endocr Rev 2022;43(2):405–36.

58. Gabel K, Cienfuegos S, Kalam F, et al. Time-restricted eating to improve cardiovascular health. Curr Atheroscler Rep 2021;23(5).

59. Crose A, Alvear A, Singroy S, et al. Time-restricted eating improves quality of life measures in overweight humans. Nutrients 2021;13(5).

60. Ben-Yacov O, Godneva A, Rein M, et al. Personalized postprandial glucose response-targeting diet versus mediterranean diet for glycemic control in prediabetes. Diabetes Care 2021;44(9):1980–91.

61. Carter P, Achana F, Troughton J, et al. A mediterranean diet improves HbA1c but not fasting blood glucose compared to alternative dietary strategies: A network meta-analysis. J Hum Nutr Diet 2014;27(3):280–97.

62. AI V, PV V, AA D. Fasting mimicking diets: A literature review of their impact on inflammatory arthritis. Mediterr J Rheumatol 2020;30(4):201.

63. Ismail S, Manaf R, Mahmud A. Comparison of time-restricted feeding and islamic fasting: A scoping review. East Mediterr Health J 2019;25(4).

64. Haigh L, Kirk C, El Gendy K, et al. The effectiveness and acceptability of Mediterranean diet and calorie restriction in non-alcoholic fatty liver disease (NAFLD): A systematic review and meta-analysis. Clin Nutr 2022;41(9):1913–31.

65. Wheaton AG, Chapman DP, Croft JB. School start times, sleep, behavioral, health, and academic outcomes: a review of the literature. J Sch Health 2016; 86(5):363–81.

66. Tackett JL, McShane BB. Conceptualizing and evaluating replication across domains of behavioral research. Behav Brain Sci 2018;41:e152.

67. Frank HR, Ubel PA, Wong CA. Behavioral economic insights for pediatric obesity: suggestions for translating the guidelines for our patients. JAMA Pediatr 2020;174(4):319–20.

68. Tremblay MS, Carson V, Chaput JP, et al. Canadian 24-hour movement guidelines for children and youth: An integration of physical activity, sedentary behaviour, and sleep. Appl Physiol Nutr Metabol 2016;41(6):S311–27.

69. Füzéki E, Engeroff T, Banzer W. Health benefits of light-intensity physical activity: a systematic review of accelerometer data of the National Health and Nutrition Examination Survey (NHANES). Sports Med 2017;47(9):1769–93.

70. Craig CL, Marshall AL, Sjöström M, et al. International physical activity questionnaire: 12-Country reliability and validity. Med Sci Sports Exerc 2003;35(8): 1381–95.

71. Hallal PC, Victora CG. Reliability and validity of the International Physical Activity Questionnaire (IPAQ) [2]. Med Sci Sports Exerc 2004;36(3):556.

72. Sriram K, Mulder HS, Frank HR, et al. The dose-response relationship between physical activity and cardiometabolic health in adolescents. Am J Prev Med 2021;60(1):95–103.

73. Kriska A, Delahanty L, Edelstein S, et al. Sedentary behavior and physical activity in youth with recent onset of type 2 diabetes. Pediatrics 2013;131(3).

74. Brazendale K, Beets MW, Armstrong B, et al. Children's moderate-to-vigorous physical activity on weekdays versus weekend days: a multi-country analysis. Int J Behav Nutr Phys Activ 2021;18(1).

75. Patel ML, Hopkins CM, Brooks TL, et al. Comparing self-monitoring strategies for weight loss in a smartphone app: randomized controlled trial. JMIR Mhealth Uhealth 2019;7(2).
76. Farage G, Simmons C, Kocak M, et al. Assessing the contribution of self-monitoring through a commercial weight loss app: mediation and predictive modeling study. JMIR Mhealth Uhealth 2021;9(7).
77. Darling KE, Sato AF. Systematic review and meta-analysis examining the effectiveness of mobile health technologies in using self-monitoring for pediatric weight management. Child Obes 2017;13(5):347–55.
78. Wright JA, Phillips BD, Watson BL, et al. Randomized trial of a family-based, automated, conversational obesity treatment program for underserved populations. Obesity 2013;21(9).
79. Quattrin T, Cao Y, Paluch RA, et al. Cost-effectiveness of family-based obesity treatment. Pediatrics 2017;140(3).
80. Goldfield GS, Epstein LH, Kilanowski CK, et al. Cost-effectiveness of group and mixed family-based treatment for childhood obesity. Int J Obes Relat Metab Disord 2001;25(12):1843–9.
81. Schmied EA, Madanat H, Chuang E, et al. Factors predicting parent engagement in a family-based childhood obesity prevention and control program. BMC Publ Health 2023;23(1):457.
82. Position of the American Dietetic Association: individual-, family-, school-, and community-based interventions for pediatric overweight. J Am Diet Assoc 2006;106(6):925–45.
83. Wilfley DE. Design of a family-based lifestyle intervention for youth with type 2 diabetes: The today study. Int J Obes 2010;34(2).
84. Janicke DM, Sallinen BJ, Perri MG, et al. Comparison of program costs for parent-only and family-based interventions for pediatric obesity in medically underserved rural settings. J Rural Health 2009;25(3):326–30.
85. Zanganeh M, Adab P, Li B, et al. Cost-effectiveness of a school-and family-based childhood obesity prevention programme in China: The "CHIRPY DRAGON" cluster-randomised controlled trial. Int J Publ Health 2021;66.
86. Heerman et al. 2017.
87. Kamath et al. 2008.
88. Fox CK, Kelly AS. Pharmacotherapy for severe obesity in children. Clin Pediatr (Phila) 2015;54(13):1302.
89. Zhao X, Wang M, Wen Z, et al. GLP-1 receptor agonists: beyond their pancreatic effects. Front Endocrinol 2021;12.
90. Drucker DJ. GLP-1 physiology informs the pharmacotherapy of obesity. Mol Metabol 2022;57.
91. Secher A, Jelsing J, Baquero AF, et al. The arcuate nucleus mediates GLP-1 receptor agonist liraglutide-dependent weight loss. J Clin Invest 2014;124(10):4473–88.
92. Tamborlane WV, Bishai R, Geller D, et al. Once-weekly exenatide in youth with type 2 diabetes. Diabetes Care 2022;45(8):1833–40.
93. Tamborlane WV, Barrientos-Pérez M, Fainberg U, et al. Liraglutide in children and adolescents with type 2 diabetes. N Engl J Med 2019;381(7):637–46.
94. Weghuber D, Barrett T, Barrientos-Pérez M, et al. Once-weekly semaglutide in adolescents with obesity. N Engl J Med 2022;387(24).
95. Lewis KH, Fischer H, Ard J, et al. Safety and effectiveness of longer-term phentermine use: clinical outcomes from an electronic health record cohort. Obesity 2019;27(4):591–602.

96. Murali S. Knowledge gaps in long-term phentermine use: making the case for maintenance. Obesity 2019;27(8):1219.
97. Ryder JR, Kaizer A, Rudser KD, et al. Effect of phentermine on weight reduction in a pediatric weight management clinic. Int J Obes 2017;41(1):90–3.
98. Becker BA. Pharmacologic activity of phentermine (phenylt-butylamine). Toxicol Appl Pharmacol 1961;3(2):256–9.
99. Khalil NY, AlRabiah HK, AL Rashoud SS, et al. Topiramate: comprehensive profile. Profiles Drug Subst Excipients Relat Methodol 2019;44:333–78.
100. Glauser TA. Topiramate. Epilepsia 1999;40(Suppl 5):s71–80.
101. CK F, KL M, KD R, et al. Topiramate for weight reduction in adolescents with severe obesity. Clin Pediatr (Phila) 2015;54(1):19–24.
102. Berman C, Naguib M, Hegedus E, et al. Topiramate for weight management in children with severe obesity. Child Obes 2023;19(4).
103. Johnson DB, Quick J. Topiramate and phentermine. StatPearls 2023. Available at: https://www.ncbi.nlm.nih.gov/books/NBK482165/. [Accessed 11 June 2023].
104. Dhillon S. Phentermine/Topiramate: Pediatric First Approval. Pediatr Drugs 2022;24(6):715–20.
105. Kelly AS, Bensignor MO, Hsia DS, et al. Phentermine/topiramate for the treatment of adolescent obesity. NEJM evidence 2022;1(6).
106. Smith SM, Meyer M, Trinkley KE. Phentermine/topiramate for the treatment of obesity. Ann Pharmacother 2013;47(3):340–9.
107. Kiortsis DN. A review of the metabolic effects of controlled-release Phentermine/Topiramate. Hormones (Basel) 2013;12(4):507–16.
108. Lei XG, Ruan JQ, Lai C, et al. Efficacy and safety of phentermine/topiramate in adults with overweight or obesity: a systematic review and meta-analysis. Obesity 2021;29(6):985–94.
109. Hsia DS, Gosselin NH, Williams J, et al. A randomized, double-blind, placebo-controlled, pharmacokinetic and pharmacodynamic study of a fixed-dose combination of phentermine/topiramate in adolescents with obesity. Diabetes Obes Metabol 2020;22(4):480–91.
110. Tek C. Naltrexone HCl/bupropion HCl for chronic weight management in obese adults: patient selection and perspectives. Patient Prefer Adherence 2016;10:751–9.
111. Ozkan B, Bereket A, Turan S, et al. Addition of orlistat to conventional treatment in adolescents with severe obesity. Eur J Pediatr 2004;163(12):738–41.
112. Chanoine JP, Hampl S, Jensen C, et al. Effect of orlistat on weight and body composition in obese adolescents: a randomized controlled trial. JAMA 2005;293(23):2873–83.
113. Caklili OT, Cesur M, Mikhailidis DP, et al. Novel anti-obesity therapies and their different effects and safety profiles: a critical overview. Diabetes Metab Syndr Obes 2023;16:1767–74.
114. Chakhtoura M, Haber R, Ghezzawi M, et al. Pharmacotherapy of obesity: an update on the available medications and drugs under investigation. EClinicalMedicine 2023;58.
115. Naltrexone/bupropion for obesity. Drug Therapeut Bull 2017;55(11):126–9.
116. Masarwa R, Brunetti VC, Aloe S, et al. Efficacy and safety of metformin for obesity: a systematic review. Pediatrics 2021;147(3).
117. Clément K, van den Akker E, Argente J, et al. Efficacy and safety of setmelanotide, an MC4R agonist, in individuals with severe obesity due to LEPR or POMC deficiency: single-arm, open-label, multicentre, phase 3 trials. Lancet Diabetes Endocrinol 2020;8(12):960–70.

118. Wabitsch M, Farooqi S, Flück CE, et al. Natural history of obesity due to POMC, PCSK1, and LEPR deficiency and the impact of setmelanotide. J Endocr Soc 2022;6(6):bvac057.
119. Ryan DH. Next generation antiobesity medications: setmelanotide, semaglutide, tirzepatide and bimagrumab: what do they mean for clinical practice? J Obes Metab Syndr 2021;30(3):196–208.
120. Bairdain S, Samnaliev PhD M. Cost-effectiveness of adolescent bariatric surgery. Cureus 2015;7(2).
121. Klebanoff MJ, Chhatwal J, Nudel JD, et al. Cost-effectiveness of bariatric surgery in adolescents with obesity. JAMA Surg 2017;152(2):136–41.
122. Xanthakos SA, Jenkins TM, Kleiner DE, et al. High prevalence of nonalcoholic fatty liver disease in adolescents undergoing bariatric surgery. Gastroenterology 2015;149(3). 623e8-634.e8.
123. Fittipaldi-Fernandez RJ, Guedes MR, Galvao Neto MP, et al. Efficacy of intragastric balloon treatment for adolescent obesity. Obes Surg 2017;27(10):2546–51.
124. Abu Dayyeh BK, Bazerbachi F, Vargas EJ, et al. Endoscopic sleeve gastroplasty for treatment of class 1 and 2 obesity (MERIT): a prospective, multicentre, randomised trial. Lancet 2022;400(10350):441–51.
125. Bazerbachi F, Vargas EJ, Rizk M, et al. Intragastric balloon placement induces significant metabolic and histologic improvement in patients with nonalcoholic steatohepatitis. Clin Gastroenterol Hepatol 2021;19(1):146–54.e4.
126. Chandan S, Mohan BP, Khan SR, et al. Efficacy and Safety of Intragastric Balloon (IGB) in Non-alcoholic Fatty Liver Disease (NAFLD): a Comprehensive Review and Meta-analysis. Obes Surg 2021;31(3):1271–9.
127. Abu Dayyeh BK, Kumar N, Edmundowicz SA, et al. ASGE Bariatric Endoscopy Task Force systematic review and meta-analysis assessing the ASGE PIVI thresholds for adopting endoscopic bariatric therapies Prepared. Gastrointest Endosc 2015;82(3):425–38.e5.
128. Alqahtani A, Elahmedi M, Alqahtani YA, et al. Endoscopic sleeve gastroplasty in 109 consecutive children and adolescents with obesity: Two-year outcomes of a new modality. Am J Gastroenterol 2019;114(12):1857–62.
129. Piester TL, Jagtap N, Kalapala R. Review of paediatric obesity and non-alcoholic fatty liver disease—A focus on emerging non-pharmacologic treatment strategies. Pediatr Obes 2023;18(10).
130. De Peppo F, Caccamo R, Adorisio O, et al. The Obalon swallowable intragastric balloon in pediatric and adolescent morbid obesity. Endosc Int Open 2017; 05(01):E59–63.
131. Lorber J. Obesity in childhood. A controlled trial of anorectic drugs. Arch Dis Child 1966;41(217):309–12.
132. Rauh JL, Lipp R. Chlorphentermine as an anorexigenic agent in adolescent obesity. Report of its efficacy in a double-blind study of 30 teen-agers. Clin Pediatr (Phila) 1968;7(3):138–40.
133. Ali Ibrahim AI, Mendoza B, Stanford FC, et al. Real-world experience of the efficacy and safety of phentermine use in adolescents: a case series. Child Obes 2022. https://doi.org/10.1089/CHI.2022.0147.
134. Fox CK, Kaizer AM, Rudser KD, et al. Meal replacements followed by topiramate for the treatment of adolescent severe obesity: A pilot randomized controlled trial. Obesity 2016;24(12):2553–61.
135. Consoli A, Çabal Berthoumieu S, Raffin M, et al. Effect of topiramate on eating behaviours in Prader-Willi syndrome: TOPRADER double-blind randomised placebo-controlled study. Transl Psychiatry 2019;9(1).

136. Kelly AS, Auerbach P, Barrientos-Perez M, et al. A randomized, controlled trial of liraglutide for adolescents with obesity. N Engl J Med 2020;382(22):2117–28.

137. Bensignor MO, Bomberg EM, Bramante CT, et al. Effect of liraglutide treatment on body mass index and weight parameters in children and adolescents with type 2 diabetes: Post hoc analysis of the ellipse trial. Pediatr Obes 2021;16(8).

138. Kelly AS, Metzig AM, Rudser KD, et al. Exenatide as a weight-loss therapy in extreme pediatric obesity: a randomized, controlled pilot study. Obesity 2012; 20(2):364–70.

139. Fox CK, Clark JM, Rudser KD, et al. Exenatide for weight-loss maintenance in adolescents with severe obesity: A randomized, placebo-controlled trial. Obesity 2022;30(5):1105–15.

The Future of Endobariatrics
Bridging the Gap

Ali Lahooti, BS, Kate E. Johnson, BA, Reem Z. Sharaiha, MD, MSc*

KEYWORDS

- Obesity • Weight loss • Endobariatrics • Endoscopic sleeve gastroplasty
- Intragastric balloons • Endoscopic bariatric therapy

KEY POINTS

- Overview of the most promising future directions in the field of endobariatrics.
- Clinical trials and international results highlighting developing tools and techniques.
- Practical, economic, and clinical considerations for adopting endobariatrics in patient care.

INTRODUCTION

The global obesity epidemic continues to escalate at an alarming rate, posing significant challenges to health care systems and individuals worldwide. In the United States alone, projections indicate that by 2030, nearly half of all adults will have obesity, with almost a quarter struggling with severe obesity.[1] Obesity is a complex, multifactorial chronic disease associated with numerous health risks, including type 2 diabetes, cardiovascular disease, and various metabolic disorders.[2] The economic consequences are staggering, with estimates suggesting annual costs exceeding $260 billion in the United States.[3,4]

Current treatment modalities for obesity, such as lifestyle modifications, pharmacotherapy, and bariatric surgery, have limitations. Lifestyle interventions, including dietary changes and increased physical activity, are the cornerstone of obesity management but often yield modest and temporary benefits.[5] The Look AHEAD trial and the Diabetes Prevention Program, 2 landmark studies, provided evidence supporting the efficacy of intensive lifestyle interventions in promoting weight loss and overall health improvements.[6,7] However, the magnitude and sustainability of weight loss achieved through these interventions remain significantly lower compared with other treatment options.

Pharmacotherapy has emerged as another tool in the fight against obesity, with several US Food and Drug Administration (FDA)-approved medications available. As

Division of Gastroenterology and Hepatology, Department of Medicine, Weill Cornell Medicine, New York
* Corresponding author. Division of Gastroenterology and Hepatology, Department of Medicine, Weill Cornell Medical College, 1305 York Avenue, 4th Floor, New York, NY 10021.
E-mail address: rzs9001@med.cornell.edu

Gastrointest Endoscopy Clin N Am 34 (2024) 805–818
https://doi.org/10.1016/j.giec.2024.07.001
1052-5157/24/© 2024 Elsevier Inc. All rights reserved, including those for text and data mining, AI training, and similar technologies.

giendo.theclinics.com

of October 2023, 7 antiobesity medications have been approved by the FDA, with an eighth, Tirzepatide (Mounjaro), currently under expedited review.[8] Although these medications have shown promise in aiding weight loss and improving metabolic parameters, their efficacy varies among individuals, and long-term adherence remains a challenge.[8,9] A detailed analysis of phase 3 and extension trials of these antiobesity agents reveals that, with the exception of Semaglutide (14.8% total body weight loss [TBWL]) and Tirzepatide (15% to 20.9% TBWL), the weight loss efficacy of the medications ranges from 6% to 10% TBWL. Even the most effective pharmacologic agents fall short when compared to the outcomes achieved with endobariatric therapies and surgical interventions.[8] Furthermore, within the subgroup of patients achieving at least 10% TBWL, there is a notable difficulty in maintaining these weight loss milestones long-term, suggesting that although these pharmacologic agents represent progress, there is a clear need for integrated management strategies to enhance and sustain therapeutic outcomes.

Bariatric surgery, including procedures such as Roux-en-Y gastric bypass (RYGB) and sleeve gastrectomy (SG), has demonstrated remarkable success in producing substantial and sustained weight loss and improving metabolic health. A randomized controlled trial examining 5-year postsurgical outcomes found that RYGB and SG yielded TBWL rates of 21.7% and 18.5%, respectively.[10] However, these procedures are not without risks and complications. Postsurgical patients commonly experience nutrient anemia or calcium and vitamin deficiencies, necessitating lifelong supplementation.[11-13] More severe complications can include micro- and macronutrient deficiencies, anastomotic stenosis, ulceration, reflux esophagitis, cholelithiasis, steatohepatitis, and altered pharmacokinetics.[11-13] Furthermore, although many patients perceive bariatric surgery as transformative, leading to weight loss, improved obesity-related health issues, and enhanced quality of life, many express concerns about the associated risks, particularly among racial minority groups.[14]

Despite the potential benefits of bariatric surgery, its utilization remains low. It is estimated that less than 1% of eligible patients opt for bariatric surgery because of concerns related to accessibility, costs, and apprehensions about both actual and perceived health risks associated with the procedure.[15,16] The limited adoption of bariatric surgery highlights the need for alternative treatment options that bridge the gap between lifestyle interventions and surgical procedures. In this context, endobariatric therapies have emerged as a promising solution, offering minimally invasive alternatives that fill the void between the often-ineffective lifestyle modifications and the invasive nature of bariatric surgery.

Looking ahead to the future of endobariatrics, it is essential to learn from the challenges of the past and apply those lessons to pave the way for success. Although previous endobariatric therapies faced obstacles such as limited market adoption, advertising constraints, reimbursement hurdles, and restricted accessibility, the future holds immense potential for therapies that demonstrate effectiveness, safety, minimally invasive approaches, reduced complication rates, shorter recovery periods, and favorable patient feedback.[17] With a clear understanding of past challenges and a commitment to innovation, the endobariatric community can enthusiastically embrace the opportunities that lie ahead.

ENDOBARIATRIC THERAPIES: THE CURRENT LANDSCAPE

Endobariatric therapies have emerged as a compelling alternative to conventional obesity treatments. By leveraging advanced endoscopic techniques and technologies, endobariatric procedures provide safer, more accessible, and less invasive options to promote weight loss and enhance metabolic health. FDA-approved therapies encompass restrictive procedures and aspiration therapy.

Restrictive endobariatric procedures aim to reduce gastric capacity and induce early satiety, leading to reduced caloric intake and weight loss. The most widely utilized restrictive procedures include intragastric balloons (IGBs) and endoscopic sleeve gastroplasty (ESG). IGBs are space-occupying devices placed endoscopically into the stomach to induce satiety and restrict food intake. Several IGBs have been approved by the FDA, including single fluid-filled balloons (Orbera and Spatz3), gas-filled balloons (Obalon), and double fluid-filled balloons (ReShape Duo, no longer commercially available).[16] The efficacy of these devices has been demonstrated across multiple studies. A meta-analysis of 5668 patients who underwent IGB placement demonstrated a mean TBWL of 11.1%, a mean excess body weight loss (EBWL) of 31.8%, and improvements in obesity-related comorbidities such as hypertension, dyslipidemia, and type 2 diabetes mellitus.[18] Randomized controlled trials and studies have shown significant weight loss results with the Orbera,[19] ReShape Duo,[20] Obalon,[21] and Spatz3[22] balloons, with each offering unique advantages such as adjustable inflation levels (Spatz3) and swallowable placement (Obalon).[23]

Whereas IGBs temporarily reduce stomach capacity, ESG offers a more durable reduction in gastric volume. ESG utilizes an endoscopic suturing device such as Apollo OverStitch to create a sleeve-like gastric pouch along the lesser curvature of the stomach, reducing its volume and altering gastric emptying. A prospective, multicenter study evaluating the long-term outcomes of ESG found a mean TBWL of 15.1% and a mean EBWL of 57.7% at 6 months, with sustained weight loss at 12 and 18 to 24 months.[24] This weight loss is sustained over a period of 2 to 5 years.[25] ESG has also been associated with improvements in hypertension, type 2 diabetes, and hyperlipidemia.[26]

Aspiration therapy involves the use of a percutaneous gastrostomy tube with an external port that allows for the removal of a portion of the ingested meal from the stomach, reducing caloric absorption. The AspireAssist system (Aspire Bariatrics) was the only FDA-approved aspiration therapy device but is no longer available.[27] In the PATHWAY trial, patients using the AspireAssist system achieved 14.2% TBWL at 1 year, 15.3% at 2 years, 16.6% at 3 years, and 18.7% at 4 years, along with improvements in HbA1c, lipid profiles, and liver enzymes.[27]

The FDA-approved TransPyloric Shuttle (TPS) positions a spherical silicone balloon between the stomach and duodenum, utilizing a ball-valve mechanism to delay gastric emptying. In the ENDO-BESITY II trial (NCT02518685), patients who received TPS achieved 9.5% TBWL at 12 months compared with 2.8% in the sham group.[28] A recent study also showed the potential for sustained weight loss following TPS removal.[29]

ADVANCEMENTS IN ENDOBARIATRIC TECHNIQUES AND DEVICES

The endoscopist's toolkit is constantly expanding as new technologies undergo rigorous testing and come to market. These emerging tools incorporate feedback from previous generations of devices and promise enhancements in safety and efficacy.

Advancements in Endoscopic Suturing and Endoscopic Sleeve Gastroplasty

The techniques and devices used in ESG are continuously advancing, leading to improvements in the outcomes of endoscopic bariatric therapies. For instance, a small single-center study using a new longitudinal compression suturing technique demonstrated superior weight loss compared with traditional suturing patterns, although this technique is not yet FDA-approved.[30]

The EndoZip is an automated suturing system designed to simplify ESG and reduce the learning curve. In a first-in-human study with 11 patients, the device achieved a percent TBWL of 16.2 plus or minus 6.0% and a percent EWL of 54.3 plus or minus 28.4%, while preliminary results from a multicenter pilot study involving 45 patients showed a percent TBWL of 13.5%.[31] Although promising, more large-scale studies are needed to demonstrate the efficacy and safety of the procedure.

Differing from ESG in the suture location and technique, the primary obesity surgery endoluminal (POSE) procedure involves the placement of full-thickness sutures in the gastric fundus and distal body, resulting in a functional gastric volume reduction and delayed gastric emptying. A meta-analysis of 613 patients who underwent POSE found a mean EBWL of 48.86% and a mean TBWL of 12.68% at 12 to 15 months, with a pooled adverse event rate of 2.2%.[32] In addition, a distal belt-and-suspenders approach for gastric plication has been proposed.[33]

Endoscopic gastric plication involves creating pleats in the stomach lining without the full-thickness sutures used in POSE. The technique employs the Endomina suturing device, which can be easily assembled with any standard flexible endoscope. Although not currently FDA-approved, initial findings from a multicenter study involving 45 patients demonstrated a 29% EBWL and a 7.4% TBWL at 12 months, with no reports of severe adverse events.[34,35]

Advancements in Intragastric Balloons

The future of IGBs includes smart balloons with adjustable inflation levels and those that do not require endoscopic removal. The Allurion Balloon (Allurion Technologies, Natick, Massachusetts) is a swallowable, self-emptying balloon that does not require endoscopic placement or removal, offering a less invasive option for patients. In a large, multicenter study of 1770 patients, the Allurion Balloon achieved a percent TBWL of 14.4% at 4 months, with a low rate of serious adverse events (0.2%). Moreover, 99.9% of patients successfully swallowed the balloon with or without stylet assistance, bolstering its technical feasibility.[36]

Malabsorptive and Metabolic Therapies: New Directions

Malabsorptive endobariatric procedures aim to reduce nutrient absorption in the small intestine, mimicking the effects of surgical bypass procedures.

One example is duodenal mucosal resurfacing (DMR), which involves the application of thermal energy to the duodenal mucosa using the Revita DMR system (Fractyl Laboratories, Lexington, Massachusetts). This leads to mucosal remodeling and alters enteroendocrine signaling, potentially improving insulin sensitivity and glucose homeostasis. An international pilot study showed that DMR significantly lowered HbA1c and improved hepatic indexes assessing fibrosis.[37] In a small pilot study (n = 16), DMR combined with GLP-1 agonist liraglutide enabled 69% of patients to discontinue insulin and maintain HbA1c levels of no more than 7.5% at 6 months.[38] US clinical trials are currently enrolling to assess the safety and efficacy of DMR (NCT04419779).

Another example is the duodenal-jejunal bypass liner (DJBL), previously known as the EndoBarrier. It is a sleeve extending from the duodenal bulb to the proximal jejunum that blocks nutrient uptake and enzymatic secretion in the duodenum. Prior to removal from the market, studies showed reductions in weight and improvements in metabolic parameters; however, these were overshadowed by the number and severity of adverse events and ultimately did not meet the ASGE/ASMBS thresholds for the treatment of obesity.[39,40] Nonetheless, a single-center Chinese study demonstrated notable weight loss and improvements in hepatic steatosis, liver enzymes, insulin resistance, and metabolic parameters in obese patients with metabolic dysfunction-associated steatotic liver disease (MASLD) after a 3-month implantation of the DJBL.[41] The device has undergone modifications, particularly to its anchoring system, resulting in FDA and institutional review board approval for the new STEP-1 pivotal trial (NCT04101669).[41,42]

Partial jejunal diversion (PJD) is an endoscopic technique that induces weight loss by creating an anastomosis between the proximal and distal small bowel using self-assembling magnets (Incisionless Magnetic Anastomosis System). A pilot study involving 10 patients with obesity and type 2 diabetes successfully created anastomosis, resulting in significant weight loss (14.6% TWBL and 40.2% EWL), reduced HbA1c levels, and a 12% reduction in alanine aminotransferase (ALT) levels at 1 year.[43]

Promising research into the hormonal activity of gastric mucosa suggests that gastric mucosal devitalization using argon plasma coagulation (APC) may achieve metabolic benefits comparable to those of bariatric surgery, as demonstrated in ex vivo human and animal studies.[44–46] The technique resulted in weight loss, an improvement in visceral adiposity, and metabolic profile.

The concept of small intestinal modulation remains an active area of research, with novel devices and techniques being developed to optimize outcomes and minimize complications. These malabsorptive endoscopic bariatric therapies enhance weight loss and insulin secretion by limiting nutrient absorption and enhancing peptide secretion from enteroendocrine cells, potentially offering a less invasive alternative to traditional bariatric surgery.

Novel Gastric Motility Interventions

Bariatric endoscopic antral myotomy (BEAM) is a novel procedure that involves the endoscopic dissection of the gastric antrum, aiming to delay gastric emptying and induce weight loss without gastroparesis. The first successful human proof-of-concept study demonstrated the potential to reduce procedure time, enhance reproducibility, minimize perioperative discomfort, and increase long-term effectiveness.[47]

Extraluminal/Pancreatic Endoscopic Metabolic Therapy

Rejuva (Fractyl) is a gene therapy platform utilizing adeno-associated virus technology to stimulate the pancreas to produce therapeutic proteins. A feasibility and safety study in a Yucatan pig model demonstrated the activity of the adeno-associated virus in up to 80% of the targeted cells, with no procedure-related pancreatitis events but some pancreatic inflammation at 3 weeks.[48] Although still in its early stages, extraluminal/pancreatic gene therapy holds promise as a research avenue for the treatment and management of diabetes.

METABOLIC BENEFITS BEYOND WEIGHT LOSS

Endobariatric therapies have demonstrated significant potential in improving metabolic health beyond their effects on weight loss alone. Several studies have shown improvements in obesity-related comorbidities, such as type 2 diabetes, MASLD, and cardiovascular risk factors following endobariatric interventions.

ESG has been associated with significant improvements in hypertension, type 2 diabetes, and hyperlipidemia.[26] In patients with MASLD, ESG has been shown to improve liver function and decrease fibrosis scores.[49] Two randomized controlled trials (RCTs) are currently underway to evaluate the effectiveness of ESG in treating nonalcoholic steatohepatitis (NASH) compared with laparoscopic sleeve gastrectomy (TESLA-NASH, NCT04060368) or a placebo procedure (NASH-APOLLO, NCT03426111).[50]

Meanwhile, POSE has been shown to improve glucose metabolism and gut hormone signaling, with a prospective study revealing significant improvements in the glucose/insulin ratio, decreased postprandial ghrelin levels, and an increase in postprandial peptide YY.[51]

In a comprehensive meta-analysis involving 5668 patients, IGBs used for up to 6 months resulted in statistically significant improvements in several metabolic parameters, including fasting blood glucose, systolic blood pressure, HbA1c levels, and transaminases.[18] As newer renditions of IGB gain FDA approval, assessing the metabolic changes accompanying weight loss will be crucial.

As research continues to unravel the complex mechanisms underlying the metabolic effects of endobariatric therapies, the concept of "metabolic endoscopy" is gaining prominence, focusing on the use of endoscopic interventions to target specific metabolic pathways and improve overall health outcomes.

ADJUNCTIVE AND COMBINATION THERAPIES

Endobariatric therapies have shown promising results as standalone treatments for obesity and related comorbidities. However, their efficacy and durability may be further enhanced through combination approaches with pharmacotherapy and bariatric surgery. These adjunctive strategies aim to optimize weight loss outcomes, prevent weight regain, and manage complications associated with obesity and its treatment.

Pharmacotherapy

The use of pharmacotherapy in conjunction with endobariatric therapies has gained attention as a potential means to augment weight loss and maintain long-term results. A recent study demonstrated that the addition of GLP-1 receptor agonists (liraglutide/semaglutide) to ESG resulted in significantly greater weight loss (23.7% TBWL) compared with ESG alone (17.3% TBWL) at 1 year.[52] This finding highlights the potential synergistic effects of combining endoscopic interventions with targeted pharmacologic agents.

In the context of IGBs, a retrospective study found that combining IGBs with currently approved pharmacotherapies did not increase weight loss at 6 months compared with IGBs and lifestyle changes alone. However, the combination approach led to greater weight loss and reduced weight regain after balloon removal at 12 months.[53] This suggests that pharmacotherapy may play a role in sustaining the benefits of endobariatric therapies beyond the initial treatment period.

Pharmacotherapy has also shown promise in managing weight recidivism following endoscopic interventions. In a study evaluating patients undergoing transoral outlet reduction (TORe) for weight regain after Roux-en-Y gastric bypass, the immediate initiation of pharmacotherapy in combination with TORe facilitated greater weight loss compared to TORe alone.[54] This finding underscores the potential of pharmacotherapy to enhance the durability of endobariatric procedures in the setting of weight recidivism.

Bariatric Surgery

The combination of endobariatric therapies with bariatric surgery has been explored to optimize outcomes and manage complications. IGBs have garnered interest as a transitional treatment preceding bariatric surgery. The hypothesis is that IGBs can facilitate presurgical weight loss, thereby streamlining surgical procedures and mitigating perioperative complications.[55] A meta-analysis assessing IGBs as bridging therapy before bariatric surgery found them to be effective, with an adequate procedural safety profile.[56] This suggests that IGBs may have a role in preparing patients for bariatric surgery and potentially improving surgical outcomes.

In the setting of failed bariatric surgery, endobariatric therapies have shown promise in addressing weight recidivism. A recent multicenter analysis demonstrated that revisional ESG is a safe and effective approach for managing weight regain in patients with dilated laparoscopic sleeve gastrectomy, leading to sustained weight loss.[57] Similarly, following Roux-en-Y gastric bypass, endoscopic procedures such as transoral outlet reduction (TORe) and argon plasma coagulation have been employed to reduce the gastrojejunal anastomosis. These techniques have been shown to be safe, reproducible, and effective in managing weight recidivism.[58,59]

Combination Therapy: Future Directions

Although the available evidence supports the potential of adjunctive and combination therapies in enhancing the outcomes of endobariatric procedures, further research is needed to establish their long-term efficacy and safety. Robust randomized controlled trials are essential to assess the effectiveness of combining endobariatric therapies with pharmacotherapy and bariatric surgery. These studies will help inform the development of evidence-based guidelines for the optimal utilization of adjunctive strategies in the management of obesity and related comorbidities.

ENDOBARIATRICS IN CLINICAL PRACTICE
Multidisciplinary Care and Patient Support

Adherence to outpatient follow-up has been recognized as the most crucial independent predictor of success, regardless of the specific type of endobariatric treatment. Currently, there is no established gold-standard for psychosocial evaluation and monitoring of patients undergoing endoscopic bariatric therapies (EBTs), potentially because of the lack of insurance coverage. In contrast, patients undergoing metabolic and bariatric surgery (MBS) are required to undergo a presurgical psychosocial evaluation to identify mental health disorders, eating disorders, and substance use problems that could impact their outcomes and to ensure patients fully understand their role in recovery.[60]

Multidisciplinary care models (MDCs) may provide a solution to this urgent problem, fostering coordinated care through integrated consultations within a single clinic space. These models have demonstrated improved clinical outcomes and patient satisfaction in other fields, such as oncology.[61,62] Patients who engage with a multidisciplinary team before and during EBT implementation are likely to benefit the most, as EBTs are often adjunctive to lifestyle changes. Consistent engagement with a support team, including dieticians, exercise specialists, and mental health professionals, can enhance adherence and improve weight loss and overall health outcomes.

Optimal management of patients undergoing endobariatric therapies requires collaboration among endoscopists, bariatric surgeons, nutritionists, psychologists, and other health care professionals. Pre-procedure evaluation should include a thorough assessment of patients' medical, nutritional, and psychological status to identify potential contraindications and optimize treatment outcomes. The POWER (Practice Guide on Obesity and Weight Management, Education and Resources) guidelines provide a framework for a comprehensive, multidisciplinary approach to obesity management.[63] This includes an assessment of obesity-related comorbidities, such as type 2 diabetes, hypertension, dyslipidemia, and obstructive sleep apnea, as well as an evaluation of patients' readiness for change and potential barriers to treatment adherence. Post-procedure follow-up is equally crucial for long-term success. Patients should receive ongoing nutritional guidance, behavioral support, and monitoring for weight loss progress and potential complications.

Training and Credentialing

As endobariatrics continues to evolve as a subspecialty, standardized training and credentialing processes will be critical to ensure high-quality care and patient safety. The development of accredited fellowship programs in endobariatrics, either as part of advanced endoscopy training or as standalone programs, will be essential to provide comprehensive education and hands-on experience with various techniques and devices.

Professional societies, including gastroenterology and surgical specialty societies, should establish credentialing guidelines for endobariatric procedures, specifying the quality metrics required to determine competency with these procedures.

The inclusion of endobariatric training in gastroenterology and surgical fellowship programs can help to build a workforce of skilled providers and promote the integration of these therapies into standard obesity management pathways.[64] As demonstrated in the bariatric surgery sphere, interprofessional education and collaboration among different specialties involved in obesity care, such as endocrinology, nutrition, and psychology, can foster a team-based approach to patient management and improve care coordination.[65]

As endobariatric procedures become more widely adopted, it is crucial to ensure that health care providers maintain competency and proficiency in these techniques. The establishment of standardized credentialing and privileging criteria for endobariatric procedures can help to ensure the quality and safety of patient care.[66] Furthermore, ongoing education and training opportunities, such as continuing medical education (CME) courses and peer-to-peer learning, can help providers stay up to date with the latest advances in the field.

Billing and Coding Frameworks

The development of specific billing codes for endobariatric procedures is essential to ensure appropriate reimbursement and facilitate access to these therapies. Currently, the lack of standardized billing codes and limited insurance coverage can create significant barriers for patients and providers.

As more long-term data on the safety, efficacy, and cost-effectiveness of endobariatric therapies become available, collaboration with payers to establish comprehensive coverage policies and reimbursement rates will be crucial in integrating these procedures into the standard of care for obesity management.

Accessibility and Insurance Coverage

Equitable access to endobariatric therapies is a global health care challenge that requires multifaceted approaches, including training health care providers in underserved regions, raising awareness of endobariatric treatments, and facilitating knowledge sharing and expertise dissemination through collaborative initiatives among international organizations, governments, and health care institutions.

Accessibility to these therapies is influenced by factors such as health care infrastructure, regulatory approvals, insurance coverage, cost, awareness, and socioeconomic conditions. Policy changes, expanded insurance coverage, heightened awareness, and ongoing research to enhance affordability and effectiveness are necessary to improve access. Continuing education for health care providers is also crucial to keep them updated on emerging technologies, best practices, and research findings, ensuring the delivery of advanced and effective treatments to patients.

Advances in cost-effective technologies and strategies are key to enhancing the affordability of endobariatric therapies, with potential cost reduction achieved through research into more economical materials and procedural techniques. Furthermore, efficient administrative processes and resource optimization can further control expenses, expanding access to these therapies.

Despite the potential benefits of endobariatric therapies, access to these procedures remains limited, largely because of the lack of insurance coverage and reimbursement. In the United States, most endobariatric procedures are not covered by insurance plans, leading to significant out-of-pocket costs for patients.[67] This lack of coverage creates a significant barrier to treatment, particularly for individuals from lower socioeconomic backgrounds who are disproportionately affected by obesity.

Efforts to expand insurance coverage for endobariatric therapies should focus on demonstrating their cost-effectiveness and long-term health benefits compared with conventional treatments. Economic evaluations, such as cost-utility analyses, can provide valuable evidence to support the inclusion of endobariatric therapies in insurance policies and health care systems. A recent cost-effectiveness analysis in the United Kingdom found that ESG was cost-effective compared to lifestyle modification for the treatment of obesity, with an incremental cost-effectiveness ratio (ICER) of £2453 (approximately $3100) per quality-adjusted life year (QALY) gained.[68]

In addition to economic evaluations, the development of standardized guidelines and quality metrics for endobariatric procedures can help to ensure their safety, efficacy, and appropriateness for patient care. The American Society for Gastrointestinal Endoscopy (ASGE) has published a position statement on the role of endoscopy in the bariatric patient, outlining key considerations for patient selection, procedure preparation, and post-procedure management.[66] The establishment of national registries and databases for endobariatric procedures could also provide valuable insights into real-world outcomes and inform clinical decision making.

Ultimately, expanding access to endobariatric therapies will require a coordinated effort among health care providers, policymakers, and patient advocates. Strategies to improve access may include increasing public awareness of endobariatric options, advocating for policy changes to expand insurance coverage, and developing innovative payment models that incentivize the adoption of cost-effective treatments.

SUMMARY

Endobariatric therapies have emerged as a transformative solution in the battle against the global obesity epidemic, bridging the gap between lifestyle interventions and bariatric surgery. These minimally invasive procedures offer a spectrum of options, including restrictive techniques, aspiration therapy, and emerging metabolic interventions, providing safer, more accessible, and less invasive alternatives to conventional treatments. As the field of endobariatrics continues to evolve, advancements in techniques, devices, and combination approaches with pharmacotherapy and bariatric surgery hold immense potential to enhance weight loss outcomes and improve overall metabolic health, offering hope to millions of individuals struggling with obesity and weight-related comorbidities.

The successful integration of endobariatric therapies into clinical practice necessitates a multidisciplinary, patient-centered approach, guided by the principles of ethics, inclusivity, and global accessibility. Collaboration among health care professionals, including endoscopists, bariatric surgeons, nutritionists, and psychologists, is crucial to ensure high-quality care and patient safety. Standardized training and credentialing processes, along with the development of specific billing codes and comprehensive insurance coverage policies, will be essential to guarantee equitable access to these innovative treatments. Ongoing research to demonstrate the long-term efficacy, safety, and cost-effectiveness of endobariatric therapies will be vital to support their widespread adoption and inclusion in standard obesity management pathways, ultimately making these life-changing treatments accessible to those who need them most, regardless of geographic or socioeconomic factors.

By embracing the principles of patient-centered care, scientific innovation, ethical responsibility, and global accessibility, and advancing the field through research and collaboration, the treatment of obesity and its related metabolic conditions can be revolutionized. The transformative potential of endobariatric therapies extends beyond individual health outcomes, promising to alleviate the burden on health care systems worldwide and improve the quality of life for countless individuals battling obesity.

CLINICS CARE POINTS

- Endobariatric modalities such as endoscopic sleeve gastroplasty (ESG) and intragastric balloons (IGBs) offer minimally invasive alternatives to traditional bariatric surgery, providing significant weight loss and improvements in metabolic health, including benefits for type 2 diabetes and non-alcoholic fatty liver disease.

- Multidisciplinary care involving endoscopists, nutritionists, and psychologists, along with regular post-procedure follow-up, is crucial for optimal long-term outcomes in endobariatric procedures.

- Clinicians should stay informed about emerging endobariatric techniques and devices through continuing education and standardized training programs.

- Limited insurance coverage remains a significant barrier to accessing endobariatric therapies, highlighting the need for advocacy and robust long-term outcome data.

- Development of specific billing codes and comprehensive coverage policies is essential to facilitate wider adoption of endobariatric procedures in clinical practice.

DISCLOSURES

R.Z. Sharaiha: Cook Medical, Boston Scientific, Olympus, Surgical Intuitive (consultant). The remaining authors have no conflicts of interest to disclose.

REFERENCES

1. The Lancet Gastroenterology Hepatology. Obesity: another ongoing pandemic. Lancet Gastroenterol Hepatol 2021;6(6):411.
2. Ward ZJ, Bleich SN, Cradock AL, et al. Projected US state-level prevalence of adult obesity and severe obesity. N Engl J Med 2019;381(25):2440–50.
3. Kim DD, Basu A. Estimating the medical care costs of obesity in the United States: systematic review, meta-analysis, and empirical analysis. Value Health 2016;19(5):602–13.
4. Cawley J, Biener A, Meyerhoefer C, et al. Direct medical costs of obesity in the United States and the most populous states. J Manag Care Spec Pharm 2021; 27(3):354–66.

5. Wadden TA, Tronieri JS, Butryn ML. Lifestyle modification approaches for the treatment of obesity in adults. Am Psychol 2020;75(2):235–51.
6. Wadden TA, West DS, Delahanty L, et al. The Look AHEAD study: a description of the lifestyle intervention and the evidence supporting it. Obesity 2006;14(5): 737–52.
7. Long-term effects of lifestyle intervention or metformin on diabetes development and microvascular complications over 15-year follow-up: the Diabetes Prevention Program Outcomes Study. Lancet Diabetes Endocrinol 2015;3(11):866–75.
8. Chakhtoura M, Haber R, Ghezzawi M, et al. Pharmacotherapy of obesity: an update on the available medications and drugs under investigation. EClinicalMedicine 2023;58:101882.
9. Tak YJ, Lee SY. Anti-obesity drugs: long-term efficacy and safety: an updated review. World J Mens Health 2021;39(2):208–21.
10. Schauer PR, Bhatt DL, Kirwan JP, et al. Bariatric surgery versus intensive medical therapy for diabetes - 5-year outcomes. N Engl J Med 2017;376(7):641–51.
11. Nuzzo A, Czernichow S, Hertig A, et al. Prevention and treatment of nutritional complications after bariatric surgery. Lancet Gastroenterol Hepatol 2021;6(3): 238–51.
12. Chevallier JM. [From bariatric to metabolic surgery: 15 years experience in a French university hospital]. Bull Acad Natl Med 2010;194(1):25–36 [discussion 36–8]. De la chirurgie de l'obésité a la chirurgie a visée métabolique. Expérience de quinze ans dans un service hospitalier universitaire.
13. Koch TR, Finelli FC. Postoperative metabolic and nutritional complications of bariatric surgery. Gastroenterol Clin North Am 2010;39(1):109–24.
14. Gulinac M, Miteva DG, Peshevska-Sekulovska M, et al. Long-term effectiveness, outcomes and complications of bariatric surgery. World J Clin Cases 2023; 11(19):4504–12.
15. Novikov AA, Afaneh C, Saumoy M, et al. Endoscopic sleeve gastroplasty, laparoscopic sleeve gastrectomy, and laparoscopic band for weight loss: how do they compare? J Gastrointest Surg 2018;22(2):267–73.
16. Stavrou G, Shrewsbury A, Kotzampassi K. Six intragastric balloons: which to choose? World J Gastrointest Endosc 2021;13(8):238–59.
17. Lahooti A, Hassan A, Critelli B, et al. Quality and popularity trends of weight loss procedure videos on TikTok. Obes Surg 2023. https://doi.org/10.1007/s11695-022-06409-x.
18. Popov VB, Thompson CC, Kumar N, et al. Effect of intragastric balloons on liver enzymes: a systematic review and meta-analysis. Dig Dis Sci 2016;61(9): 2477–87.
19. Courcoulas A, Abu Dayyeh BK, Eaton L, et al. Intragastric balloon as an adjunct to lifestyle intervention: a randomized controlled trial. Int J Obes (Lond) 2017; 41(3):427–33.
20. Ponce J, Woodman G, Swain J, et al. The REDUCE pivotal trial: a prospective, randomized controlled pivotal trial of a dual intragastric balloon for the treatment of obesity. Surg Obes Relat Dis 2015;11(4):874–81.
21. Mion F, Ibrahim M, Marjoux S, et al. Swallowable Obalon® gastric balloons as an aid for weight loss: a pilot feasibility study. Obes Surg 2013;23(5):730–3.
22. Uyak D. Tu1913 CLINICAL STUDY OF A NEW / AN ADJUSTABLE INTRAGASTRIC-BALLOON (SPATZ 3) WITH 110 PATIENTS(MEDICAL ONE HAMBURG/ GERMANY). Gastrointest Endosc 2018;87(6):AB608.
23. Kim SH, Chun HJ, Choi HS, et al. Current status of intragastric balloon for obesity treatment. World J Gastroenterol 2016;22(24):5495–504.

24. Hedjoudje A, Abu Dayyeh BK, Cheskin LJ, et al. Efficacy and safety of endoscopic sleeve gastroplasty: a systematic review and meta-analysis. Clin Gastroenterol Hepatol 2020;18(5):1043–53.e4.

25. Sharaiha RZ, Hajifathalian K, Kumar R, et al. Five-year outcomes of endoscopic sleeve gastroplasty for the treatment of obesity. Clin Gastroenterol Hepatol 2021;19(5):1051–7.e2.

26. Abu Dayyeh BK, Bazerbachi F, Vargas EJ, et al. Endoscopic sleeve gastroplasty for treatment of class 1 and 2 obesity (MERIT): a prospective, multicentre, randomised trial. Lancet 2022;400(10350):441–51.

27. Thompson CC, Abu Dayyeh BK, Kushnir V, et al. Aspiration therapy for the treatment of obesity: 4-year results of a multicenter randomized controlled trial. Surg Obes Relat Dis 2019;15(8):1348–54.

28. Rothstein RI, Kopjar B, Woodman GE, et al. Randomized double-blind sham-controlled trial of a novel silicone-filled endoscopically placed device for weight loss. Techniques and Innovations in Gastrointestinal Endoscopy 2024;26(1):21–9.

29. Puri S, Chevalier JI, Rothstein RI. S1031 long-term weight loss outcomes of endoscopic treatment with the baronova transpyloric shuttle: a prospective observational cohort study. J Ame Coll Gastroenterol 2021;116.

30. Glaysher MA, Moekotte AL, Kelly J. Endoscopic sleeve gastroplasty: a modified technique with greater curvature compression sutures. Endosc Int Open 2019;7(10):E1303–e1309.

31. Lopez-Nava G, Asokkumar R, Rull A, et al. Safety and feasibility of a novel endoscopic suturing device (EndoZip) for treatment of obesity: first-in-human study. Obes Surg 2020;30(5):1696–703.

32. Singh S, Bazarbashi AN, Khan A, et al. Primary obesity surgery endoluminal (POSE) for the treatment of obesity: a systematic review and meta-analysis. Surg Endosc 2022;36(1):252–66.

33. Jirapinyo P, Thompson CC. Gastric plications for weight loss: distal primary obesity surgery endoluminal through a belt-and-suspenders approach. VideoGIE 2018;3(10):296–300.

34. Huberty V, Boskoski I, Bove V, et al. Endoscopic sutured gastroplasty in addition to lifestyle modification: short-term efficacy in a controlled randomised trial. Gut 2020. https://doi.org/10.1136/gutjnl-2020-322026.

35. Vincent H, Ivo B, Vincenzo B, et al. Endoscopic sutured gastroplasty in addition to lifestyle modification: short-term efficacy in a controlled randomised trial. Gut 2021;70(8):1479.

36. Ienca R, Al Jarallah M, Caballero A, et al. The procedureless Elipse gastric balloon program: multicenter experience in 1770 consecutive patients. Obes Surg 2020;30(9):3354–62.

37. van Baar ACG, Beuers U, Wong K, et al. Endoscopic duodenal mucosal resurfacing improves glycaemic and hepatic indices in type 2 diabetes: 6-month multicentre results. JHEP Rep 2019;1(6):429–37.

38. van Baar ACG, Meiring S, Smeele P, et al. Duodenal mucosal resurfacing combined with glucagon-like peptide-1 receptor agonism to discontinue insulin in type 2 diabetes: a feasibility study. Gastrointest Endosc 2021;94(1):111–20.e3.

39. Betzel B, Drenth JPH, Siersema PD. Adverse events of the duodenal-jejunal bypass liner: a systematic review. Obes Surg 2018;28(11):3669–77.

40. Yvamoto EY, de Moura DTH, Proença IM, et al. The effectiveness and safety of the duodenal-jejunal bypass liner (DJBL) for the management of obesity and glycaemic control: a systematic review and meta-analysis of randomized controlled trials. Obes Surg 2023;33(2):585–99.

41. Ren M, Zhou X, Yu M, et al. Prospective study of a new endoscopic duodenal-jejunal bypass sleeve in obese patients with nonalcoholic fatty liver disease (with video). Dig Endosc 2023;35(1):58–66.
42. Simons M, Sharaiha RZ. Updates in metabolic bariatric endoscopy. Dig Endosc 2024;36(2):107–15.
43. Machytka E, Bužga M, Zonca P, et al. Partial jejunal diversion using an incisionless magnetic anastomosis system: 1-year interim results in patients with obesity and diabetes. Gastrointest Endosc 2017;86(5):904–12.
44. Fayad L, Oberbach A, Schweitzer M, et al. Gastric mucosal devitalization (GMD): translation to a novel endoscopic metabolic therapy. Endosc Int Open 2019;7(12): E1640–e1645.
45. Oberbach A, Schlichting N, Heinrich M, et al. Gastric mucosal devitalization reduces adiposity and improves lipid and glucose metabolism in obese rats. Gastrointest Endosc 2018;87(1):288–99.e6.
46. Kumbhari V, Lehmann S, Schlichting N, et al. Gastric mucosal devitalization is safe and effective in reducing body weight and visceral adiposity in a porcine model. Gastrointest Endosc 2018;88(1):175–84.e1.
47. Thompson CC, Trasolini R, Jirapinyo P. Bariatric endoscopic antral myotomy: first-in-human proof of concept of a novel therapeutic method to delay gastric emptying and induce weight loss. iGIE 2023;2(2):102–6.
48. Thompson C, Wainer J, Liou A, et al. Initial feasibility and safety of a novel endoscopic ultrasound-guided local delivery system for AAV-based pancreatic gene therapy. Gastrointest Endosc 2023;97(6):AB819.
49. Hajifathalian K, Mehta A, Ang B, et al. Improvement in insulin resistance and estimated hepatic steatosis and fibrosis after endoscopic sleeve gastroplasty. Gastrointest Endosc 2021;93(5):1110–8.
50. Lavín-Alconero L, Fernández-Lanas T, Iruzubieta-Coz P, et al. Efficacy and safety of endoscopic sleeve gastroplasty versus laparoscopic sleeve gastrectomy in obese subjects with non-alcoholic steatohepatitis (NASH): study protocol for a randomized controlled trial (TESLA-NASH study). Trials 2021;22(1):756.
51. Espinós JC, Turró R, Moragas G, et al. Gastrointestinal physiological changes and their relationship to weight loss following the POSE procedure. Obes Surg 2016;26(5):1081–9.
52. Jirapinyo P, Jaroenlapnopparat A, Thompson CC. 703 endoscopic sleeve gastroplasty with anti-obesity medications: analysis of combination therapy, optimal timing and agents. Gastroenterology 2023;164(6):S–145.
53. Mehta A, Shah S, Dawod E, et al. Impact of adjunctive pharmacotherapy with intragastric balloons for the treatment of obesity. Am Surg 2023;89(4):707–13.
54. Lahooti A, Critelli B, Hassan A, et al. 701 A randomized, double-blind, two-way crossover study to evaluate the efficacy of liraglutide treatment in patients undergoing transoral outlet reduction endoscopy. Gastroenterology 2023;164(6 Supplement):S–144.
55. Van Nieuwenhove Y, Dambrauskas Z, Campillo-Soto A, et al. Preoperative very low-calorie diet and operative outcome after laparoscopic gastric bypass: a randomized multicenter study. Arch Surg 2011;146(11):1300–5.
56. Loo JH, Lim YH, Seah HL, et al. Intragastric balloon as bridging therapy prior to bariatric surgery for patients with severe obesity (BMI $\geq$ 50 kg/m2): a systematic review and meta-analysis. Obes Surg 2022/02/01 2022;32(2):489–502.
57. Maselli DB, Alqahtani AR, Abu Dayyeh BK, et al. Revisional endoscopic sleeve gastroplasty of laparoscopic sleeve gastrectomy: an international, multicenter study. Gastrointest Endosc 2021;93(1):122–30.

58. Gurian GC, Watanabe LM, Nonino CB, et al. Efficacy of the argon plasma coagulation in patients with weight regain after gastric bypass: a randomized control trial. Endosc Int Open 2023;11(01):E43–51.

59. Vargas EJ, Bazerbachi F, Rizk M, et al. Transoral outlet reduction with full thickness endoscopic suturing for weight regain after gastric bypass: a large multicenter international experience and meta-analysis. Surg Endosc 2018;32(1): 252–9.

60. Mechanick JI, Apovian C, Brethauer S, et al. Clinical practice guidelines for the perioperative nutrition, metabolic, and nonsurgical support of patients undergoing bariatric procedures - 2019 update: cosponsored by American Association of Clinical Endocrinologists/American College of Endocrinology, The Obesity Society, American Society for Metabolic and Bariatric Surgery, Obesity Medicine Association, and American Society of Anesthesiologists. Obesity 2020;28(4): O1–o58.

61. Sundi D, Cohen JE, Cole AP, et al. Establishment of a new prostate cancer multidisciplinary clinic: format and initial experience. Prostate 2015;75(2):191–9.

62. Zhang J, Mavros M, Cosgrove D, et al. Impact of a single-day multidisciplinary clinic on the management of patients with liver tumours. Curr Oncol 2013; 20(2):123–31.

63. Acosta A, Streett S, Kroh MD, et al. White paper AGA: POWER - practice guide on obesity and weight management, education, and resources. Clin Gastroenterol Hepatol 2017;15(5):631–49.e10.

64. Jirapinyo P, Thompson CC. Training in bariatric and metabolic endoscopic therapies. Clin Endosc 2018;51(5):430–8.

65. Eisenberg D, Lohnberg JA, Kubat EP, et al. Systems innovation model: an integrated interdisciplinary team approach pre- and post-bariatric surgery at a Veterans Affairs (VA) medical center. Surg Obes Relat Dis 2017;13(4):600–6.

66. Sullivan S, Kumar N, Edmundowicz SA, et al. ASGE position statement on endoscopic bariatric therapies in clinical practice. Gastrointest Endosc 2015;82(5): 767–72.

67. Dave N, Dawod E, Simmons OL. Endobariatrics: a still underutilized weight loss tool. Curr Treat Options Gastroenterol 2023;21(2):172–84.

68. Kelly J, Menon V, O'Neill F, et al. UK cost-effectiveness analysis of endoscopic sleeve gastroplasty versus lifestyle modification alone for adults with class II obesity. Int J Obes 2023;47(11):1161–70.

UNITED STATES POSTAL SERVICE ®

Statement of Ownership, Management, and Circulation
(All Periodicals Publications Except Requester Publications)

1. Publication Title	2. Publication Number	3. Filing Date
GASTROINTESTINAL ENDOSCOPY CLINICS OF NORTH AMERICA	012 – 603	9/18/2024

4. Issue Frequency	5. Number of Issues Published Annually	6. Annual Subscription Price
JAN, APR, JUL, OCT	4	$392.00

7. Complete Mailing Address of Known Office of Publication (Not printer) (Street, city, county, state, and ZIP+4®)

ELSEVIER INC.
230 Park Avenue, Suite 800
New York, NY 10169

Contact Person: Malathi Samayan
Telephone (Include area code): 91-44-4299-4507

8. Complete Mailing Address of Headquarters or General Business Office of Publisher (Not printer)

ELSEVIER INC.
230 Park Avenue, Suite 800
New York, NY 10169

9. Full Names and Complete Mailing Addresses of Publisher, Editor, and Managing Editor (Do not leave blank)

Publisher (Name and complete mailing address)

Dolores Meloni, ELSEVIER INC.
1600 JOHN F KENNEDY BLVD. SUITE 1600
PHILADELPHIA, PA 19103-2899

Editor (Name and complete mailing address)

KERRY HOLLAND, ELSEVIER INC.
1600 JOHN F KENNEDY BLVD. SUITE 1600
PHILADELPHIA, PA 19103-2899

Managing Editor (Name and complete mailing address)

PATRICK MANLEY, ELSEVIER INC.
1600 JOHN F KENNEDY BLVD. SUITE 1600
PHILADELPHIA, PA 19103-2899

10. Owner (Do not leave blank. If the publication is owned by a corporation, give the name and address of the corporation immediately followed by the names and addresses of all stockholders owning or holding 1 percent or more of the total amount of stock. If not owned by a corporation, give the names and addresses of the individual owners. If owned by a partnership or other unincorporated firm, give its name and address as well as those of each individual owner. If the publication is published by a nonprofit organization, give its name and address.)

Full Name	Complete Mailing Address
WHOLLY OWNED SUBSIDIARY OF REED/ELSEVIER, US HOLDINGS	1600 JOHN F KENNEDY BLVD. SUITE 1600 PHILADELPHIA, PA 19103-2899

11. Known Bondholders, Mortgagees, and Other Security Holders Owning or Holding 1 Percent or More of Total Amount of Bonds, Mortgages, or Other Securities. If none, check box ► ☐ None

Full Name	Complete Mailing Address
N/A	

12. Tax Status (For completion by nonprofit organizations authorized to mail at nonprofit rates) (Check one)
The purpose, function, and nonprofit status of this organization and the exempt status for federal income tax purposes:
☒ Has Not Changed During Preceding 12 Months
☐ Has Changed During Preceding 12 Months (Publisher must submit explanation of change with this statement)

PS Form **3526**, July 2014 (Page 1 of 4 (see instructions page 4)) PSN: 7530-01-000-9931 PRIVACY NOTICE: See our privacy policy on www.usps.com.

---

13. Publication Title	14. Issue Date for Circulation Data Below
GASTROINTESTINAL ENDOSCOPY CLINICS OF NORTH AMERICA	JULY 2024

15. Extent and Nature of Circulation		Average No. Copies Each Issue During Preceding 12 Months	No. Copies of Single Issue Published Nearest to Filing Date
a. Total Number of Copies (Net press run)		105	98
b. Paid Circulation (By Mail and Outside the Mail)	(1) Mailed Outside-County Paid Subscriptions Stated on PS Form 3541 (Include paid distribution above nominal rate, advertiser's proof copies, and exchange copies)	47	46
	(2) Mailed In-County Paid Subscriptions Stated on PS Form 3541 (Include paid distribution above nominal rate, advertiser's proof copies, and exchange copies)	0	0
	(3) Paid Distribution Outside the Mails Including Sales Through Dealers and Carriers, Street Vendors, Counter Sales, and Other Paid Distribution Outside USPS®	33	26
	(4) Paid Distribution by Other Classes of Mail Through the USPS (e.g., First-Class Mail®)	8	8
c. Total Paid Distribution (Sum of 15b (1), (2), (3), and (4))	►	88	80
d. Free or Nominal Rate Distribution (By Mail and Outside the Mail)	(1) Free or Nominal Rate Outside-County Copies included on PS Form 3541	17	17
	(2) Free or Nominal Rate In-County Copies Included on PS Form 3541	0	0
	(3) Free or Nominal Rate Copies Mailed at Other Classes Through the USPS (e.g., First-Class Mail)	0	0
	(4) Free or Nominal Rate Distribution Outside the Mail (Carriers or other means)	1	1
e. Total Free or Nominal Rate Distribution (Sum of 15d (1), (2), (3) and (4))	►	18	18
f. Total Distribution (Sum of 15c and 15e)	►	105	98
g. Copies not Distributed (See Instructions to Publishers #4 (page #3))	►	0	0
h. Total (Sum of 15f and g)	►	105	98
i. Percent Paid (15c divided by 15f times 100)	►	83.33%	81.63%

* If you are claiming electronic copies, go to line 16 on page 3. If you are not claiming electronic copies, skip to line 17 on page 3.

PS Form **3526**, July 2014 (Page 2 of 4)

16. Electronic Copy Circulation		Average No. Copies Each Issue During Preceding 12 Months	No. Copies of Single Issue Published Nearest to Filing Date
a. Paid Electronic Copies	►		
b. Total Paid Print Copies (Line 15c) + Paid Electronic Copies (Line 16a)	►		
c. Total Print Distribution (Line 15f) + Paid Electronic Copies (Line 16a)	►		
d. Percent Paid (Both Print & Electronic Copies) (16b divided by 16c × 100)	►		

☒ I certify that 50% of all my distributed copies (electronic and print) are paid above a nominal price.

17. Publication of Statement of Ownership
☒ If the publication is a general publication, publication of this statement is required. Will be printed in the OCTOBER 2024 issue of this publication. ☐ Publication not required.

18. Signature and Title of Editor, Publisher, Business Manager, or Owner

Malathi Samayan — Malathi Samayan - Distribution Controller

Date: 9/18/2024

I certify that all information furnished on this form is true and complete. I understand that anyone who furnishes false or misleading information on this form or who omits material or information requested on the form may be subject to criminal sanctions (including fines and imprisonment) and/or civil sanctions (including civil penalties).

PS Form **3526**, July 2014 (Page 3 of 4) PRIVACY NOTICE: See our privacy policy on www.usps.com.

Moving?

Make sure your subscription moves with you!

To notify us of your new address, find your **Clinics Account Number** (located on your mailing label above your name), and contact customer service at:

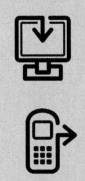

Email: **journalscustomerservice-usa@elsevier.com**

800-654-2452 (subscribers in the U.S. & Canada)
314-447-8871 (subscribers outside of the U.S. & Canada)

Fax number: **314-447-8029**

Elsevier Health Sciences Division
Subscription Customer Service
3251 Riverport Lane
Maryland Heights, MO 63043

*To ensure uninterrupted delivery of your subscription, please notify us at least 4 weeks in advance of move.

Printed and bound by CPI Group (UK) Ltd, Croydon, CR0 4YY

08/05/2025

01864724-0007